The
Cancer Experience

Nursing Diagnosis and Management

The Cancer

Nursing Diagnosis

Doris L. Carnevali, RN, MN
Associate Professor Emeritus
Community Health Care Systems
School of Nursing
University of Washington
Seattle, Washington

Ann C. Reiner, RN, MN, OCN
Clinical Director—Oncology Nursing
Virginia Mason Medical Center
Seattle, Washington

J.B. LIPPINCOTT COMPANY
Philadelphia

Grand Rapids   London
New York   Sydney
St. Louis   Tokyo
San Francisco

Experience

and Management

Acquisition/Sponsoring Editor: David Carroll
Coordinating Editorial Assistant: Amy Stonehouse
Project Editor: Virginia Barishek
Manuscript Editor: Linda Stewart
Indexer: Katherine Pitcoff
Design Coordinator: Ellen C. Dawson
Interior and Cover Designer: Ellen C. Dawson
Cover Art: Origins I by Martha Slaymaker
      36" × 55"
        Porcelain, mixed media on plywood
Production Manager: Caren Erlichman
Production Coordinator: Pamela Milcos
Compositor: Circle Graphics Inc.
Printer/Binder: R.R. Donnelley & Sons Company

1 3 5 6 4 2   QZ 200.1

Library of Congress Cataloging-in-Publication Data   0011340

Carnevali, Doris L.
  The cancer experience: nursing diagnosis and management / Doris
L. Carnevali, Ann C. Reiner.
    p.   cm.
  Includes bibliographical references.
  ISBN 0-397-54726-9
  1. Cancer–Nursing. I. Reiner, Ann. II. Title.
  [DNLM: 1. Activities of Daily Living. 2. Nursing Assessment.
3. Oncologic Nursing.   WY 156 C289c]
  RC266.C37   1990
  610.73'698–dc20
  DNLM/DLC
  for Library of Congress   89-13777
                                            CIP

*This book is dedicated
to the young ones who entered our lives
during the writing of this book:*

Granddaughters

*Julia Lynn and Maria Ann
Carnevali*

and daughter

Diana Kathryn Martin

Preface

Cancer is a disease, but it is also a series of experiences that profoundly affect the daily living of both the person who has the cancer and those who share the experiences. Given the dual perspectives for viewing cancer, diagnosis and treatment can be similarly divided into those directed at the neoplastic processes and those concerned with the problems and issues in managing daily living throughout the cancer experience. Other cancer nursing books have thoroughly covered the knowledge and expertise required by nurses to make clinical judgments and carry out skills associated with management of the neoplastic processes. This book focuses instead on the knowledge and expertise needed by the nurse to diagnose and treat the daily living dimensions of the cancer experience. It uses knowledge of pathology, pathophysiology, psychopathology, medical prognosis, and medical treatment as part of the knowledge base needed to generate nursing diagnoses and treat cancer-associated problems in daily living.

In each topic the distinctive perspectives of the medical and nursing disciplines are described. (Medical references were used as a basis for describing the medical perspective.) This division was made not to set arbitrary boundaries in clinical practice for either nurses or physicians, but to heighten awareness of potential differences in each discipline's focus and priorities. The distinction is also intended to help nurses make conscious, smooth transitions between the demands for knowledge and skill in the medically oriented elements of their practice and their primary accountability for expert diagnosis and treatment in the nursing domain.

Because of its daily living focus, the book has been organized by the phases of the experience rather than by the type or location of the cancer. It begins with issues and problems associated with risk reduction and self-monitoring in daily living and moves through the phases of living with diagnosis, treatment, post treatment, survival, recurrence, and advancing cancer. The intent is to provide knowledge about problems in daily living and functioning that are common to all phases. In the clinical situation, patients may not experience every phase, or with recurrence they may have quite different experiences as they again live with medical diagnostic and treatment activities. Furthermore, it is anticipated that many of the challenges patients experience in one phase may spill over into the next phase. Some problems, for example, oncologic emergencies, sexuality, role changes, or burnout, can occur during several of the phases, but are covered only once in the book because the diagnoses and treatment tend to be the same in any phase. Others, such as pain, fatigue, and eating problems, are addressed as an acute problem in the initial treatment phase and again as a chronic problem of increasing severity in the chapter on advancing cancer. The underlying mechanisms, nursing diagnoses, prognoses, and treatment are modified depending on the phase in which they occur.

The content of the book is not based solely on the opportunities nurses have to encounter the patient or family for diagnosis and treatment. (Some phases of the cancer experience provide for extensive nursing encounters, while others provide for minimal contact.) Instead, the content is based on common or high-risk problems and issues that may occur during a phase. It is anticipated that, if nurses can predict the problems, they can use some nursing time during high-contact periods to prepare patients and families to cope more effectively with potential problems in daily living that they may experience when nursing contacts are less frequent. It is also expected that knowledge of the risks and manifestations of the problems will prepare the nurse to identify any existing problems should there be a contact (e.g., a phone call or clinic visit) with patients or family members during a low-contact time, such as the survival phase.

This book is based on earlier work on diagnostic reasoning. The underlying assumption in organizing the information is that a consistent format, highlighting features such as risk factors and manifestations, would foster effective problem sensing and recognition. Consistent presentation of knowledge about underlying mechanisms, prognostic variables, and possible complications could assist in shaping treatment decisions. The hope is that this consistent approach that takes information processing strategies into account will expedite storage of knowledge and retrieval for diagnostic and treatment purposes.

This book is written for practicing nurses in a wide variety of professional settings who encounter adult patients and families experiencing cancer. Its content crosses clinical specialties. Nurses care for patients in active treatment for their cancers not only on oncology units and clinics, but also on general medical, surgical, urologic, gyne-cologic, and orthopedic units. The book should also prove useful across levels of care: in intensive and acute care units in hospitals; in ambulatory care, both in specialty and general practice; in home care nursing; and in long-term care settings. It can also serve as an excellent companion reference for students who include the care of patients and families experiencing cancer in any of these clinical settings.

The authors welcome comments and suggestions from readers. Correspondence may be sent to Doris Carnevali, 3250 36th Avenue SW, Seattle, WA 98126.

Doris Carnevali, RN, MN
Ann Reiner, RN, MN, OCN

Acknowledgments

We gratefully acknowledge individuals who so generously shared their expertise, clinical wisdom, and resources:

Barbara Beasley, BS, RD, Dietician for Oncology Patients, Virginia Mason Medical Center

Shirley Beresford, PhD, Assistant Professor, Epidemiology, School of Public Health and Community Medicine, University of Washington

Noel Chrisman, PhD, Professor, Community Health Care Systems, University of Washington; Affiliate, Public Health Program, Fred Hutchinson Cancer Control Research Unit

Jane Cornman, RN, PhD, Research Assistant Professor, Parent–Child Nursing, University of Washington; Private practice in Individual and Family Therapy involving a clientele that includes cancer patients and their families

Judith Fihn, RN, BSN, Staff Nurse, Oncology Unit, Virginia Mason Medical Center; Formerly, Oncology Home Care Nurse

Scott Davis, PhD, Assistant Professor, Epidemiology, School of Public Health and Community Medicine, University of Washington; Associate Member, Programs in Public Health Sciences, Fred Hutchinson Cancer Research Center

Ann Gensler, Pharm.D., Staff Pharmacist, Virginia Mason Medical Center

Laura Heard, RN, MS, CRRN, Clinical Nurse Specialist in Rehabilitation Nursing, Virginia Mason Medical Center

Margaret Heitkemper, RN, PhD, Associate Professor, Physiological Nursing, University of Washington

Connie Horton, RN, BSN, Staff Nurse, Oncology Unit, Virginia Mason Medical Center; Formerly Oncology Home Care Nurse

Ryan Iwamoto, RN, CS, MN, Clinical Nurse Specialist in Radiation Oncology, Virginia Mason Medical Center

JoAnn Kowalski, RN, BS, OCN, Staff Nurse, Oncology Unit, Virginia Mason Medical Center

Paula Leudke, BS, RT, Inpatient and Home Respiratory Therapy, Manager—Home Respiratory Therapy Service, Virginia Mason Medical Center

Patricia Milburn, RN, MN, MS, Nursing Computer Systems Coordinator, Swedish Hospital Medical Center

Merle Mishel, RN, PhD, Associate Professor, Division Coordinator, Psychiatric Mental Health Nursing, University of Arizona

Doris Molbo, RN, MA, Associate Professor Emeritus, Physiological Nursing Department, University of Washington; First American Cancer Society Clinical Professor of Oncology Nursing

Kathleen Stetz, RN, PhD, Research Associate, Community Health Care Systems, School of Nursing, University of Washington

Mary Durand Thomas, RN, MN, PhD, Research Assistant Professor, Psychosocial Nursing Department, University of Washington; Private practice

Martha Tyler, RN, MN, RRT, Assistant Professor, Physiological Nursing Department, Adjunct Assistant Professor, Medicine, Respiratory Disease Division, University of Washington

Our thanks go also to the many nursing clinicians who drew from their long experience in caring for patients, survivors, and families during all phases of the cancer experience and who shared their expertise with us. Their ideas, their questions, and their "stories" contributed immeasurably to the practical aspects of the book.

We are also grateful to the patients and families who shared their experiences, responses, successes, and concerns with us. Two former patients, Murl Cox, CPA, and Josie Stevenson, MSW, deserve a special thanks for their review of the manuscript on survivorship. They brought a background of their own day-to-day experiences with the challenges of survival as well as those they learned through their long-term participation in cancer support groups.

We also thank Martha Slaymaker, the artist who created *Origins I*, the work of art featured on the cover of this book. A cancer survivor, she has been active in support groups, helping other cancer survivors live through the experience.

Contents

1

A Daily Living—Functional Health Status Perspective for Diagnosis and Treatment of the Cancer Experience for Patients and Their Families

Cancer is a complex and often mysterious group of diseases characterized by uncontrolled growth and spread of immature, undifferentiated cells. New knowledge about cancer is emerging daily, so there is a sense that there is more yet to be learned than is already known.

Cancer is a pervasive cluster of diseases, touching the lives of many individuals and families. It can occur in persons of all ages, both sexes, and all socioeconomic groups, cultures, and geographic areas. In the United States, when accidents and suicide are removed from the statistics, cancer is the first cause of death among females of all ages up to age 75; it is first among males up to age 15 and second for all other male age categories (Silverberg and Lubera, 1989). In addition to those who have died, there are more than 5 million Americans who are living with a history of cancer—the survivors (American Cancer Society, 1989). Family members, friends, and acquaintances of persons who have had cancer or who died from it provide an additional pool of people who have had an experience with cancer. Further, advertisements, fiction and nonfiction books, plays, movies, television programs, and health promotion programs in community, school, and work settings introduce thoughts of cancer, cancer surveillance activities, or concerns about symptoms to millions of others. Thus, almost any person whom nurses contact in their professional practice will have had some type of encounter with the reality or possibility of cancer. This could then be a factor in their response to the presenting health situation, even when cancer is not a primary concern.

Major Perspectives in Research and Treatment of Cancer

Cancer can be viewed from two major perspectives. Malignant neoplasms can be addressed in terms of their pathogenesis, pathology, and responsiveness to forms of intervention. Cancer can also be studied, diagnosed, and treated in terms of the experience of cancer.

The human experience with cancer includes both emotional and physical components. The *intensity* of the cancer experience can vary from almost no impact to the significant stress of managing daily living with threatening disease in oneself or a family member or friend. The *nature* of the experience can be an abstract relationship associated with hearing or reading about cancer when one is presumably cancer-free and has few recognized risks. It can also be a dominating force in daily living when the disease and its treatment involve a person's own body appearance and functioning or that of a close relative or companion.

Professional Nursing Role in Cancer

A health care professional's primary perspective in approaching cancer is usually discipline-specific. The medical perspective tends to give primacy to pathology for both research and clinical practice, if one judges by the focus of medical taxonomy related to malignant neoplasia, oncologic literature, and medical practice. Nursing's perspective of cancer is made more complex by the dual clinical role responsibilities of carrying out the delegated medical observation and treatment of the patient and diagnosing and treating phenomena that fall within the nursing domain.

Medical Component of the Nursing Role

The medical element of professional cancer nursing practice holds an important place in professional nursing roles in hospital, clinic, and home settings; patient well-being depends on it. Nurses carry out the crucial delegated medical functions of case finding with referral for medical diagnosis and treatment, implementation of prescribed medical treatments, and monitoring patient response to the cancer and the medical treatment. A solid understanding of pathology and medical treatment plus skills in applying that knowledge to patient observation and technical activities is required. This use of knowledge when the patient is being viewed from the medical perspective is shown in Figure 1-1.

Knowledge of Pathogenesis Pathology Treatment options	➡	Differential diagnosis and staging of the tumor	➡	Medical treatment of the tumor

Figure 1-1.   *Medicine's oncologic knowledge base for diagnosis and treatment.*

Use of Medical Knowledge in the Nursing Domain

The perspective of pathology and knowledge of oncologic therapeutics are important elements in the nursing domain as well. However, the way in which these pieces of information are used in nursing diagnosis and treatment is quite distinct from the way they are used for diagnosis, treatment, and monitoring from the medical perspective, whether that medical care is given by physicians or nurses.

The nursing perspective concerns itself with different phenomena and relationships, with the result that knowledge and data from other disciplines are used in nursing's discipline-specific way. In the nursing domain, knowledge of pathology, medical diagnosis, treatment, and patient response are not the end point. Instead, they are a point of departure for a second generation of knowledge for nursing diagnosis and treatment, as can be seen in Figure 1-2. Knowledge about the pathogenesis of cancer is also used by nurses in dealing with risk reduction, as can be seen in Figure 3-1.

These assumptions about nursing's discipline-specific perspective for diagnosis and treatment form the basis for this book's approach to the use of knowledge about pathology, pathophysiology, and medical treatment. The reader will find that these topics are integrated as parts of the underlying dynamics of phenomena that are central to the nursing domain. One example is that cancer pathogenesis becomes one part of the underlying dynamics for understanding nursing diagnosis and treatment of problems people have in incorporating cancer risk reduction into daily living. A second example is use of the pathophysiology of nausea, fatigue, or pain and their physiologic linkage with particular forms of cancer or medical treatment in identifying the basis for the resultant areas of dysfunction and in specifying the impact on daily living.

Medical knowledge provides *part* of the knowledge base nurses use to understand phenomena they diagnose and treat within the nursing domain. It contributes to an awareness of certain risks and problems. It becomes one variable in considering prognosis. It also contributes to the rationale for some forms of nursing treatment. Knowledge from the medical domain is important in the nursing domain; however, it not the entirety of the body of knowledge needed for nursing diagnosis and treatment.

Nursing Domain for Diagnosis and Treatment

The perspective for nursing diagnosis, prognosis, and treatment used in this book is a variation on several of the major conceptual frameworks currently used to describe nursing. It is not incongruent with the theoretic frameworks of self-care, adaptation,

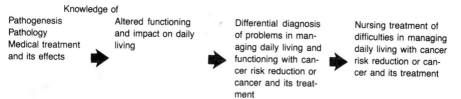

Knowledge of

| Pathogenesis Pathology Medical treatment and its effects | ➡ | Altered functioning and impact on daily living | ➡ | Differential diagnosis of problems in managing daily living and functioning with cancer risk reduction or cancer and its treatment | ➡ | Nursing treatment of difficulties in managing daily living with cancer risk reduction or cancer and its treatment |

Figure 1-2. *Nursing's knowledge base for diagnosis and treatment.*

and human response to actual or potential health problems. It structures their common themes in a slightly different way. Most of the diagnostic areas in the book will address:

Self-care and the factors that affect it

Various forms and levels of adaptation that patients and families face and issues of available resources

Human responses that individuals and families make to the particular health situations they face

The diagnostic areas identified in this book tend to be more specific than the categories currently available within the taxonomy of the North American Nursing Diagnosis Association (NANDA). However, there is no question that any of the diagnostic areas can be placed into one or more of the NANDA taxonomic categories below the "Impaired" or "Altered" levels, at the reader's discretion (Fitzpatrick et al, 1989; Hurley, 1986).

Daily Living and Functional Health Status as a Perspective for Nursing Diagnosis and Treatment of the Cancer Experience

One way of viewing the human experience with cancer, whether one deals with risk reduction, self-monitoring, or any of the phases of the disease and its treatment, is to consider it from the perspective of two basic categories of phenomena—daily living and functional health status. In this conceptual framework, daily living and functional health status are always viewed in relationship to each other. Thus, one always looks at daily living not in isolation, but as it affects or is affected by functional health status. Functional health status, in turn, is always seen in terms of its effect on managing the requirements of daily living or the impact that daily living has on functional capacity. Figure 1-3 illustrates this relationship.

General concepts of daily living and functional health status are not peculiar to nursing. However, nursing does concern itself with particular dimensions of both daily living and functioning. These become evident when the subcategories of these major areas are considered. These subcategories are operationally defined below.

Daily Living Factors

Daily living related to functional health status, as it is of particular concern in nursing, can be described in five subcategories.

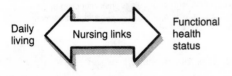

Figure 1-3. Domain for nursing diagnosis and treatment. (After Carnevali D, Patrick M. Nursing management for the elderly. 2nd ed. Philadelphia: JB Lippincott, 1986:5.)

Activities in Daily Living

Included in the category of Activities in Daily Living is anything that the person being diagnosed (e.g., patient, family member, care giver, friends, etc.), actually does that is relevant to the presenting health situation. These activities may reflect a usual pattern or may be unusual. They may take place in the home or community or in any type of institutional setting. They may occur often during a day or on a daily, weekly, or less frequent basis. The activities may be related to prescribed health care (e.g., participating in a treatment) or may be personal in nature (e.g., decisions concerning sexual activity, childbearing, or diet as a part of cancer risk reduction).

TIME FRAME. Nursing perspectives on activities in daily living have a time frame consideration. *Past* activities may affect the present responses of the patient or family (e.g., having been a primary care giver for a parent or child with advanced cancer can affect expectations and physiologic responses to one's own cancer and its treatment). *Present* activities must be managed within current capacities and external resources (e.g., self-care of suctioning, maintaining nutrition in the face of anorexia, or being transported to and from the treatment site when one has problems of vomiting or diarrhea). *Future* activities are identified in terms of the challenges they will offer to the patient or care giver—taking into consideration their predicted functional status and external resources (e.g., the patient's return to work with the diagnosis of cancer or visible side-effects of treatment; the care giver's planning meals for the person who is expected to experience severe esophagitis from radiation treatment).

SIGNIFICANCE. The importance of any particular activity varies with the individual. Nursing is often concerned with altering activities and patterns in daily living. Whenever change is contemplated, the significance of the activity to the individual having to make that change is an important consideration. Unimportant activities can be changed more easily than those whose current patterns have real significance to those involved (e.g., a department head who values his current position and salary postpones, on several occasions, scheduled surgery to have suspicious "moles" removed because his employer continues to set up deadlines that must be met).

Events in Daily Living

Events are occurrences, usually of some importance. They may be of a personal nature (e.g., anniversaries, travel, social events, births, deaths) or they may be related to the health care situation (e.g., a new diagnosis of cancer, news of remission or recurrence, the next chemotherapy series, placement or removal of tubes in the body).

TIME FRAME. Like activities, events too have a time frame. *Past* events can affect current responses. Knowledge or skills acquired in previous participation in an event can increase competence and confidence in subsequent participation in similar events. Memories of past events can affect both mood and physiology (e.g., anticipatory nausea and vomiting as one approaches the later cycles of a cisplatin series, or anxiety prior to the next oncologic checkup in the survival phase). *Present* events are approached with the aim of incorporating them into daily living, within the parameters of the internal and external resources of the individual and family. *Future* events are approached as effectively as possible, given the predicted resources of the patient and family.

SIGNIFICANCE.   Events, too, may vary in the degree of importance to the individual or family—or to health care providers. Data on significance of an event or incongruence of significance among those who are concerned with it can be an important area for diagnosis and treatment. Such findings can also serve as a prognostic variable. For example, the physician may be interested in having this case included in current research on protocol response; thus, adherence of the patient to the protocol is highly significant to him. The patient may assign more significance to attending a child's wedding than to coming for a treatment according to a protocol schedule.

Demands in Daily Living

Demands are the expectations regarding activities, behaviors, or attitudes that affect the individual's behavior or emotions. Demands arise from three sources: *self* (e.g., expectations of control over one's responses or lifestyle, body image, competence, participation), *others* (e.g., family members, employers, colleagues, social group, health care providers, third party payers), and *one's possessions* (e.g., home, car, pets).

Engaging with the health care system for the diagnosis and treatment of cancer places many new and stringent demands on patients and families, in both the short and long term. The consequences of complying or failing to meet those demands for tests, treatment protocols, and changes in daily living patterns can be seen as affecting life and death outcomes. Patients who choose courses of action that are incongruent with the expectations of the health care team may experience negative sanctions from health care providers, such as anger, guilt-producing behavior, or even risk of rejection or abandonment. There are many pressures for patients and families to comply with the demands of others.

Environment in Daily Living

The environment in daily living, as it concerns nursing, involves *the physical, sensory, and interpersonal milieu within which the person's daily living is taking place.* It may be the lead-shielded radiation treatment room; the narrow tube of the magnetic resonance imaging machine; laminar airflow rooms with personnel who are masked, gowned, and gloved; the bedlam of a home with young children clamoring for attention; a kitchen filled with cooking odors; or a work setting with employers and colleagues who are solicitous or fearful. The environment may include barriers to effective management of daily living (e.g., one bedroom with a double bed shared by the patient with advanced disease and a spouse who must continue to work; stairs or too long a distance to the toilet for the person with severe diarrhea; inconvenient laundry facilities; or the distance to the grocery store).

Nursing's concern with the environment addresses elements that have potential for a positive or negative impact for the patient, family, or care giver as they try to manage daily living with their specific health situation and personal needs, wherever that daily living is occurring.

Values and Beliefs

Values and beliefs of concern in the nursing domain are those that play a part in the choices, feelings, actions, and interactions associated with the cancer experience. They can involve values and beliefs held by the patient, family, personal care givers, health care providers, employers, colleagues, and society. Examples of values and beliefs that often have relevance in the cancer experience include beliefs about sick roles and illness roles; contagion and cancer; assignment of blame or guilt; the person's right to die; informed consent; the right to know one's diagnosis and prognosis; and the right to choose freely.

Nursing assessment, diagnosis, and treatment in value- and belief-related areas often address those that interfere with effective management of daily living with cancer risk reduction or with the cancer and its treatment. These may include conflict of values among patient, family, care givers, and health care providers. Conflicting values and beliefs are often at the core of health care providers' dissatisfaction with the status of patient incorporation of treatment into daily living. For example, a judgment of "noncompliance" might well have been predicted and possibly better managed with an earlier nursing diagnosis that identified:

1. Specific incongruencies between patient and health care provider values
2. The potential effect on patient participation
3. Health care providers' predicted or resultant attitudes and behavior

Functional Health Status

Functional health status, seen in relationship to daily living, can be operationally defined in terms of nursing's discipline-specific perspective. Consideration of functional health status in the nursing domain involves three general categories of functional health as well as specific functional areas that affect one's capacity to manage requirements in daily living. The three major functional areas are:

Age-related psychobiologic status: This aspect of functional health status involves the effect of one's biologic age on normal physiologic, cognitive, and psychologic capacity to function.

Developmental task achievement: Developmental task achievement in the nursing domain is viewed from the past, present, and future. *Past* developmental task achievement affects the present capacity to function (e.g., trust, autonomy, intimacy, generativity, and integration). Nursing also considers the effect of the patient's *present* health experiences on maintenance or achievement of *current and future* developmental tasks (e.g., lack of desired help from oncology nurses or physicians and resultant loss of trust; the impact of disfigurement on intimacy; pelvic radiation's impact on generativity as it concerns having children; functional losses and the task of integration).

Pathology and associated medical diagnostic and treatment activities: From the nursing perspective, the pathology and associated medical activities are viewed in terms of the way in which their magnitude and trajectory affect functional capacities to manage the requirements of daily living. In this book the focus is on cancer pathology and oncologic diagnosis and treatment.

These three factors are then applied to specific functional capacities as the nurse assesses them in relationship to the current and future requirements of the patient's daily living. Specific functional health status areas in nursing perspective go beyond the first generation of functions, such as respiration, circulation, neurologic integrity, and digestion, to a second generation of the actual capacities required to manage daily living (see Fig. 1-2). These are translated into such capacities as physical and emotional strength and endurance, cognitive capacities, mobility, flexibility, motivation, mood, capacity to take risks, and ability to communicate.

External Resources

The capacity to manage the requirements of daily living is affected not only by functional capacities (internal resources), but also by the status of one's external resources, which may either enhance or diminish one's functional capacity. Examples of external resources include the personal support network of family, friends, and care givers; pets; financial resources; available housing and furnishings; transportation; communication facilities (phone, postal system); equipment and supplies; and available health services and technology, as well as other types of services and the status of support organizations in the community.

Daily Living–Functional Health Status as a Balance

The nursing perspective may be seen as assessing, diagnosing, and treating the patient or family's capacity to achieve a satisfactory balance between the requirements in their daily living and their internal and external resources for managing those require-ments. This is shown in Figure 1-4.

Nursing Goals in Diagnosis and Treatment

Nursing's overall goals in diagnosing and treating daily living and functional health status in health-related areas are comparable to the goals of medicine in diagnosing and treating pathology. Nurses diagnose and treat phenomena in order to:

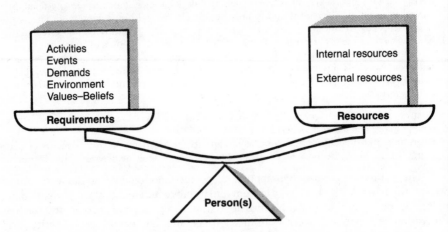

Figure 1-4. A model for nursing's data base and diagnostic/treatment orientation. (After Carnevali D. Daily living and functional health status: a perspective for nurs-ing diagnosis and treatment. Archives of Psychiatric Nursing 2(6):330, 1988. Used with permission.)

Prevent, minimize, or delay problems in daily living and functioning when this is possible

Cure those diagnosed problems of dysfunction or daily living that can be resolved with nursing treatment

Palliate those diagnosed problems in daily living and functioning that can be neither prevented nor cured

Areas for Nursing Diagnosis and Treatment in the Daily Living–Functional Health Status Focus

Four major areas for nursing diagnosis and treatment emerge with the use of the daily living–functional health status focus:

Functional status that limits effective management of the requirements of daily living and health maintenance (Functional health status may be affected by normal developmental status, pathology, or medical diagnostic and treatment activities.)

Daily living that fails to promote health or produces dysfunction or ill health

Difficulties in incorporating health behaviors or treatment regimens into daily living

Inadequate or inappropriate external resources that create barriers to effective and satisfying management of daily living in health-related areas

Application of the Nursing Perspective to Diagnosis and Treatment Planning

Effective oncologic treatment of malignancies is based on accurate, precise diagnosis and prognostic clinical judgments. Effective nursing treatment of daily living and functional health problems during the cancer experience is also based on accurate, precise diagnostic and prognostic judgments.

Expertise in nursing diagnosis and treatment planning is a blend of theoretic and experiential knowledge (Benner and Tanner, 1987; Tanner, 1987). Such knowledge enables nurses to sense potential problems, recognize existing problems, make prognostic judgments, predict complications, decide on treatment, and monitor response to treatment. In keeping with this assumption, the knowledge needed for each of these aspects of clinical judgments and treatment decisions is addressed in a consistent format in this book. In the remainder of this chapter the elements of nursing judgments and treatment decisions are discussed as a rationale for the approach to the content in each of the subsequent clinical chapters.

Sensing Risks of Potential Problems

An important function of diagnosis and treatment is prevention. Here nurses seek to sense and identify potential or incipient problems before they occur or become full-blown. Such sensing is based on recognition of a pattern of risk factors present in the patient, environment, medical treatment, and support network. Nursing treatment is prescribed and implemented to modify either the situation, the environment, or the person in order to avoid, delay, or minimize the potential problem.

Risks can range in occurrence from the absence of risk to the presence of inevitable risk. For example, with an absolute neutrophil count of less than 500, even in the most protected of environments, infection of some sort almost always occurs. Nursing treatment of the immunosuppressed patient and the environment seeks to limit the number and kind of exogenous pathogens to which the patient is exposed in daily living, to protect the body areas from opportunities for entry, and to limit the sensory deprivation such environments engender. (See Chapter 6 sections on Vulnerability to Infection and Social Isolation for illustrations of risk factors.)

Knowledge of three areas concerning the patient and the health problem is needed to discern the possible risk of a problem in daily living associated with the cancer experience:

1. The usual functional capacity and lifestyle of the patient and the family or support network
2. The pathology or the treatment as they may affect the patients and families and their capacity to function
3. The nature of past, present, and future daily living—the patterns, requirements, values and beliefs, and environment, and the status of an individual's support network and external resources

Among the risk factors listed for problem areas covered in subsequent chapters the reader will see illustrations of specific findings in each of the three perspectives.

Diagnosis

Sensing that an individual is having a problem in the cancer experience involves an awareness of the *presence of a pattern of cues* suggesting that something is not as it should be. These patterns of cues often include risk factors, stressors in the clinical or personal situation in daily living, and evidence of inadequate functional capacities or external resources for managing the requirements of daily living.

. When clinicians sense or observe these clusters of cues, they also usually experience a retrieval (not necessarily conscious) from long-term memory of several possible explanations or other similar situations. This recall of possible diagnoses or similar situations carries with it knowledge of patterns of features or findings. At some level of consciousness comparisons are made between what is observed and what is known and previously experienced. Certain possible explanations or comparisons are ruled out while others are retained for further consideration and refinement.

When the findings in the present situation are similar to that which is recalled—in both the presence *and* absence of cues, then that diagnosis or clinical judgment is accepted as the best description or categorization of the presenting situation. It is helpful to remember that a conscious or unconscious nursing diagnosis tends to precede and form the basis for almost any independent nursing action. Having some awareness of the basis for one's nursing activities with patients and families would seem to be the more professional approach.

In order to best utilize the clinical judgment that has been made, the sometimes fuzzy findings and the related clinical judgments need to be translated into words— *nursing diagnoses.* These communicate the reality and the nuances of the situation, both to the nurse and to colleagues (Carnevali, 1983). Documentation of nursing diagnoses is a requirement in most institutions and agencies; however, most importantly, a valid, specific, precisely verbalized diagnosis serves as the foundation for a sound, individualized treatment plan that can be carried out in a consistent manner by all nursing care givers.

In this book, the diagnostic areas offered suggest some ideas to the reader about problem areas in daily living and functioning that are associated with particular phenomena. The designation of diagnostic areas is deliberate. They are intended to give only an initial structure or direction. To be translated into actual diagnoses for a patient they must be refined and made precise by integration of data from the individual patient and family as they participate in the cancer experience.

Prognostic Judgments

Treatment, both of the cancer and of individuals whose daily living involves experiencing the cancer, is based on prognosis as well as diagnosis. Oncology nursing does not have the precise staging categories and criteria that oncology medicine uses to determine prognosis and treatment protocols. Nevertheless, the development of a data-supported prognosis is as crucial for effective nursing therapy as staging is for medical therapy.

It is important for nurses caring for patients who have cancer to separate medical from nursing prognoses. The medical prognosis identifies the predicted course the pathology will take without treatment and with the various treatment protocols. *Nursing prognosis deals with the course of events and outcomes that is likely in terms of managing daily living and functioning, given the presenting health and treatment situation and the reality of the patient's daily living and resources. Satisfaction with quality of life is also a consideration in nursing prognosis.* Thus, the nursing prognosis has a related but quite different focus from the medical prognosis for the same patient (Carnevali, 1983).

The medical diagnosis, prognosis, and patient data are important elements in the nursing prognosis, but they are only part of the variables needed to generate a nursing prognosis. Nursing also considers the requirements and patterns of daily living, environment, values and beliefs, functional capabilities, and external resources.

Nursing and medical prognoses need not be identical; in fact, they may move in opposite directions. Two patients with the same medical prognosis can have quite different prognoses for how effectively they will manage daily living. Both may be survivors of the cancer and its treatment, but one may effectively manage the tasks of living with survival from cancer while the other may not. In another situation, two patients may have end-stage metastatic disease. One patient's daily living situation and resources may enable that individual and family to manage daily living with advancing cancer in a way that is effective and relatively satisfying to them. The other patient may have a daily living situation and resources that make the management of symptoms and requirements of daily living a miserable experience for all involved.

Medicine cannot eradicate and cure every malignant tumor. Nor can nursing cure all of the problems in daily living and functioning associated with living with cancer. And, just as oncologic treatment is different for localized versus metastasized tumors, so nursing treatment is different when daily living and functional problems can be resolved versus those that cannot. It is important for the nurse to be realistic and to make prognostic judgments based on data, not on wishful thinking.

Prognoses and Realistic Goals

Data on prognostic variables need to be considered *before* goals can be considered and negotiated with the patient, care giver, or family. The goals or desired outcomes identified in standard care plans establish areas for goals that are *ideal outcomes* associated with a particular phenomenon or treatment. Standardized goals should serve only as a point of departure for considering feasible and desirable goals for the individual patient or family, given the prevailing circumstances. The *working goals* that form the basis for treatment and evaluation take into account data on the strengths and deficits of the patient's daily living, functioning, and resources. They can look quite different from the ideal or standard goals and outcomes, but they have the merit of being realistic, having been based on patient data.

Goal setting with patients whose daily living and functioning are inadequate or deteriorating is much more difficult than with patients for whom things are going well. Yet, realistic goal setting for nursing treatment at these times can make a difference in the quality of life the patients and families experience.

Prognostic Approaches in this Book

The reader will find prognostic variables identified for each phenomenon in the clinical chapters. It can be noted that daily living and resources tend to take predominance over the medical oncologic prognostic variables among the variables used in determining the nursing prognosis.

Where the nursing prognosis suggests that the individual or family are not going to manage daily living or function well, nursing treatment may be directed toward improving the prognosis. However, under some circumstances nurses will need to accept the likelihood that a patient's or family's circumstances will not permit a better prognosis. Such nursing prognoses should cause nurses to:

Set realistic, prognosis-supported goals rather than "pie-in-the-sky," desired, or standard outcomes often seen in standard care plans.

Prescribe preventive, curative, or palliative nursing interventions that fit the specific diagnosis and prognosis.

Avoid anger, fear, or guilt-producing nurse behavior when nursing problems with poor prognoses do not respond to curative nursing interventions. The patient has not "failed the nursing protocol"; the problem and prognosis did not lend themselves to cure.

Set reasonable evaluation criteria that are commensurate with the prognosis-related outcomes and goals.

Complications in the Nursing Domain

There can be sequelae associated with failure to manage daily living and functional deficits. There also can be undesired side-effects to nursing interventions or failure to intervene. Nursing treatments, prescribed or unprescribed, planned or unplanned, are not innocuous. They have an effect. What the nurse does or does not do, when it is done, and how it is done can have negative as well as positive consequences for the patient or family. It is important for nurses to consider possible complications and iatrogenic responses within the nursing domain just as in the medical domain.

A section on complications has been developed for each of the phenomena discussed in the book. As with so many other areas of nursing knowledge, this area has not been well researched, so the information found under the heading Complications has been derived empirically. It behooves the reader to take this into account and validate or modify the ideas and to remain alert for complications and iatrogenic responses to nursing care that have not been identified.

Nursing Treatment

Treatment within the nursing domain, at this stage of the profession's development, tends to be spontaneous and idiosyncratic to the individual nurse rather than cohesively and rationally planned. Standard nursing care plans and general treatment protocols are available (Reiner, 1988; McNally et al, 1985). Prescribed, documented individualization of these guidelines into treatment plans for the individual patient that would be comparable, for example, to the fine localizations made prior to individualizing radiation therapy is relatively rare. Yet, the well-being of patients and families depends on nursing treatment that has been rationally and specifically developed to address the difficulties in the individual patient's situation so that it can be implemented in a consistent manner in all subsequent nursing contacts. The goal of this book is to promote this type of individualized treatment.

Nursing treatment addresses the requirements of daily living, its environment (institution, clinic, home, work), the functional capacities of the person, and the external resources. The plan provides directions for nursing action in specific areas in which data show that patients and families are having difficulty maintaining a balance between identified requirements in daily living and the available capacities and external resources.

Rationale for Nursing Treatment

While nursing research is increasing at a rapid pace, much of the underlying rationale for nursing therapy is yet to be developed. Ideally, prescribed nursing treatment is based on an understanding of:

1. The underlying mechanisms of the phenomenon or situation that has been diagnosed
2. Actions that can be predicted to alleviate the difficulties or support the patient when they cannot be resolved

For example, with a panic level of anxiety, the cerebral circuitry is presumed to be already overloaded with internal stimuli. Therefore, the treatment seeks to minimize the magnitude of external stimuli and demands on the patient. One does not subject the severely anxious patient to heavy teaching or expect the patient to engage in problem solving. It is a time for protection of the patient, for advocacy, for serving as a surrogate for the patient, and for controlling threatening stimuli in the environment.

In each clinical problem area in this book the reader will find supporting knowledge from the medical and nursing fields in two sections—Nature of the Phenomenon and Underlying Mechanisms. Knowledge about the effects of the tumor and the various forms of medical treatment is linked to the functional health status and affected areas in daily living. Additionally, areas in daily living and functioning may be disrupted by factors not related to the tumor or medical treatment; these too are identified. In the future, new research may permit closer links between underlying dynamics and the interventions that are intended to modify them.

Nurse–Patient Collaborative Decision Making

Though much of the planning of nursing treatment takes place within an institutional setting (inpatient or outpatient), most of the daily living and functioning in the cancer experience tends to take place outside of institutions. It is therefore essential that nursing treatment decisions incorporate patients' and care givers' capacities and willingness to participate. Another important consideration is the feasibility of the planned treatment within the patient's and care giver's daily living and its environment.

A *participative perspective* is the dominant mode for treatment planning and implementation in the nursing domain (in contrast to a compliance perspective). This requires collaborative decision making on treatment between nurses and patients, care givers, and families. The treatment builds on documented strengths and available resources in the patient's situation. (Note that these capabilities and resources can increase or decrease rapidly at times.)

The reality of the environment (institution or home) is a crucial consideration. The functioning values and beliefs that will shape the behavior and actions of the patient, family, close associates, employers, and co-workers also are significant elements in nursing treatment plans. Treatment plans that will be effective are based on accurate data about the patient's actual situation and resources, not on some wishful ideal or standard.

In addition to collaborating with patients, families, and care givers, nurses bring their daily living—functional health status perspective to their collaborative practice with physicians. This is particularly true in the area of symptom management, but it can occur in scheduling of diagnostic and treatment activities as well.

Treatment Guidelines

The Treatment Guidelines sections in this book are meant to suggest options for the nurse to consider. Like the Diagnostic Areas sections, guidelines are intended to serve only as points of departure for individualizing the care to the patient or family based on specific, up-to-date data about strengths, resources, deficits, and desires.

Each set of guidelines is linked to a specific diagnostic area rather than to general phenomena, so they go a step beyond many standard care plans or guidelines. The step yet to be taken in using these guidelines in clinical practice is to fine-tune them to address the treatment needed for the precise diagnosis and prognosis made for individual patient situations.

Evaluation

Nursing treatment is undertaken because it is supposed to affect patient or family outcomes. Therefore, the response to prescribed and implemented nursing interventions is observed and judgments are made as to whether to continue, discontinue, or modify any or all parts of the treatment plan.

Some of these evaluations take place during the intervention. For example, observation that the patient or family member is "shutting down" during a teaching session suggests the need to discontinue the activity or at least to stop long enough to determine what is going on and whether the person is capable of learning at this point in time. Other evaluation observations take place at points in time when the effects of the treatment are likely to have taken place and therefore can be observed or reported on by the patient. Many of the responses to nursing intervention involve the patient's or family members' actual functioning in daily living during institutional stays or at home. Due to shorter hospital stays and the fact that most cancer management takes place on an outpatient basis, patient and family or care giver feedback will most often involve self-reporting verbally or in writing. Unless structure and opportunities for this evaluative reporting are planned between the person and the nurse, they are likely to be absent, sporadic, or ineffective. There are, of course, objective data as well that validate or modify interpretation of the reported data. These can reflect some aspects of effectiveness in managing daily living with cancer and its treatment (e.g., weight, blood and serum findings, facial expression and body language, movement, vital signs, grooming, speech).

Since the eye does not see what the mind does not know, it is important to have an observational shopping list in mind for each patient follow-up contact in terms of evaluating response to nursing as well as medical treatment. It is also important to document the findings and judgments in order to see patterns of patient or family response and to determine subsequent nursing treatment.

Determination of response to nursing treatment is important as a basis for retaining or modifying the plan and documenting the patient's and family's course of events. Areas for evaluation are identified for each problem area in the book.

Summary

Cancer is not only a pathologic problem, it is a challenge to the patient's and family's capacities to manage the requirements in daily living and personal lifestyle. Nursing diagnosis and treatment of issues and problems associated with daily living to reduce cancer risks, to engage in appropriate self-monitoring, or to live with the disruptions and discomforts of cancer and its treatment can be as important to a person's survival and quality of life as the medical treatment. It cannot be valued less merely because daily living and its management are mundane compared to the high drama of the bone marrow transplants, head and neck dissections, and other obvious and aggressive elements of the medical perspective. Effective diagnosis and management of daily living issues and personal responses to the cancer experience can have important consequences to both well-being and survival.

The goal of this book is to present knowledge needed to make sound clinical judgments in the nursing domain. Thus, knowledge of pathogenesis, pathology, pathophysiology, medical treatment, and host response are considered primarily as factors affecting daily living and functional capacity for managing its requirements, rather than as they are used within the medical domain. This is not in any way intended to diminish the importance of the nurse's role in expertly implementing delegated medical functions.

The format and organization of each of the clinical chapters of the book are consistent for each problem area, such as dyspnea, pain, sexuality, and role. The titles and the focus of each of the sections are shown in Table 1-1. It is hoped that this approach to nursing knowledge and the consistent pattern of organization will expedite the readers' storage and use of knowledge for efficient nursing diagnosis and treatment.

Table 1-1. Organization of Content in Each Problem Area

Introduction
Phenomenon and its linkage to daily living
Medical perspective
Nursing perspective

Nature of Phenomenon
Description of problem area and elements in it

Underlying Mechanisms
Description of factors that effect changes in functioning or daily living from the perspectives of:

Pathophysiology and factors related to medical treatment. Includes tumor-related factors and factors associated with surgery, chemotherapy, radiation therapy, biologic response modification, and pharmacologic treatment.

Areas of daily living affecting and affected by phenomenon (varies with phenomenon). Includes activities in daily living, events in daily living (personal, health-related), demands in daily living (self-expectations, demands of others and of possessions), environmental features in either institutional or home and community setting, and values and beliefs.

Areas of functional health status affecting and affected by the phenomenon. Varies with phenomenon but often includes strength and endurance for physical, emotional, and intellectual work; cognition; motivation; courage; communication; and mood.

Nursing Diagnosis and Treatment

Diagnostic Targets
Focus for assessment and diagnosis. Targets always include patients and their presenting situation. Other frequent diagnostic targets include critical family members, companions, care givers, co-workers, sexual partners, or employers when these individuals have an impact on patient's well-being.

Risk Factors
Cues in presenting situation that suggest higher potential for occurrence of problems in daily living, dysfunction, inadequate capacity to manage the requirements of daily living, or deficits in external resources

Diagnostic Areas
Specific diagnostic categories that identify problem areas and related factors. They focus on daily living, areas of dysfunction, or status of resources that impairs effective management of daily living in the presenting situation.

Manifestations
Signs and symptoms that tend to be associated with the phenomenon identified in the diagnostic area; findings that give evidence that daily living is adversely affecting the situation or that deficits in functioning or external resources interfere with effective management of daily living. (Note: Data on strengths in patterns of daily living, functional capacity, and external resources are used as a means of ruling out problems and as elements in decisions about treatment strategies.)

Prognostic Variables
Variables that predict the course of events, trajectory, and outcome in the diagnosed problem areas and the likelihood of satisfaction with the resultant quality of life

Complications
Sequelae associated with failure to manage daily living, functioning or external resources effectively; iatrogenic effects of particular nursing interventions

Table 1-1.   Oragnization of Content in Each Problem Area (continued)

Treatment Guidelines
Strategies prescribed to help the patient, family, or others modify daily living, or their functional capacity or use their external resources in such a way as to promote more effective and satisfying daily living

Evaluation
Variables in which data are collected on an ongoing basis to measure changes in daily living (in any of the relevant subcategories), in functioning, or in availability or use of external resources.

Bibliography

American Cancer Society. Cancer facts and figures—1989. Atlanta: American Cancer Society, 1989.

Benner P, Tanner C. Clinical judgment: how expert nurses use intuition. Am J Nurs 1987;87:23.

Carnevali D. Daily living and functional health status: a perspective for nursing diagnosis and treatment. Archives of Psychiatric Nursing 1988;2:330.

Carnevali D. Nursing care planning: diagnosis and management. 3rd ed. Philadelphia: JB Lippincott, 1983.

Carnevali D, Patrick M: Nursing management for the elderly. 2nd ed. Philadelphia: JB Lippincott, 1986.

Fitzpatrick JJ, Kerr ME, Saba VK et al. Nursing diagnosis: translating nursing diagnosis into ICD code. Am J Nurs 1989;89:493.

Hurley ME, ed. Classification of nursing diagnoses. Proceedings of the Sixth Conference of the North American Nursing Diagnosis Association. St Louis: CV Mosby, 1986.

McNally JC, Stair JC, Sommerville ET, eds. Guidelines for cancer nursing practice. Orlando: Grune & Stratton, 1985.

Reiner A. Manual of patient care standards. Rockville, MD: Aspen Publishers, 1988.

Silverberg E, Lubera JB. Cancer statistics, 1989. CA 1989;39:3.

Tanner C. Theoretical perspectives for research on clinical judgments. In: Hannah KJ, Reimer M, Mills C, Letourneau S, eds. Clinical judgment and decision making: the future with nursing diagnosis. New York: John Wiley & Sons, 1987.

Families and the Experience of Cancer

Individuals who are diagnosed as having cancer are not alone in this experience. They are always a part of some type of a family unit that has a past history, established patterns of relating in normal and crisis times, and a current situation that incorporates much more than a cancer diagnosis for one of its members (Lewis, 1983). The individual with cancer cannot be viewed in isolation from the family, even within the narrow perspectives of physiology and pathophysiology. Here too there is opportunity for the family to affect patient response (Wright and Leahey, 1987; Reiss et al, 1986).

Families have important influences on genetic and lifestyle cancer risks for their members. Past generations contribute to the genetic pool and familial tendencies for the occurrence of cancer.* Family members in the current generation provide an environment and lifestyle that often determines the nature of cancer risks in daily living. The family also tends to establish the values and belief system associated with health and health care, and thus can affect both self-monitoring and use of the health care system.

The family as an entity and the individuals in it will be affected by the occurrence of cancer in a family member. Individuals will vary in their responses to the experience and in their ongoing capacity to relate to the patient, and will alter patterns of daily living to accommodate new roles and functions. In turn, these responses will affect them as individuals, the family as a unit, and, of course, the patient as a member of that family unit.

In subsequent clinical chapters, specific problems faced by family members in a variety of cancer-related situations are identified. Areas for diagnosis are offered and treatment guidelines are proposed. This chapter addresses some basic perspectives for viewing the family as it affects and is affected by cancer in daily living.

---

* See Chapter 5 for more information about genetic factors and family tendencies as well as risk factors in daily living.

Nature of the Family and its Relationship to the Cancer Experience

Families can be viewed in several ways. Each will be important in addressing daily living from the perspectives of risk reduction, cancer detection, and management of issues and problems associated with diagnosis, treatment, survival, advancing disease, and death.

Genetic Families

Individual family members are linked genetically to previous and subsequent generations. Thus, genetic risk factors and familial tendencies are part of the data base when the nurse considers risk management in daily living and priorities for self-monitoring and use of professional health services (Kelly, 1987). When genetic factors or familial tendencies are known factors in the patient's disease, the nurse will want to be alert to emotional responses associated with anger or guilt in the patient, parents, and grandparents. There can also be fear or concern about transmission of the tendency among family members who have children or are contemplating having them.

Family as a Social Unit

Today's configurations for the family as a social unit encompass so many forms that a narrow definition is ineffective for a nursing perspective. Two descriptions will serve as the perspectives used in this book. Family Service of America (1984, p. 7) defined a family as "two or more people joined by bonds of sharing and intimacy." A second description could be that the family is what the patient says it is.

Functions of the Family as a Social Unit

The family as a social unit has several functions (Wright and Leahey, 1987). These include providing for its members:

Support for physical and health needs

A locus of love, intimacy, and motivation

Sociologic and psychologic roots

The family is also an important setting within which developmental or maturational tasks are accomplished.

When a family member has been diagnosed as having cancer, the family assumes some particular functions (Lewis, 1986). Family members:

1.   May contribute to the way in which the patient evolves a personal meaning, purpose, and sense of self-worth as the implications of the cancer diagnosis are assimilated
2.   Take on and are affected by the new demands, stresses, and role realignments imposed by the illness and its contingencies

Family as an Environment

The patient is a product of family environments. Adult patients can bring to the cancer experience a background of both past and current family environments. The environments of childhood will have generated certain beliefs, values, and attitudes toward health and health care, and contributed to some health practices. There can also be a current family environment that is quite different from the childhood environment. This second family environment may involve a partner or solo lifestyle, children, in-laws, older dependent parents, and a different home setting. This current family environment creates current demands, tensions, and supports in daily living. Both earlier and current family environments are factors in diagnosing and treating responses to cancer risk reduction, self-monitoring, and the experience of cancer and its treatment.

Health Teams as Family

It has been proposed that, in life-threatening illness, the treatment team also can come to be seen as family—a therapeutic family (Bahnson, 1987). When cancer becomes a chronic, life-threatening illness, the treatment family may take over some of the functions of the family having to do with physical and health needs. It can also serve as a locus of support and motivation. In many instances the professionals develop emotional bonds with both the patient and some members of the patient's family. These bonds, in turn, affect the team member's responses to changes in the patient's and the family's physiologic and psychosocial responses.

Nurses as an Element in the Patient Family

Nurses and nursing personnel are a source of support for the patient's family during the active treatment and advanced cancer stages. They are an integral part of daily living in the institution and sometimes in the home—sharing the good times and the bad. They learn about family and home strengths and weaknesses as well as the issues of current concern. Nurses are often the bearers of tidings about the cancer experience, bringing good or bad news about test results or response to treatment. While the physician may give the initial information, it is often the nurse who translates and gives meaning to the findings and how they will affect the patient and the daily living of the patient and family. Nurses assist patients and families to prepare for movement to the next step, whether that step is survival with cancer remission or living with advancing disease.

When patients and families are between hospital stays, nurses often receive phone calls or letters reporting progress and gains or problems. Sometimes nurses are contacted for support before or after a particularly frightening visit to the oncologist. Nurses become strong allies—sources of information and support, during hospital contacts and at home.

It is not unusual for nurses who have shared the patient's and family's daily living with the cancer experience over extended periods of time and in a particularly close way to attend the funeral when the patient dies. Both patients and families often see "their nurse" as a part of their extended family during the cancer experience.

Relationships Between the Treatment Family and the Patient Family

Mutual support can evolve as the patient's family and the treatment family attempt to negotiate their priorities and roles around the patient's daily living with cancer. However, it is also possible for tensions to arise between the patient's family and the treatment team as each seeks to provide care to the patient. Attitudes and emotions (whether within the patient or treatment family) are contagious; they can affect the patient's reaction to treatment, to adjustment to the illness, and to rehabilitation. Therefore, awareness of tensions and nontherapeutic responses in either patient or treatment family are important.

Factors Affecting the Family's Adaptation to Stress

Family capacity to adapt to stress has been linked to the interaction between three variables:

The accumulation of demands being made on the family unit—the current stressors, associated hardships, other current events, normal transitional stressors, and any prior strains within the family. These include maturational crises (e.g., children leaving home and creating the empty nest stage, retirement, or becoming an in-law or a grandparent), and situational crises (e.g., job changes, moving, divorces, or accidents) (Lewis et al, 1985).

The internal tensions within the family (e.g., teenagers acting out, problems in managing finances, parenting difficulties). Special effort is needed to manage the family resources and the capacities of individual members. Thought and energy are needed to manage linkages between the family and external resources.

The family's interpretation of the event, its perception of all other demands being placed on the family, and its determination of the actions to be taken in order to balance the requirements with its resources (Mays, 1988; McCubbin and Patterson, 1983). It is important to consider ethnic and religious factors that help to shape both the family's interpretation of events and the types of actions it decides to take.

Difficulties occur when specific or total requirements exceed the available resources. Adaptation occurs with the availability of sufficient total resources and functional capacities and external resources specific to the demands of the situation. Adaptation or coping is a dynamic, fluid state that requires regular nursing assessment, diagnosis, and treatment as requirements and resources change during the course of the cancer experience.

Sources of Family Strains in the Cancer Experience

The experience of cancer within a family presents some common challenges. They affect both individual members and the family unit.

Emotional Strains

Feelings of anxiety, uncertainty, guilt, powerlessness, helplessness, anger, and egocentricity can be generated by events or perceptions of events. Some of the stressors include:

Difficulties in accepting a diagnosed, life-threatening illness and its implications for the family

Occurrence of a cancer in a family member associated with a known genetic origin or familial pattern, leading to feelings of guilt in parents or grandparents, anger in the patient, fear in other offspring

Occurrence of a cancer that is linked to a lifestyle that another family member has tried unsuccessfully to change (e.g., smoking or use of smokeless tobacco, unsafe sexual practices)

Failure to recognize early symptoms of the cancer or to convince the patient to seek prompt medical attention

Discrepancies between health care system and family values or expectations regarding the oncologic treatment of the patient

Occurrence of signs and symptoms associated with the tumor or the treatment that cause suffering, suggest negative outcomes, or are difficult to manage

Inability of family members to offer support to the patient related to difficulties in getting beyond their own discomfort

Loss of the ability to work of a person on whom the family depends for income or care giving

Impending death and the actual death of the family member

Role Realignments and Altered Family Lifestyles

When one member of the family is diagnosed as having cancer and undergoes cancer therapy, it affects the roles and lifestyles of other family members. Roles that are relinquished or only partially filled can disrupt basic areas of family functioning. These can involve critical roles such as homemaker, parent, sexual partner, companion, income producer, or care giver. Often nurses see the male patient's wife continuing to do everything involved in her role before the illness, plus picking up essential activities formerly carried by the patient and adding the burdens of care giving. The increase in physical and emotional demands is tremendous.

Sometimes family members become attached to their new roles and functions or to the changed relationships and power base. When the patient recovers energy and well-being and seeks to return to former roles and relationships, other family members may be reluctant to return to the former patterns.

Priorities and plans may change; for example, a family member may take an early retirement, quit a job, or shift responsibility for care of an older family member to an institution in order to give time and energy to the care of a younger member in the family (Lovejoy, 1986).

New roles are often adopted in the care of the patient, such as helper, companion, watchdog, or advocate. Sometimes one sees the oldest daughter, who is still a child, take on housekeeping and parenting chores, thus hastening the transition into adult roles.

The intensity of preoccupation with the patient may be such that some family members, particularly spouses, become totally "immersed," to the point of neglect of other roles, self-neglect, and, eventually, exhaustion (Lovejoy, 1986). Nurses often recognize this condition when they have assured themselves and the family members that the patient's symptoms are under control, yet the family members still feel unable to leave the bedside to attend to their own needs for rest and respite.

In chronic, life-threatening illness, new sets of rules emerge for interpersonal relationships between the patient and other members of the family. The nature of role relationships changes, even within roles that continue to be fulfilled. For example, the patient may have enough energy to keep working, but have no energy for continuing to do the usual tasks at home. Sometimes these changes in role relationships between family members are openly negotiated. More often they are silently adopted, with varying degrees of satisfaction with the modifications. Communication patterns can change. There may be less willingness and comfort in discussing either physical status or emotional reactions to the situation; or, there may be the reverse—a total preoccupation with the cancer experience to the exclusion of all else. Dissatisfactions with role relationships that are unaddressed can create problems (see sections on Role and Sexuality in Chapter 6.)

Care Giver Roles in the Family

The assignment and implementation of direct care giver roles in the family can be another source of family difficulties. One person may become the care giver by default or be assigned the role—often because of geographic considerations or other factors that seem to make the role a logical one. That person may be comfortable with the role, or may feel "put upon" or "used" by other family members. On the other hand, there may be competition for the dominant care giver or decision maker role; this too can cause problems. Some family members may feel guilty at not contributing "their fair share." Still others may wish to serve as consultants and advice givers, without being involved with assuming any direct responsibility. This latter behavior has been known to create serious anger and resentment for the person who actually delivers the care.

In addition to the intrafamily tensions associated with the care giver respon-sibilities, there can be disagreements between the family care giver and the treatment team. The care giver may sense that new symptoms mean a progression of the cancer, but the treatment team may ignore the reports. On the other hand, the oncologists may want to give more treatment than the family thinks is desirable. Sometimes the patient and the family will have made formal "Physician Directives,"† expecting that no further treatment other than comfort measures will be prescribed. Some physicians will respect this directive as it applies to the cancer, yet still aggressively treat iatrogenic complica-tions in the terminally ill patient. Discrepancies in role expectations, priorities, and values can occur, with resultant tensions and discomfort.

Unfinished Family Business

Sometimes the crisis of the cancer experience brings new life and urgency to previously unresolved, possibly long-dormant, family situations. Unfinished family

---

† A patient and family decision that only palliative treatment be given and that no resuscitative measure be employed—formerly called a "Living Will." For a sample, see Figure 11-1.

business can affect relationships between the patient and family members or between family members. Some examples of unresolved situations are an argument that was never settled satisfactorily; a hurt that was either never disclosed or that was disclosed but never forgiven; a parenting style that affected the child's life negatively; guilt at not living up to another's expectations; or wanting to live long enough to see closure on the part of a family member's achievements, such as seeing a child finish college or get married.

Uncertainty in Providing Comfort to the Patient

Family members may be uncertain and uncomfortable about comforting the patient in his or her physical and emotional suffering. The technical skills, prerequisite knowledge, observational skills, and physical demands of direct care may exceed family resources. Nurses see some families in which the available care givers are incapable of delivering care to the patient. Instead of receiving care at home the patient has multiple hospital admissions—fine discharge plans are doomed to failure.

Feelings of helplessness, guilt, or anger can emerge when the best efforts of the care giver fail to bring comfort, patient acceptance, or a therapeutic outcome. For example, the patient rejects well-prepared, attractively served meals that include favorite foods time after time; efforts to become closer emotionally are rebuffed; pain relief measures fail to bring comfort; or the patient appears to be giving up despite an apparently positive prognosis.

Some family members no longer know how to act toward the patient (Cooper, 1984; Lovejoy, 1986). They don't know what to talk about or how to express their concern—or their discomfort—with the situation.

Concerns About the Meaning of Life, Dying, and Death

The diagnosis of a life-threatening disease such as cancer in a family member can heighten the personal sense of vulnerability or mortality among the others. Fear of the patient's dying occurs at the time of diagnosis and recurs at all transitional points in the course of the disease or treatment (Lewis, 1986).

Some families have a clear need for family structure and relief from tension. For these families, unpredictable treatment results or patterns of remission and relapse characteristic of cancer's chronic stage can be intolerable (Bahnson, 1987). In families that are emotionally close, the patient's suffering and need for care becomes a tremendous burden. Death may then be the contribution the patient makes to the family, so that it can return to a more normal way of life (Reiss et al, 1986; Rolland, 1984).

There are varying degrees of openness in discussion about the issues and problems of daily living with cancer and its consequences for the patient, individual family members, and the family as a unit.

Professionals have seen open discussion of illness-related issues as essential (Northouse, 1984; Lewis, 1986). However, families tend to continue to use earlier communication patterns, and sometimes these patterns have involved avoidance of discussions of emotional issues. When family members have been asked whether openness or avoidance in discussion of existential issues made a difference, they varied in their opinions as to the need for more explicit discussions of the meaning of the cancer and the risks or reality of dying. Some indicated that more open discussions would have made life easier; others thought that it would have made no difference (Welch, 1981; Vachon, 1977; Hinton, 1981).

Nonconvergent Needs

The pace at which the patient and members of the family cognitively and emotionally assimilate the patient's current situation can vary markedly. A corollary to this assumption is another: The needs of patients and those of the family as they seek to manage daily living with a cancer experience are not necessarily congruent. Priorities of concerns, fears, and desired relationships have been found to be quite different (Lewis, 1986). It is crucial, therefore, to gather data from the patient and from the most involved family members about their status of integration of the medical diagnosis and treatment and their needs and not to make unsupported assumptions. It also reinforces the importance of setting realistic nursing goals that take into account the *current* patient and family data base.

Summary

People who have cancer cannot be diagnosed and treated effectively without giving consideration to their family context, past and present. Patient well-being often depends on family well-being. In subsequent chapters, specific issues associated with patients, care givers, family members, companions, and partners will be addressed. Diagnostic areas and treatment guidelines will be offered for them. In addition, patient diagnoses and treatment guidelines that concern relationships with family members and others will also be covered. Daily living with cancer and its treatment, of necessity, involves patients, their family heritage, and their current family situations. Nursing diagnosis, prognosis, and treatment incorporate all of these.

Many families have remarkable capacities for righting themselves as they manage daily living with health-related crises. Nurses can often make a contribution by their judicious help and their "informed and affirming" presence (Lewis, 1983).

Bibliography

Bahnson CB. The impact of life-threatening illness on the family and the impact of the family on illness: an overview. In: Leahey M, Wright LM, eds. Families and life-threatening illness. Springhouse, PA: Springhouse Corp, 1987.

Cooper ET. A pilot study on the effects of the diagnosis of lung cancer on family relationships. Cancer Nurs 1984;7:301.

Family Service of America. The state of families, 1984–85. New York: Family Service America, 1984.

Hinton J. Sharing or withholding awareness of dying between husband and wife. J Psychosom Res 1981;25:337.

Kelly PT. Risk counseling for relatives of cancer patients: new information, new approaches. Journal of Psychosocial Oncology 1987;5:65.

Lewis FM. Family-level services for the cancer patient: critical distinctions, fallacies and assessment. Cancer Nurs 1983;6:193.

Lewis FM. The impact of cancer on the family: a critical analysis of the research literature. Patient Education and Counseling 1986;8:269.

Lewis FM, Ellison ES, Woods NF. The impact of breast cancer on the family. Seminars in Oncology Nursing 1985;1:206.

Lovejoy NC. Family responses to cancer hospitalization. Oncology Nursing Forum 1986;13:33.

Mays RM. Family stress and adaptation. Nurse Pract 1988;13:52.

McCubbin HI, Patterson JM. The family process: the double ABC-X model of adjustment and adaptation. In: McCubbin HI et al, eds. Social stress and the family: advances and developments in family stress theory and research. New York: Haworth Press, 1983.

Northouse L. The impact of cancer on the family: an overview. Int J Psychiatry Med 1984;14:215.

Reiss D et al. Family process, chronic illness and death: on the weakness of strong bonds. Arch Gen Psychiatry 1986;43:795.

Rolland JS. Toward a psychosocial typology of chronic and life-threatening illness. Family Systems Medicine 1984;2:245.

Vachon MLS, Freedman K, Formo A, et al. The final illness in cancer: the widow's perspective. Can Med Assoc J 1977;117:1151.

Welch D. Planning nursing interventions for family members of adult cancer patients. Cancer Nurs 1981;4:365.

Wright LM, Leahey M. Families and life-threatening illness: assumptions, assessment and intervention. In Wright LM, Leahey M, eds. Families and life-threatening illness. Springhouse PA: Springhouse Corp, 1987.

3

Managing Daily Living With Cancer Risk Reduction

Nursing's perspective in cancer prevention is to assist individuals and groups in finding ways of managing daily living in order to limit exposure to known cancer risk factors and to maintain optimum immune status. Figure 3-1 illustrates the utilization of knowledge of the pathogenesis of cancer as a basis for nursing diagnosis and treatment planning in this field.

At present, many factors are thought to contribute to the development of cancers. It is not possible to control some risks; however, there are many variables in patterns of daily living that are thought to influence the development of cancers over which individuals can exert some control.

The nursing perspective for diagnosis and treatment addresses reduction of cancer risks in daily living. Diagnosis involves:

Determining the risk areas in this person's daily living

Diagnosing any deterrents in the presenting situation that will interfere with the person adopting a lifestyle to reduce cancer risk factors

Treatment involves:

Helping individuals and families make informed decisions about their lifestyle as it relates to cancer risks, and teaching them how lifestyle choices can promote a competent immune system

Helping individuals or families develop strategies for making lifestyle changes that will reduce cancer risk

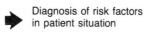

| Knowledge of pathology/ risk factors | | Diagnosis of risk factors in patient situation | | Rx: Changes in daily living/functioning/ environment |

Figure 3-1. *Knowledge needed to diagnose and treat individuals and groups so as to reduce known cancer risks in daily living.*

29

Description of Cancer Risk Reduction

Five areas of concern in cancer risk reduction include:

Genetic background

Nature of exposure to carcinogens in past daily living

Current exposure to risks and the options for risk avoidance in daily living

Maintenance or support of immune system through maintaining an adequate diet, engaging in safe sexual practices, and possibly by responding to stress in as healthy a way as possible

Factors that deter individuals or families from incorporating risk reduction activities and behavior into patterns of daily living

The body of knowledge about factors that contribute to development of cancers and host responses is growing and changing rapidly. There is much that is not known, and what seems true today may not be true tomorrow. Effective nursing diagnosis and treatment to reduce cancer risks relies on a regularly updated knowledge base.

Underlying Mechanisms

Research shows that the appearance of a cancer may represent a multistage pathophysiologic response at the cellular level to exposure to a variety of insults over time (Groer, 1987). Individuals are generally exposed to multiple, rather than single, risks. An example of this is a person who has worked at an occupation involving exposure to asbestos; smokes; drinks alcohol; eats a high fat, low fiber diet with marginal amounts of beta carotene and vitamins A, C, and E; hates vegetables in the cabbage–cauliflower family; has parents and siblings who have had cancer; and is in his fifties.

Less than 20% of cancers are presently attributed to genetic factors. Thus, the bulk of cancers seem to result from lifestyle exposure to carcinogenic factors and some failure in the immunocompetence of the host for surveillance and control of cell alterations (Pitot, 1986).

Pathophysiology

The transformation from normal to malignant cell takes place in several stages involving initiators and promoters, mutations, and changes in gene expression. The change from a normal to malignant cell is thought to be accomplished in three possible ways (Groer, 1987):

Mutagenic change: Genetic information is introduced into the DNA, and there is a resultant somatic mutation that is not adequately repaired. The mutation is continued through transmission to daughter cells in every mitotic division.

Direct action on the cell: A carcinogen may act enzymatically directly on cellular RNA. The enzymatic action modifies the template for the production of DNA, resulting in alteration of the genetic code.

Damage to cellular protein: This alteration results in repression of bits of genetic information that can, in turn, lead to changes in cell characteristics that are associated with malignancy.

Once normal cells have been transformed into a malignant state, body resources involving the host defense system come into play. Nonimmunologic processes, such as endocrinologic and biochemical controls, can interfere with tumor growth and metastasis. Immunologic cancer defenses involve specifically and nonspecifically stimulated cytotoxic T lymphocytes, macrophages, and natural killer (NK) lymphocytes. Research shows that immunocompetence can be diminished by clinical syndromes involving immunologic deficiency. Nutritional status, in general and in specific ways, may influence immune status. Excessive calories, deficiencies in zinc and selenium, and excessive unsaturated fatty acids may be linked to reduced immunocompetence, while vitamin C may enhance the immune system (Creasey, 1985).

Risk Factors for Cancers in Daily Living

Risk factors can be divided into two major categories: host characteristics and host lifestyle, including the environment in which the host's daily living takes place.

Host Characteristics

The host's genetic makeup and other internal variables may play an important role in modification of carcinogens that are encountered (Pitot, 1986).

AGE. Certain cancers occur with greater frequency at differing ages, for example, Wilms' tumors in children, testicular tumors in young men, prostatic tumors in aging men, and Hodgkin's disease, which has a bimodal pattern of higher incidence in the 25- to 34-year and over 55-year age groups. Incidence of cancers increases with aging, possibly related to decreasing immunocompetence or opportunity for more exposure to carcinogens over a longer lifespan.

ETHNICITY. Ethnic groups in the United States tend to show differing patterns of incidence of cancers. There is some question as to whether these differences reflect genetic differences or differences in lifestyle and environment.

Ethnic or Religious Group	Cancer Incidence
Blacks	Increased incidence of lung, prostate, cervical, colon, esophageal, pancreatic, stomach cancers
	Lower incidence of skin cancer
Native Americans	Increased incidence of cervical, gallbladder, pancreatic, stomach cancers
Jews	Increased incidence of ovarian cancer
	Lower incidence of cervical cancer
Mormons	Increased incidence of colon cancer
	Decreased incidence of cervical cancer
Seventh Day Adventists	Decreased incidence of colon and breast cancers
Hispanics	Increased incidence of cervical, gallbladder, liver, stomach cancers
	Lower incidence of breast and colon cancers
White Americans	Increased incidence of bladder, breast, colorectal, larynx, lung, ovarian, prostate, testis, uterus cancers

HEREDITY.   At least 50 hereditary conditions have been linked to the occurrence of particular cancers (Pitot, 1986). Further, family cancer syndromes have been identified that occur in succeeding generations. These cancers are characterized as having a commonality of site, occurring at an earlier age, occurring in multiple sites and paired organs, and showing a narrower range of histologic expression (Oleske and Groenwald, 1987).

PERSONALITY TRAITS.   While the research findings are mixed, a review of reported research suggests that two traits may have some association with the incidence of cancer. These are loss of or lack of an important person in one's early years (e.g., death of a parent) and an inability to express hostile feelings (Cox and MacKay, 1982).

PREVIOUS DISEASES.   Some previously experienced diseases place an individual at greater risk for subsequent cancers.

Type of Cancer	Previous Disease	Strength of Risk
Breast	Obesity	S
	Previous breast cancer	S
Cervical	Cervical dysplasia	K
	Herpes simplex type 2	S
	Papilloma virus	K
Colon	Adenomatous polyps	K
	Crohn's disease	K
	Ulcerative colitis	K
Endometrial	Obesity	S
Hepatoma	Hepatitis B	S
	Cirrhosis	S
Lymphoma	Epstein-Barr virus	S
	Malaria	S
	AIDS	K
Mouth	Leukoplakia	K
Sarcoma	AIDS	K
Skin	Keratosis	S

K: known risk; S: speculated risk
(Oleske and Groenwald, 1987; Pitot, 1986)

PRIOR MEDICAL TREATMENT.   Prior medical treatment of pathology can influence the subsequent occurrence of cancers. Persons who were subjected to the following prescribed medical treatments have greater risks of specific forms of cancer.

Medical Treatment	Form of Cancer
Radiation for enlarged thymus or thyroid glands or tinea capitis	Cancers of head and neck
Radiation for benign gynecologic conditions	Leukemias and tumors in pelvic region
Estrogen for post-menopausal symptoms	Endometrial cancer

(continued)

Medical Treatment	Form of Cancer
Radiation of fetus in utero	Increased cancer incidence in offspring
Immunosuppressive therapy	Reticuloendothelial system cancers
Alkylating agents (cyclophosphamide, melphalan)	Bladder cancer
Diethylstilbesterol to prevent loss of a pregnancy	Vaginal adenocarcinomas in offspring

GENDER.   Certain cancers are obviously linked to a specific sex, for example, ovarian cancers in women and prostatic cancers in men. However, beyond this it has been found that men, overall, have a higher incidence of cancer and a lower survival rate (Silverberg and Lubera, 1989).

STRESS   There is some speculation that links may exist between stress, coping, and cancers (Borysenko and Borysenko, 1982; Ersek, 1986; Locke, 1982). Scientific strategies for discovering these linkages are difficult and findings have been inconsistent. However, pathways have been hypothesized (Riley et al, 1981), and future work may offer greater insight.

SUMMARY.   Background circumstances and events alter the host environment for carcinogens and neoplastic changes. Many factors are beyond the control of the individual. Data on hereditary background and earlier life events that increase cancer risks are important from a nursing perspective, since they may signal a need for more careful self-monitoring and monitoring by medical professionals.

Host Behavior and Lifestyle

It has been estimated that about 80% of cancers can be linked to exogenous factors. Many of these fall well within the control of the individual, families, and groups (DeWys et al, 1986; Doll and Peto, 1981).

ALCOHOL CONSUMPTION.   Alcohol consumption alone has been linked to increased risk for esophageal and liver cancers. As a cocarcinogen with smoking it greatly increases the risk for cancers of the mouth, larynx, throat, esophagus, and liver (American Cancer Society, 1989; Tuyns, 1979; Tuyns et al, 1982).

USE OF TOBACCO.   Tobacco, whether smoked, placed in the mouth, chewed, or used as snuff, is carcinogenic to the lungs and the oral and nasal cavities. It has been estimated that 85% to 90% of lung cancer and 30% of all other cancers in the United States are directly connected to tobacco smoking (Doll and Peto, 1981). Use of tobacco has also been implicated as a risk factor in cancers of the mouth, pharynx, larynx, esophagus, pancreas, cervix, and bladder (American Cancer Society, 1989).

Exposure to the sidestream smoke of cigarette smokers (passive smoking) in enclosed spaces such as home and work environments has been under study since the mid 1970s. There seems to be agreement that passive smoking does carry some degree of cancer risk (Saracci, 1986).

DIET.   Some dietary characteristics currently are thought to increase the risk of cancer, while some others may reduce the risk (American Cancer Society, 1989; Byers and Funch, 1984; Cohen, 1987; United States Public Health Service, 1988; Willett and MacMahon, 1984).

Dietary Characteristics	Site of Possible Increased Cancer Risk
High fat	Colon, endometrium, breast, prostate
High fat, low fiber	Colon
High fat, high unsaturated fats	Breast, lung
High alcohol intake	Mouth, larynx, esophagus, liver
Excessive calories (women)	Breast, endometrium
Charred or browned foods	Stomach, esophagus
Smoked foods—nitrates, nitrosamine	Bladder, stomach, esophagus
Moldy foods—aflatoxin (contaminated peanuts, corn, cottonseed, cheese)	Liver, esophagus

(American Cancer Society, 1989; United States Public Health Service, Office of the Surgeon General, 1988)

Dietary Characteristics	Site of Possible Reduced Cancer Risk
Regular intake of vegetable, fruit, and cereal fiber and lowered fat intake	Colon
Regular intake of cruciferous vegetables	Colon
Vitamin C	Bladder, colon, esophagus, mouth, lung
Vitamin A (beta carotene, retinol)	Bladder, esophagus, larynx, lung, mouth
Vitamin E (antioxidant)	General protection

(American Cancer Society, 1989; Cohen, 1987; Craddock, 1983; Creasey, 1985; Doll and Peto, 1981; Yamanaka, 1987)

Iron supplementation resulting in high body iron stores has been reported to increase cancer risk in men; it may have the same effect in women (Stevens et al, 1988). Iron serves as an oxidant, and may interact with other agents (e.g., radiation) to magnify their effects. Iron supplementation is considered unwise for those who are not anemic.

Regular inclusion of certain foods in the diet and use of specific manners of food preparation can either increase cancer risks or provide protection. Current guidelines suggest:

Regular inclusion of fruits, vegetables, and whole grains to provide adequate fiber—20 to 30 g per day, but not more than 35 g

Regular inclusion of cruciferous vegetables—broccoli, cabbage, kale, cauliflower, and brussels sprouts

Regular inclusion of fresh carrots, peaches, apricots, and squash (i.e., yellow fruits and vegetables) and broccoli for their beta carotene (Menkes et al, 1986)

Regular inclusion of fruits and vegetables high in vitamin C—citrus fruits, cantaloupe, strawberries, red and green peppers, broccoli, and tomatoes

Restrictions in use of smoked, salt-cured, brined, and nitrite-cured foods

Restriction of fat to 30% or less of total caloric intake

Restriction of calories to attain or maintain an optimum weight for height and age

Restrictions in foods that have been charred or burnt in their cooking

Avoidance of cheeses or foods that have developed molds on them during storage

Moderation in the intake of alcoholic beverages

Careful washing of fruits and vegetables grown in areas of industrial pollution

EXPOSURE TO SUNLIGHT. Exposure to ultraviolet rays from the sun has been known to increase the incidence of skin cancers, both melanomas and nonmelanomatous tumors. Lighter skin, hair, and eye color; duration of exposure; exposure between 10 AM and 3 PM; being closer to the equator; and the presence of dysplastic moles (i.e., moles displaying asymmetry, border irregularity, color that is not uniform, or having a diameter greater than 6 mm) or senile keratoses all increase the risks. Solar radiation risks may be increasing for humans generally. For each percentage point of decrease in the stratospheric ozone layer around the earth, a 4% or greater increase in the number of nonmelanomatous skin cancers is predicted (Schottenfeld and Fraumeni, 1982).

It has been speculated that ultraviolet light may enhance rather than initiate melanomas (Viola and Houghton, 1982), or may alter the host immunologic status in such a way as to enhance neoplastic growth (Kripke, 1979).

HOUSING. Carcinogenic pollutants associated with housing are being considered as a possible risk factor in daily living.

Radon gas, a natural byproduct of radium and uranium in the soil, has received increasing attention as a contributor to lung cancer, not only for uranium miners, but also for the general population. In the outdoors radon is thought to be diluted to nondangerous levels; however, it has been found to accumulate in buildings. In some homes and other buildings levels of radon have been found to exceed the 4 picocuries per liter (pCi/L) recommended by the Environmental Protection Agency. Studies are in progress to determine the extent of the cancer risk posed by radon levels exceeding this standard. Current positions on the risk vary widely (American Cancer Society, 1989; Council on Scientific Affairs, American Medical Association, 1987). In the meantime, individuals who are concerned can obtain home testing kits. There are strategies to reduce the radon entering a building and to vent any entering radon from the home. Information on the most updated technology can be obtained from the U.S. Environmental Protection Agency, Center for Environmental Information, 26 W. St. Clair Street, Cincinnati, Ohio 45268.

There are other possible risk factors. Carcinogenic chemicals in drinking water may be a matter for concern (Beresford, 1986). Carcinogenic links have also been suggested associated with living under high-tension wires (Savitz, 1985). Living in the prevailing wind pattern from nuclear plants, where accidental releases of radiation can occur, may increase risks of subsequent cancer development. While these are matters for community action rather than individual action in most instances, such action needs to be founded on a sound base of knowledge.

OCCUPATION.   Exposure to carcinogens in the work environment is receiving increasing attention. Some substances have a questionable linkage with cancer, but for others the evidence for carcinogenicity is sufficient. Among the latter are:

Carcinogen or Industry	Associated Cancers
Aromatic amines and nitroamines (paint manufacturers, leather and shoe workers)	Bladder
Arsenic (tanners, smelters, vintners, plastic workers, insecticide makers, sprayers)	Lung
Abestos (asbestos users)	Lung
Benzene (benzene, explosives, and rubber cement workers)	Leukemia
Bis—choromethyl ether (chemical workers)	Lung
Chromium (glass, pottery, and linoleum makers)	Lung
Coal dust (hematite miners)	Lung
Isopropyl alcohol (manufacturers)	Paranasal
Hardwood dust (manufacturers using hardwoods)	Nasal
Ionizing radiation (radiologists, radium dial painters)	Leukemia, osteosarcoma
Leather dust (shoe manufacturers and repairers)	Nasal
Nickel (nickel smelters, mixers, and roasters, electrolysis workers)	Lung, nasal
Rubber (rubber manufacturers)	Leukemia, bladder
Soot, tars, and oils (asphalt, coal, tar, and pitch workers, gas strokers)	Skin, lung, bladder, gastrointestinal tract
Vinyl choloride used in manufacturing of plastics	Liver

(Pitot, 1986)

SEXUAL ACTIVITY PATTERNS.   Some patterns of sexual activity have been linked to increased incidence of cancer. Women who become sexually active early and have multiple partners are at greater risk of cervical cancer. Nulliparous women, those who do not breast-feed, and those who have their children after the age of 30 have increased risk of breast cancer. Women who have multiple sexual partners and fail to require effective condom use or who are married to men who are bisexual or are intravenous drug users risk acquired immunodeficiency syndrome (AIDS) and the associated Kaposi's sarcoma or non-Hodgkin's lymphomas. Children born of human immunodeficiency virus (HIV)-positive or AIDS-infected mothers also face risks of being born HIV positive. Men who are sexually active with other men, particularly those who have multiple partners and those who do not use condoms consistently and effectively, are at high risk for AIDS and the associated cancers.

SOCIOECONOMIC STATUS.   A few cancers have been linked to socioeconomic status. Cervical and stomach cancers have a higher incidence among individuals of low economic status, and colon cancers among people of higher economic status (Oleske and Groenwald, 1987).

SUMMARY.   It would be impossible to order one's daily living to avoid all of the presently known cancer risk factors. People who are survivors inevitably age and have greater risk for cancer. One's parents and genetic heritage are a given. One's initial socioeconomic status, cultural and religious background, and geographic area and housing during childhood are all controlled by others. To a major extent, so are air and water quality and the placement of industries, power lines, and nuclear facilities. However, there is a growing awareness of the power that people in a community can have when they unite to control developments they see as harmful. This is represented by the new acronym, NIMBY, meaning "not in my backyard." Informed decision making regarding cancer risk factors is being extended from the individual focus to local, regional, and international communities.

Dynamics of Introducing Changes in Daily Living

There is no question that individuals and groups must have usable information on the current status of known cancer risk factors in order to make informed decisions about their lifestyle and the environment in which they live. However, while necessary, the availability of information is only one variable that influences health behavior in daily living.

Other factors that have been found to influence individuals' willingness to modify their daily living to include specific health-related behaviors include (Janz and Becker, 1984; Redecker, 1988; Rosenstock, 1974):

Belief in personal susceptibility to a disease

Belief that the disease would have at least moderately severe consequences for some aspect of daily living and quality of life

Belief that the proposed behavior change will reduce the health threat

Belief that the benefits outweigh the personal costs of the behavior to be undertaken

The amount of change in behavior involved

Duration of the required change in behavior or patterns in daily living

The difficulty involved in changing behavior or patterns in daily living

Social and cultural cues that are strong enough to trigger a person to take action and to maintain the behavior

Self-concept of the person who is considering making the changes

Locus of control in the person who is considering making the changes

All of these dynamics should be considered in the nursing diagnosis and treatment of problems individuals and families encounter as they contemplate changes in daily living to reduce cancer risks or promote resistance.

Daily Living Factors

There are specific areas in daily living and particular elements within these areas that are involved with managing daily living in order to reduce cancer risks. Cancer risk can be reduced by applying knowledge and understanding of the underlying dynamics addressed in the previous section of the chapter to relevant areas of daily living. Examples of applications follow.

Activities in Daily Living	Reading labels for possible carcinogens (e.g., food additives) in prepared foods when shopping

Avoiding food preparation that involves charring or burning

Developing patterns of food selection that include appropriate levels of vegetable, cereal, and fruit fiber; a low fat content; and adequate amounts of beta carotene and vitamins A and C

Discarding moldy cheese, bread, and other foods

Not smoking and avoiding passive cigarette smoke in enclosed spaces as much as possible

Limiting exposure of the skin and eyes to solar radiation through use of clothing, grade 15 or higher sunscreen protection, effective sunglasses (see the sun protection rating on the glasses and select protection adequate for the proposed activity), restriction of sun exposure between 10 AM and 3 PM, and avoidance of artificial tanning devices or medications

Engaging in "safe" sexual practices—abstinence, monogamy, effective condom use

Maintaining an awareness of carcinogens in the workplace, using protective devices, and advocating for adequate control of or protection from carcinogens

Gathering information on carcinogenic risks associated with housing prior to renting or purchasing. Monitoring for radon in buildings in high risk areas and using currently available technology to reduce risks

Participating in activities (reading, listening, watching, discussing) to expand knowledge of current perspectives on cancer prevention

Events in Daily Living

Awareness of past events that may have increased one's risks for cancer, and thus require greater care in self-monitoring and monitoring by medical professionals (e.g., exposure to radiation fallout or severe sunburn in childhood, with risk for subsequent melanoma)

Avoidance of future events that may carry unusual risks of exposure to carcinogens

Participation in activities to help others to reduce cancer risks

Participation in elections, hearings, and petition drives in which carcinogenic risks are an issue

Demands in Daily Living

Self-expectations

Status of an individual's or family's self-expectations for engaging in daily living in such a way as to incorporate cancer risk reduction without developing cancer phobia

Status of self-expectations for conformity with the demands of others (see below) versus taking action for personal well-being and that of others

Others' expectations

Expectations of developers, industrialists, employers, governments, and agribusinesses that they be allowed to increase risks related to carcinogens or that regulations be set for standards that reduce or eliminate unacceptable cancer risks

Demands of others that one engage in or continue behaviors that create a risk for cancer (e.g., unsafe sexual activity or occupational activities)

Environment for Daily Living

Reducing the presence of known carcinogens in one's personal environment

Avoiding areas where carcinogens are known to exist, or taking appropriate precautions

Being politically active in monitoring and controlling carcinogens in the environment

Promoting resources in the community for keeping abreast of changing knowledge on cancer prevention

Values and Beliefs

Status of values related to a lifestyle that minimizes known cancer risks versus a previously preferred lifestyle in eating, sunbathing, use of tobacco and alcohol, sexual practices, occupation, or housing

Functional Health Status

Certain areas of functional capacity are crucial to effective management of daily living to reduce cancer risks. Examples of these follow.

Cognition

Capacity to learn about cancer prevention

Ability to evaluate one's own life situation in terms of cancer risks

Understanding of strategies for changing established behavior or addictive patterns

Motivation

Status of desire to make adaptations in daily living activities, values, and environment in order to reduce cancer risks

Willingness to initiate changes in lifestyle

Endurance

Capacity to persist in lifestyle changes once they have been introduced

Communication

Verbal skills to discuss ideas and issues related to cancer risk reduction in lifestyle and environment

Verbal skills to negotiate with others regarding new needs and changes in behavior and role relationships associated with cancer risk reduction in one's daily living

Nursing Diagnosis and Treatment

Nursing diagnosis, prognosis, and treatment address data-supported difficulties and problems that individuals, families, and groups are having, or are predicted to have, in reducing cancer risks in their daily living. The focus also addresses means to promote health and make the host more resistant to the insults of unavoidable carcinogens.

Diagnostic Targets

Individuals, families, and groups who need or want assistance in either of the following:

Understanding why they need to change their daily living to reduce cancer risks

Developing workable strategies for making changes in daily living to reduce cancer risks

Risk Factors

Individuals and families at risk of not incorporating risk reduction into daily living include those whose:

Health beliefs do not link patterns in daily living and the environment to risks of malignancy

Preference for or addiction to current lifestyle and environment override concern about risk reduction for cancers ("It can't happen to me")

Working knowledge of risk factors in daily living is insufficient to offer a foundation for informed decision making regarding daily living and cancer risks, due to lack of either opportunity or ability to learn

Life situation and resources do not permit the changes needed to reduce cancer risks

Diagnostic Areas

Decreased ability to make informed decisions related to (R/T) lack of exposure to knowledge in a usable form regarding risk factors in daily living

Decreased ability to make informed decisions R/T limitations in capacity to understand the available information about cancer risks as it applies to their daily living

Inadequate ability to change patterns in daily living and environment to reduce cancer risk factors R/T having only recall level, rather than application level, of understanding

Inability to incorporate knowledge of cancer risk factors into daily living R/T health belief system that does not permit linking risk factors in daily living to the occurrence of cancer

Lack of willingness to acquire knowledge about cancer risks in daily living R/T sense of own immortality, which negates any need to have such information

Limited motivation to initiate lifestyle changes R/T preference for present lifestyle and environment over those associated with cancer risk reduction

Difficulty in changing lifestyle R/T addiction to a cancer risk activity

Inability to alter (specified) risk factors in daily living R/T constraints of life situation or external resources

Manifestations   Impaired ability to reduce cancer risks, or daily living that does not incorporate cancer risk reduction can be manifested in a variety of ways:

Reported or observed lack of exposure to cancer risk information in a form that can be comprehended or used

Observed lack of available sources of information on cancer risk reduction and health promotion that take into consideration:

The person's first language

The appropriate level of vocabulary, sentence structure, and illustrations

A visual or auditory form that is usable for persons who are illiterate, preliterate, or who have visual or hearing impairments

The cultural variables for expression of concepts, use of words, and illustrations

Person recalls information about cancer risks in daily living, but reports or is observed not to have patterns of daily living that reflect this knowledge. Reports that he or she doesn't know how to make the changes.

Person reports no concern about cancer: "There is no cancer in my family" or "I know many old people who have smoked all their lives and don't have cancer" or "If you're going to get the 'big C,' you're going to get it—no sense worrying about it all the time."

Member of a culture (ethnic, religious) whose belief system does not link cancer to the currently identified risk factors. Evidence of membership in such a group or the person reports such a health belief system

Person gives evidence of adequate knowledge of risk factors in own daily living, but continues to engage in activities or behavior that contain risks. Indicates a preference to continue current lifestyle, for now.

Daily living includes activities or substances that are known to be physiologically or psychologically addictive, and patterns of these activities and use of substances reflect addiction, with its associated values and norms

Evidence of constraints in life situation that do not permit incorporation of selected risk reduction—limited financial resources, sanctions from personal network, job obligations, obligation in care for others, dependence on others in living situation, and limited control over geographic location, housing, diet, or other elements of lifestyle

Prognostic Variables

A good prognosis for the person adapting his or her lifestyle and environment to incorporate cancer risk reduction is associated with:

Being female (Disch, 1987)

Being part of or having been part of a family in which the norms support a cancer risk reduction lifestyle and active participation in positive health related behaviors

Having access to current information in a form that is usable to the individual or group

Having readily available and acceptable assistance in translating knowledge into strategies for making adaptations in lifestyle that might otherwise be difficult (e.g., stop smoking programs, dietary changes adapted to previous patterns and ethnic norms, radon monitors, asbestos removal programs, gay groups promoting safer sexual practices, community programs offering bleach packets to intravenous drug users)

Ongoing exchanges or discussions that may enable the individual to integrate cancer risk reduction ideas and values into personal philosophy

Personal characteristics of intellectual ability, adaptability, strong health motivation, and capacity to influence others who control elements of his or her life

Complications

Failure to reduce known cancer risks can result in the appearance of malignancies (e.g., smoking and lung cancer, tanning and skin cancers, intravenous drug use with shared needles and AIDS and then cancers).

Incorporation of changes in lifestyle that are alien from one's family or social group can result in alienation and social isolation.

Sense of quality of life may be reduced by the changes in lifestyle or environment that are adopted in reducing cancer risks.

Cancer phobia may develop that dominates lifestyle and decreases quality of life.

Treatment Guidelines

Lack of availability of cancer risk reduction information

Refer to a reliable resource for information.

Provide information in a form that is usable to the person.

Work with organizations to develop materials to meet the needs of individuals and groups who require adjustments from currently available written, audio, and visual resources.

Work with organizations to make resources about cancer risk reduction accessible to individuals and groups who may not fit mainstream norms.

Learning difficulties

Gather data on the nature and history of learning difficulties. Make a prognostic judgment as to the likelihood of the person being able to assimilate cancer risk reduction information into his or her thinking and lifestyle. Undertake a treatment plan that realistically incorporates the specifics of the prognosis.

Refer to resources or provide information in forms that circum-vent or minimize the learning difficulty.

Offer occasions for the person to safely and comfortably discuss his or her perception or interpretation of the information and receive validating or modifying feedback.

Learning limited to recall rather than application level

Gather data to make a prognostic judgment as to the ability of the person to utilize cancer risk reduction information in mak-ing appropriate adjustments in lifestyle. Adjust treatment strat-egies to prognostic judgment.

Gather data on cancer risk reduction regarding one area of current patterns of daily living (e.g., eating, smoking, alcohol use, sexual activity). Ask the person to give examples of how this knowledge can be used as a basis for modifying patterns of daily living in that area. If the person has difficulty, model the application of knowledge to daily living (in one's own or his or her situation). Explore potential problems and alternative strat-egies for resolving them.

Health belief system precludes incorporation of cancer risk reduction into daily living

Gather data on the nature of the beliefs that have an impact on cancer risk reduction. Make a judgment as to whether there is any way to integrate any of the concepts of carcinogenesis and risk reduction into the existing belief system.

If there seems to be a possibility, neutrally offer the ideas or concepts in a way that utilizes the elements and words of the existing belief system. Ask whether there is congruence be-tween these ideas and the belief system.

If the health belief system seems to preclude an integration of cancer risks, indicate the legitimacy of differences in perspec-tive and offer to serve as a resource, should the person have questions or wish to explore the ideas further at a future time.

"Not me" syndrome

Gather information on the basis for the lack of interest in minimizing cancer risks.

Explore relevant areas of daily living in which adjustments could be made that would be minimally disruptive.

Introduce the idea of informed decision making in control of one's lifestyle.

Identify resources for information on cancer risks and risk reduction for use should an interest or concern arise at a later date.

Preference for, or addictions within, present lifestyle

Gather data on daily living patterns that currently incorporate cancer risk reduction and those that do not. Give positive recognition to current lifestyle patterns that include risk reduction.

In areas of daily living in which modifications might further reduce cancer risks, gather information to distinguish those areas that may be open to change versus those that are currently too valued or addicted to be changed. Acknowledge that change is not easy.

Explore options and strategies for introducing risk reduction changes in areas that do not fall within the currently unchangeable category.

In areas of daily living that are currently too valued or addicted to be changed, provide information regarding cancer risks, but only as a basis for the person's informed decision making—not as a threat.

Identify resources for information and for support in making lifestyle changes that may be difficult to do in isolation (e.g., stop smoking programs, drug rehabilitation programs, weight reduction programs).

Life circumstances preclude incorporation of specific risk reduction activities

Gather data on areas of daily living in which risk reduction is in place and those in which further risk reduction would be advisable. Give positive recognition for current achievements in cancer risk reduction.

Gather data on the barriers in areas of cancer risk reduction that the person or family desires to make (e.g., lack of money for proper nutrition, inability to change occupations or housing, inability to escape passive cigarette smoke at home or in the work setting).

Refer to, or mobilize, resources that may enable the person or family to gain greater control over the risk area. Explore ways to minimize risk and promote health within the factors that cannot be changed.

Evaluation   Response to the nursing interventions to help individuals or families to modify daily living to reduce cancer risk factors can be evaluated in terms of the status of:

Availability of resources for learning about cancer risks in forms that the person or group can use and assimilate

Capacity to learn

Ability to identify verbally the cancer risk factors in daily living

Ability to describe the cancer risk factors as they apply to personal daily living—current behavior and environmental factors that are protective or risk reducing and those that produce risks

Ability to plan and implement strategies to change behavior and environment to reduce cancer risks

Willingness to entertain the possibility of future changes in lifestyle to reduce cancer risks

Awareness of resources for gaining information about cancer risks and forms of support for making changes in lifestyle

Possibilities for integrating concepts of carcinogenesis and daily living for cancer risk reduction with existing health belief system

Insight into the influence that currently held beliefs and values are having on daily living as it relates to cancer risk reduction

Access to resources for overcoming barriers to making cancer reduction changes in lifestyle or environment

Summary

At present it is believed that the majority of cancers are linked to lifestyle and environment. Many of these cancer risk factors are within the control of the individual, family, group, or community. The nursing perspective for diagnosis, prognosis, and treatment in cancer risk reduction addresses individuals' daily living patterns and environment as these interact with their internal and external resources. The goal is to effect the implementation of a lifestyle that promotes protective factors and removes risk factors.

Bibliography

American Cancer Society. Cancer facts and figures—1989. Atlanta: American Cancer Society, 1989.

Beresford SA. Epidemiologic assessment of health risks associated with organic micropollutants in drinking water. In: Ram NM, Calabrese E, Christman RF, eds. Organic carcinogens in drinking water. New York: John Wiley & Sons, 1986.

Borysenko M, Borysenko J. Stress behavior and immunity: animal models and mediating mechanisms. Gen Hosp Psychiatry 1982;4:59.

Byers T, Funch D. Towards the dietary prevention of cancer: contributions of epidemiology. Cancer Detect Prev 1984;7:135.

Cohen LA. Diet and cancer. Sci Am 1987;257:42.

Council on Scientific Affairs, American Medical Association. Radon in homes. JAMA 1987;258:668.

Cox T, MacKay C. Psychosocial factors and psychophysiological mechanisms in the aetiology and development of cancers. Soc Sci Med 1982;16:381.

Craddock VM. Nitrosamines and human cancer: proof of an association? Nature 1983;306:618.

Creasey WA. Diet and cancer. Philadelphia: Lea & Febiger, 1985.

DeWys WD, Malone WF, Butrum RR, Sestili MA. Clinical trials in cancer prevention. Cancer 1986;58:1954.

Disch J. Factors affecting health behavior. In: Groenwald S, ed. Cancer nursing: principles and practice. Monterey, CA: Jones & Bartlett, 1987.

Doll R, Peto R. The causes of cancer: quantitative estimates of avoidable risks of cancer in the United States today. Oxford: Oxford University Press, 1981.

Ersek M. Stress and cancer: elusive connections. Oncology Nursing Forum 1986;13:49.

Groer MW. Risk factors and theories of carcinogenesis. In: Groenwald S, ed. Cancer nursing: principles and practice. Monterey, CA: Jones & Bartlett, 1987.

Janz N, Becker M. The health belief model: a decade later. Health Educ Q 1984;11:1.

Kripke M. Speculations on the role of ultraviolet radiation in the development of malignant melanoma. Journal of the National Cancer Institute 1979;63:541.

Locke SE. Stress adaptation and immunity: studies in humans. Gen Hosp Psychiatry 1982;4:49.

Menkes MS, Comstock GW, Vuilleumier JT et al. Serum beta-carotene, vitamins A and E, selenium and the risk of lung cancer. N Engl J Med 1986;315:1250.

Oleske D, Groenwald S. Epidemiology of cancer. In: Groenwald S, ed. Cancer nursing: principles and practice. Monterey, CA: Jones & Bartlett, 1987.

Pitot HC. Fundamentals of oncology. 3rd ed. New York: Marcel Dekker, 1986.

Redecker NS. Health beliefs and adherence in chronic illness. Image 1988;20:31.

Riley V, Fitzmaurice MA, Spackman DH. Immunocompetence and neoplasia: role of anxiety, stress. In: Levy S, ed. Biological mediators of behavior and disease: neoplasia. New York: Elsevier Biomedical, 1981.

Rosenstock IM. Historical origins of the health belief model. In: Becker MH, ed. The health belief model and personal health behavior. Thorofare, NJ: Slack, 1974.

Saracci R. Passive smoking and lung cancer. International Agency for Research on Cancer Science Publication 1986;74:173.

Savitz DA. Human studies of carcinogenic, reproductive and general human health effects of ELF fields. In: Biological and human health effects of extremely low frequency (ELF) electromagnetic fields: post-1977 literature review. Washington, DC: American Institute of Biological Sciences, 1985.

Schottenfeld D, Fraumeni JF. Cancer epidemiology and prevention. Philadelphia: WB Saunders, 1982.

Silverberg E, Lubera JB. Cancer statistics, 1989. CA 1989;39:2.

Stevens RG, Jones Y, Micozzi MS, Taylor PR. Body iron stores and the risk of cancer. N Engl J Med 1988;319:1047.

Tuyns AJ. Epidemiology of alcohol and cancer. Cancer Res 1979;39:2840.

Tuyns AJ, Pequignot G, Gignoux M, Valla A. Cancers of the digestive tract, alcohol and tobacco. Int J Cancer 1982;30:9.

United States Public Health Service, Office of the Surgeon General. The surgeon general's report on nutrition and health. PHS #88-50210. Washington DC: United States Department of Health and Human Services, Public Health Service, 1988.

Viola MV, Houghton AN. Solar radiation and cutaneous melanoma. Hosp Pract 1982;17:97.

Willett WC, MacMahon B. Diet and cancer: an overview. Parts I and II. N Engl J Med 1984;310:663, 697.

Yamanaka WK. Vitamins and cancer prevention: how much do we know? Postgrad Med 1987;82:149.

4

Incorporation of Self-Monitoring for Cancer Into Daily Living

Self-monitoring and the decision to seek regular physical examinations in maintaining an awareness of one's health status is currently seen as the approach of choice for early detection and effective treatment for cancer. However, large numbers of individuals do not incorporate these health monitoring behaviors into daily living.

Nature of Self-Monitoring

Incorporating behaviors of self-surveillance and use of professional health care services to monitor for the earliest signs of cancer involves several components. These include knowledge of risk factors and earliest manifestations of cancers, body awareness, physical capabilities needed for self-observation, skills in self-monitoring, availability of professional and financial resources to seek regular health care, and values and beliefs that influence decisions and behavior.

Knowledge of Cancer Risk Factors and Early Manifestations

Incorporation of cancer surveillance behaviors into daily living seems to occur most consistently when the individual feels threatened by the disease (Rutledge, 1987; Blesch, 1986). Thus, knowledge of cancer risks and identification of factors in one's family history and lifestyle that increase the risk of cancer can be important forces in motivating self-monitoring behavior. (See Chapter 3 for a description of cancer risks.) Such knowledge also influences the person's decision to see a physician if suspicious signs or symptoms are noted. It may cause the person to seek help promptly, but it can also cause delay if the person is extremely fearful of a confirmation of a diagnosis of cancer.

Knowledge of early manifestations of cancer is crucial to effective self-monitoring and the decision to seek professional health care. Without knowing what specific cues to observe, efficient self-monitoring is not possible.

Body Awareness

Awareness of cues in the body that indicate changes in structure or functioning is an essential component of self-surveillance. The importance attached to the body's signals is another.

Some individuals pay more attention to their body signals than others do. Hypochondriasis or cancer phobia represents the extreme of the person who may attribute any change in appearance or any symptom to cancers. Individuals at the other end of the continuum tend to ignore body signals as being harmless, transitory, or amenable to the human body's own repair capability. As in any continuum, most individuals fall within these extremes, tending to pay attention to signs or symptoms or tending to minimize them with some degree of a wait-and-see attitude. Data on the usual pattern of individual and family response to signs and symptoms is important in nursing diagnosis and treatment of presenting situations involving promotion of effective self-surveillance for cancer.

Functional Capability for Self-Monitoring

Functional capability can have a major impact on the person's capability for self-surveillance. The senses, particularly vision, touch, and pain sensation, are involved in recognition of body changes. Cognitive capability to assign meaning and significance to sensory cues is also essential. At times obesity and deficits in body flexibility and mobility of parts can be factors that impede self-examination.

Skills of Self-Monitoring

Self-examination involves not only motivation, knowledge, and capability, but also skills, if it is to be done well. Crucial skills involve positioning, lighting, techniques of palpation and examination, and developing a feel and visual image of what is normal in one's own body tissue and what constitutes a significant change.

Values and Beliefs

Both societal and individual beliefs and values can influence the extent to which individuals participate in self-monitoring. They can also influence the kind of sanctioning or support that families and others offer to this health behavior.

In some cultural and religious groups, the examination of one's own body, particularly breasts and genitalia, is not acceptable behavior. Permission of a male relative or spouse must be given before females may legitimately engage in breast or vulvar self-examination in some cultures. Religious beliefs that may influence self-monitoring and seeking of professional health care include the belief that any condition or situation occurs because it is the will of God, belief in predestination or fate, and the belief that disease will not occur in individuals whose faith in the Supreme Being is sufficient. Some people believe that cancer truly is incurable so there is little point in early discovery. Stereotypes about older persons not getting cancer or not being suitable candidates for treatment can affect their access to effective self-surveillance and professional assistance (Frank-Stromberg, 1986). All of these beliefs can affect the manner in which individuals incorporate self-surveillance for cancers into daily living patterns.

Beyond societal beliefs are the individual's values and priorities. At particular stages in life, particularly among the young, there is a stronger belief in one's invulnerability or immunity to danger. Important role responsibilities and priorities in daily living (e.g., care of a dependent family member or the demands of a valued job) may give rise to a sense that the demands of current daily living do not permit a person to be ill with a disease such as cancer at this time; this can influence a person to avoid behavior that might call signs and symptoms to attention.

Some individually held beliefs about cancer and its diagnosis and treatment are thought to form a positive attitude toward participation in self-surveillance, professional screening, and diagnostic procedures (Disch, 1987). These include beliefs that:

It is possible to have the disease and be asymptomatic.

Certain symptoms can indicate a specific disease.

Early diagnosis improves prognosis.

Techniques are available that can detect both symptomatic and asymptomatic disease.

The forces of beliefs and values can be at the core of the nature of an individual's incorporation of self-surveillance and monitoring into daily living (see also Chapter 3).

Availability of Professional and Financial Resources

The status of availability of both professional services and financial resources are two other phenomena that can influence self-surveillance behavior.

The exposure to professionally provided support and training for learning about self-surveillance for cancers varies in different communities. Poor access (e.g., geographic, transportation, and cultural barriers) to professional services and technology can be a major deterrent. In settings where the number of health professionals is very low (e.g., rural areas or the inner city), the attitudes of a small number of health care providers and the importance they assign to self-monitoring can be a major influence on incorporation of self-monitoring into daily living patterns.

Information and health care services that are offered in a setting or in a language or style of presentation that does not reflect the language and cultural norms of a group limits their access to that learning.

Lack of money for health care may deter individuals from learning about self-monitoring. There may be a feeling of futility: "What is the use when there is no money for treatment if anything is found?" Absolute poverty or inability to afford health insurance may limit both exposure to information and access to professional assistance.

Standards for Monitoring

Recommendations for Monitoring for Early Detection of Cancer

The American Cancer Society has made the following age-related recommendations for self-monitoring and professional monitoring for early detection of cancer (1989).

AGE 20–40

Cancer-related check-up every 3 years, including procedures listed below and examination for cancers of the thyroid, testes, prostate, mouth, ovaries, skin, and lymph nodes

For women:

Breast self-examination (BSE) monthly

One baseline mammogram between ages 35 and 40

After age 18 or when sexually active, an annual pelvic examination and Pap test. (Pap tests may be done less frequently at the discretion of the physician after three consecutive normal annual tests.)

OVER 40

Cancer-related check-up every year, including procedures listed below and examination for cancers of the thyroid, testes, prostate, mouth, ovaries, skin, and lymph nodes

For women:

Breast self-examination monthly and examination by a physician every year

Mammogram every year after age 50

Annual pelvic examination and Pap test. (Pap tests may be done less frequently at the discretion of the physician after three normal annual tests.)

An endometrial tissue sample at menopause for women at risk

For colon or rectal cancer:

A digital rectal examination every year

A stool blood test every year after age 50

A proctoscopic examination every 3 to 5 years after two initial negative tests one year apart

Oral examinations associated with regular dental care as well as self-inspection of the oral cavity and palpation for neck nodes are important (White, 1986). Self-monitoring of changes in moles, nevi, or other skin manifestations and for women, changes in external genitalia also are important elements of an early detection regimen.

Maintenance of this kind of personal and professional surveillance for early detection of cancer requires initiative and persistence over a lifetime. Some authorities question the cost-effectiveness of this regimen (Frank-Stromberg, 1986).

Warning Signs of Cancer

Seven warning signs of cancer have become the standard for self-surveillance:

Any unusual bleeding or discharge

A lump or thickening in the breast or elsewhere

A sore that does not heal

Change in bowel or bladder habits

Hoarseness or a cough

Indigestion or difficulty in swallowing

Change in a wart or mole

    More specific guidelines of early signs and symptoms according to the age of the patient and the presenting risks are provided for professionals (White, 1986; Frank-Stromberg, 1987).

Nursing Diagnosis and Treatment

Risk Factors   Certain individuals and groups are at greater risk for not being able to effectively acquire and use knowledge of cancer risks and self-monitoring skills. Included are those who:

See themselves as invulnerable

Are unable to read, due to illiteracy, visual handicap, cognitive deficits, or psychoses

Come from cultures or religious groups in which there are special taboos associated with looking at or touching parts of the body or beliefs excluding self-examination

Are women whose mores dictate that they must seek permission from their husband or another man in the family in order to participate in self-monitoring

Are chronic alcohol or other substance abusers

Have difficulty with color discrimination

Have musculoskeletal restrictions in hands and shoulders or decreased sensory discrimination in fingertips

Live alone and have lesions in areas that are difficult to see without the help of another person

Lack the equipment needed to visualize the areas to be observed (e.g., small mirrors for the mouth, larger mirrors for breast and skin)

Lack areas of privacy for self-inspection

Diagnostic   Difficulties in incorporating self-surveillance behavior into
Areas   daily living may be related to (R/T):

Lack of knowledge or skill to carry out self-monitoring

Lack of access to *usable* knowledge and skill training

Lack of valuing of self-monitoring

Fear of findings that may indicate a malignancy

Denial of risk

Constraints from cultural norms or belief systems

Manifestations   Lack of knowledge and skills for self-monitoring for cancer may be difficult to discern because self-monitoring tends to be a private activity. Findings that may indicate nonparticipation in this health behavior include:

Verbal indications that the person does not engage in self-monitoring because he or she does not know about it, does not know how to do it, or prefers not to do it*

Findings that the prevailing language of the health care professionals and literature is poorly understood (e.g., instructions are written or spoken in a different language or use jargon or a level of vocabulary that is inappropriate to the client)

Reported or observed lack of participation in classes in which the knowledge and skills are being taught

Initial attendance at a class or clinic with failure to return or failure to maintain requested records on monitoring data

Indications that self-examination is not "accepted behavior" in the family, culture, or religious group

Lack of availability of classes in the geographic area

Sensory, cognitive, or musculoskeletal deficits that limit effective self-monitoring

Heavy responsibilities in daily living (e.g., a demanding job or being primary care giver to ill or dependent persons) that result in giving low priority to or lacking energy for self-care

Reported overriding fear of discovering cancer and an associated unwillingness to self-monitor

Prognostic   Factors that suggest a poor prognosis for acquiring the knowl-
Variables   edge and skills needed for effective self-monitoring include:

Ambivalence about facing up to the risks (e.g., family history of cancer)

A sense that it is not important because of their age group (the very young and the very old)

Reluctance to violate cultural norms of viewing and touching certain parts of their body

Indication that they probably would not carry out the procedures or would not seek professional health care if they

*The person may report participation in self-monitoring in order to avoid disapproval by the nurse.

encountered abnormal findings, and that they wish to avoid exposure to the knowledge and skills in order to avoid guilt feelings

Substance abusers

Complications

There are complications associated with failure to learn the knowledge and skills needed for appropriate self-monitoring. The most obvious complication is later recognition of a neoplasm and the possibility that treatment will be less effective than if it had been discovered earlier.

There also can be iatrogenic complications associated with nurses' behavior. Unwanted side-effects of nurses' behavior are associated with the use of scare tactics or efforts to produce guilt. Such nursing strategies seem to have a negative effect on long-term incorporation of the health behavior involved (Blainey, 1986).

Treatment Guidelines

In order to help individuals to move to a point where they are willing and able to incorporate the knowledge and skills of self-monitoring into their lives, selected approaches from the following suggestions can prove useful.

Avoid using words, behaviors, and attitudes that generate feelings of fear or guilt in the individual.

Promote their taking the initiative in planning the schedule and strategies for incorporating the behavior into their daily living pattern. Provide resources and support sources, but keep the initiative with the person who has the responsibility.

With young adult men, provide information about the higher risk years (20 to 34) and the high cure rate of testicular cancer with early detection. With young women stress the development of health patterns that include breast self-examination.

Explore areas in their daily living and self-concept in which self-monitoring has value (e.g., as a role model of health practices for other members in their family or friends they care about).

Help them to identify cultural constraints to self-monitoring and to consider options of acceptable strategies for neutralizing them. (Some known constraints include the need for getting the husband's permission to do breast self-examination and restrictions on touching oneself or visually examining parts of one's body—breast or testicular self-examination.)

Identify the activity as having a focus of health promotion rather than an illness orientation.

Demonstrate, redemonstrate, and receive return demonstrations of the skills until they:

Recognize the feel and appearance of differing types of their own normal tissue

Have confidence in their abilities with this recognition

Provide information using language and demonstrations that are compatible with the person's or group's capacity to learn (e.g., ask members of the group to write their own materials so that they incorporate any subtle language differences that may assist others like them to learn).

Provide the teaching in settings acceptable to the person or the group (e.g., store front health care settings versus hospital clinic environment; the dress of the teacher—nursing uniform versus casual dress).

Consider the specific readership when developing flyers either giving information or announcing teaching sessions. Where there may be cultural differences, obtain assistance in selecting the color of the paper, the words used, and the pictures of models or anatomic drawings.

For breast examination, give consideration to the need for privacy. In group sessions:

Have multiple mirrors available.

Provide covering, such as paper capes or towels.

Suggest the covering of one breast while the other is being examined.

Position the group during the self-examination learning experience so that there is minimal opportunity to see others or be seen by them. Figure 4-1 illustrates positioning of tables and women to increase the sense of privacy while learning breast self-examination.

For women whose menstruation is irregular or has ceased, suggest using the date of arrival of a monthly bill (e.g., a utility bill), as the reminder to do the breast self-examination.

Provide record forms for participants to document their self-monitoring activities and findings. Review them with the person at each contact.

Evaluation   Observe the participants' responses to the idea of inclusion of self-monitoring into daily living and the teaching of the knowledge and skills. Do they appear interested? Do they ask questions? Do they participate in the activities?

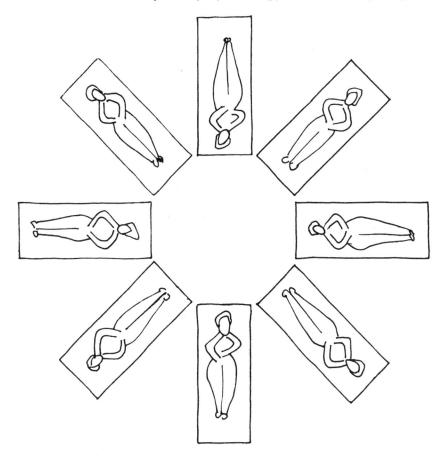

Figure 4-1. *Suggested patient placement for group instruction in breast self-examination.* (Drawn by Jerry Martin.)

Evaluate actual participation in subsequent contacts in which the person reports activities, issues, and any difficulties or problems. Evaluate the level of knowledge and skill in self-monitoring the person demonstrates at this time.

Observe to see if the self-monitoring record has been completed and if it appears to have been written at different times.

Next Steps

Suspicious findings can emerge in two ways—during examination by a physician or during self-surveillance. Differing problems can arise for the patient depending on the source of the discovery.

Two extremes in physician behavior can cause difficulties for the patient. On the one hand, the physician may be less concerned about the findings than the patient is and may suggest waiting or doing nothing. On the other hand, the physician may seem to rush into major surgery or other oncologic treatment before the patient is satisfied with the diagnosis. Where the nurse has contacts with patients who are uneasy about next steps, one safe option is to indicate to the patient that seeking a second opinion is an ethical and useful strategy.

When the patients themselves have noticed the findings that may indicate a possible malignancy, the problem tends to involve the decision as to whether and when to seek the diagnostic expertise of a physician. Delay is not uncommon when fear of a diagnosis of cancer is involved.

Factors that can have an influence on seeking professional help to rule out or confirm a diagnosis of cancer include:

Ethnicity and social class (Vernon et al, 1985; Samet et al, 1988)

Level of education (Samet et al, 1988)

Pattern of regular health check-ups by a physician (Samet et al, 1988)

Knowledge about cancer (Samet et al, 1988)

Site of the cancer and symptoms (Temoshok et al, 1984; Samet et al, 1988)

Confidence that the health care providers have the capability of providing effective treatment if cancer is diagnosed (Berkanovic, 1982; Vernon, 1985)

A positive relationship with the physician (Berkanovic, 1982; Henderson, 1965; Henderson et al, 1958)

Finances, third party payers to cover the costs of health care (Samet et al, 1988)

Support from family or personal network (Berkanovic, 1982)

Priority for self-care that permits placement of other role obligations to a lower priority if the diagnosis and treatment demand it

Nursing diagnosis of undue delay in seeking professional assistance and the factors that contributed to this delay tends to occur after the fact, since individuals tend to wrestle with these decisions privately. However, evidence of a lag time between the patient's noticing of suspicious findings and the seeking of professional health care (when other causes have been ruled out) can alert the nurse to the possibility of avoidance or denial in coping patterns that may need to be taken into account when the nurse assists the patient and family to deal with the cancer experience.

Summary

Self-surveillance and the use of professional health care screening services is currently seen by many authorities as the best means of early detection and cure for cancer. Incorporation of these behaviors and activities into daily living is influenced by a variety of factors. Nursing diagnosis and treatment can, at a minimum, enable individuals to make informed choices and have available the knowledge and skills should they choose to use them.

Bibliography

American Cancer Society. Cancer facts and figures—1989. Atlanta: American Cancer Society, 1989.

Berkanovic E. Seeking care for cancer relevant symptoms. J Chronic Dis 1982;35:727.

Blainey C. Diabetes mellitus. In: Carnevali D, Patrick M, eds. Nursing management for the elderly. 2nd ed. Philadelphia: JB Lippincott, 1986.

Blesch KS. Health beliefs about testicular cancer and self-examination among professional men. Oncology Nursing Forum 1986;13:29.

Disch J. Factors affecting health behavior. In Groenwald SL, ed. Cancer nursing: principles and practice. Monterey, CA, Jones & Bartlett, 1987.

Frank-Stromberg M. Cancer detection and screening. In Groenwald SL, ed. Cancer nursing: principles and practice. Monterey, CA: Jones & Bartlett, 1987.

Frank-Stromberg M. The role of the nurse in early detection of cancer: population sixty-six years of age and older. Oncology Nursing Forum 1986;13:66.

Henderson JG, Wittkower ED, Lougheed MN. A psychiatric investigation of the delay factor in patient to doctor presentation in cancer. Journal of Psychosomatic Medicine 1958;3:27.

Henderson JG. Denial and repression as factors in the delay of patients with cancer presenting themselves to the physician. Ann NY Acad Sci 1965;125:856.

Redeker NS. Health beliefs and adherence in chronic illness. Image 1988;20:31.

Rutledge D. Factors related to women's practice of breast self-examination. Nurs Res 1987;36:117.

Samet J, Hunt W, Lerchen M, Goodwin JS. Delay in seeking care for cancer symptoms: a population-based study of elderly New Mexicans. Journal of the National Cancer Institute 1988;80:432.

Temoshok L, di Clemente RJ, Sweet DM, et al. Factors related to patient delay in seeking medical attention for cutaneous malignant melanoma. Cancer 1984;54:3048.

Vernon SW, Tilley BC, Neale AV, et al: Ethnicity, survival and delay in seeking treatment for symptoms of breast cancer. Cancer 1985;55:1563.

Welch-McCaffrey D, Dodge J: Planning breast self-examination programs for elderly women. Oncology Nursing Forum 1988;15:811.

White N. Cancer prevention and detection: from twenty to sixty-five years of age. Oncology Nursing Forum 1986;13:59.

5

Daily Living in the Diagnostic Phase of the Cancer Experience

The diagnostic phase of the cancer experience is relatively short, lasting from a few days to a few weeks. The exceptions are those cases in which there are no initial organic findings to explain the patient's symptoms. Here the search for a diagnosis can last for several months. The diagnostic phase begins when the patient and family enter the health care system for attention to suspicious signs and symptoms or when a physician discovers an asymptomatic lesion, for example, in a routine physical examination. It ends when cancer is ruled out or when a malignancy has been definitively diagnosed. At this point the patient has been informed of the nature of the cancer, its implications, and the recommendations of the physician for its treatment. The patient then makes a choice about what treatment (if any) to accept. The cancer itself may be in an early or a highly advanced stage at the time of diagnosis.

Although this time period is not long for most patients, the intensity of stress is extremely high because matters of life and death hang in the balance. Even though family and friends may gather around to share the experience, it tends to be a time of lonely waiting and sustained uncertainty for the patient, with many hours spent contemplating possible life changes (Mullan, 1985). Family members and close friends also experience a sense of personal isolation as they too consider the patient's situation and the implications it may have for their own future daily living.

The diagnostic phase is a time of conflicting demands on the patient and family. A need for self-protection may cause the patient or family members to insulate themselves from the possibility of a negative diagnosis by avoiding unwanted information, ignoring body cues, and distorting input (Mishel, 1988a). It can also be a time when the patient and family protect each other by maintaining brave facades and continuing in their normal roles and routines as much as possible. The diagnostic phase is a time of being in limbo—suspended in one's thoughts from ordinary life. Conversely, at the end of the diagnostic phase, there is an urgent need for taking action by making a significant decision about the course of treatment. This decision making requires the opposite of the self-protective mechanisms that may have been used by the patient and family as a defense against anxiety. Ideally, informed consent requires assimilating the reality of the diagnosis, prognosis, and treatment options as well as the implications each option has for the patient and family in terms of the quality of their lives during and after the treatment phase. This decision making involves complex cognitive processing (Scott et al, 1984). Some patients will seek information and participate actively in the choices. Others are so devastated by the impact of learning of the diagnosis that their usual need for control collapses and they accept the doctor's recommendation or mandate, regardless of the projected impact on quality or length of life.

Medical Perspective

From the medical perspective, the diagnostic phase is a critical period of data gathering and decision making. There is concern for scheduling of proper tests; correct preparation of the patient to assure accurate, clear test results; appropriate and effective collection and processing of required body tissues or fluids; and discriminative analysis of the samples to determine whether or not a malignancy is present. If a malignancy is found, the pathology of the cells, stage of local or regional invasion, and distant metastasis (i.e., the TNM cancer staging criteria) are determined as a basis for selecting appropriate treatment protocols.

The final medical task of the diagnostic stage is to inform the patient (and possibly the family) of the nature of the cancer and the options for treatment, giving the information in such a way as to enable them to make informed choices. The medical profession's expectation is that the physician will place the emphasis on cure and will advocate doing all that is necessary to ablate the malignant process (D'Angio and Ross, 1981). The literature recommends that physicians place potential late complications into "proper" perspective, that is, they will occur only if the initial treatment is successful and the patient becomes a survivor. It is seen as unwise for physicians to provide information that would create fear of late consequences and thus cause the patient to decide against oncologic treatment deemed medically to be essential (D'Angio and Ross, 1981).

Nursing Perspective

Nursing's perspective involves the diagnosis and treatment of issues and problems in daily living and functioning associated with the stresses and tasks of the diagnostic phase. Both the patient and the family become the focus of attention (Mullan, 1985). Nurses' diagnosis and treatment of patient and family can involve:

Role competence for participation in:

The formally designated sick role, even though the patient may be asymptomatic at the time of diagnosis

Preparations for diagnostic tests

Diagnostic procedures and any post-test regimens

Decision making regarding treatment options

Strategies for coping with the waiting during many tests and procedures and the delays involved in scheduling of the procedures and receiving the laboratory results from both local and distant laboratories

Management of uncertainty, anticipatory grieving, and the barriers that self-protective behavior may create to achieving "informed" decision making

Assimilation of the diagnosis and its implications into one's self-concept, including recognition of the possible need to change one's vision of the future

Difficulties in decision making about courses of action to take about proposed treatment or treatment alternatives, given the possible impaired information processing abilities (Mandler, 1979)

Decisions about sharing information involving who to tell, the timing of sharing the information, and the best words to use

Family relationships as these are altered by the disruptions of diagnostic tests and the possible implications of outcomes

Nature of the Phenomena

At least three major phenomena are involved in managing daily living during the diagnostic phase of the cancer experience. The first and most dominant phenomenon is the *uncertainty* associated with the possibility of a confirmed diagnosis of cancer. Two secondary phenomena are concerned with relationships with the health care system. These include the demands of the health care system and decision making regarding oncologic treatment.

Threat of a Malignancy and Its Implications

Uncertainty, the inability to determine the meaning of events and to predict outcomes accurately, is a major phenomenon in the diagnostic phase (Mishel, 1984). Since cancer is seen as a life-threatening disease, the associated uncertainty carries a strong sense of danger (Campbell, 1986).

The possibility that a malignancy will be confirmed brings with it threats to a way of life, to one's appearance, and to one's ability to function. The possibility of death is present (Mullan, 1985).

Even the threat of a malignancy that is ruled out causes a certain loss of innocence—one can no longer take health status and usual daily living for granted; one can no longer ignore the reality that death comes to all (Mullan, 1985). Death is no longer abstract and distant, but real and personal.

The diagnostic procedures themselves reflect physicians' opinions that the initially reported symptoms or other findings are significant enough to warrant further examination; this increases their threat. These diagnostic procedures can involve surgery and complex tests. Patient and family concerns are heightened. Thoughts go to the nature of changes in immediate and long-term daily living and one's relationships with others. Existential questions arise (e.g., What is the meaning and purpose of my life? What of me and my contribution to the world will survive? If I have a limited time to live, how will I use that time—what is important to me?). Anticipatory grieving may begin even before a malignancy has been diagnosed or ruled out. Those who are most fearful may begin to "put their lives in order" by making their wills and arranging their affairs.

Demands of the Health Care System

Entry into the health care system for neoplastic diagnosing carries with it demands on the patient and family that alter both daily living and functioning. The pace of the diagnostic activities, the pre-test preparations, the delays and intervals between the tests, and, finally, the relaying of the findings by the physician all contribute to the patient's and family's anxiety level.

The health care system and health care providers are organized to provide cost-effective services concurrently to many people. The schedules and strategies that enable health care providers to deliver services efficiently appear bureaucratic. The patient and family usually find themselves accommodating the system. They appear in the prescribed clinics or departments at the scheduled times, provide the information requested, and function in ways demanded by the system's administrative and diagnostic protocols, while assuming the expected role behaviors. In this process the patient and the family tend to experience several losses, such as loss of control over their daily living, a decrease in sense of competence (Braden, 1986), and loss of privacy. For some individuals these losses are not difficult; for others they constitute another major stressor.

Decision Making About Oncologic Treatment

The third major phenomenon in managing daily living during the diagnostic phase is that of receiving the information about the confirmed diagnosis and making decisions regarding the treatment the oncologists recommend. Some patients and family members find that receiving a definite diagnosis is a relief, the end of uncertainty. As one patient said, "They acted as if all these symptoms were in my head. Now I know I wasn't crazy." More often the diagnosis either confirms acknowledged signs and symptoms and the patient's worst fears or comes as a total shock (e.g., finding an unexpected malignancy during surgery for another purpose).

There are two arenas of expertise involved in decision making about oncologic treatment. Medical expertise addresses therapeutic options for controlling the cancer (Schoene-Seifert and Childress, 1986). The patient and the family are experts in their requirements and resources for managing daily living and in their own values and priorities (Lynn, 1986). Unlike physicians, whose expertise in decision making is undiminished by the events of the diagnostic phase, patients' and families' capacities to take in and process important information and to factor in their own situation is often drastically reduced by the experiences of the diagnostic phase. This creates a situation in which it is difficult to make an informed decision. There is a particular amount of stress involved if the patient's decision does not coincide with what the medical team feels is the best approach to treating the cancer (Lynn, 1986).

Underlying Mechanisms

The diagnostic phase tends to suspend normal life for patients and those who share their daily living. It is a period of sustained uncertainty, vigilance, and waiting in which it is impossible to relax. The waiting is punctuated by scheduled tests and diagnostic procedures that are alien and usually uncomfortable. The waiting then resumes during the interval needed for the results to become known. In the end the physician presents the findings. If cancer is present, the patient is asked to consider usually unfamiliar, often frightening information about the nature of the pathology, prognostic variables, treatment options, and recommendations. An informed decision is then needed in order to move ahead with oncologic treatment. In addition, the patient and family must consider concurrent financial, employment, and other role responsibility issues.

The underlying dynamics of managing daily living and functioning with these tasks and stresses become the knowledge base for nursing's problem sensing, diagnosis, and treatment of patients and families.

Coping Strategies

Strategies for coping with situations vary with individuals and families. There is no ideal way of coping. Effectiveness of coping is observed in terms of outcomes (Folkman and Lazarus, 1980).

Coping begins with an initial appraisal of whether the uncertainty in the presenting situation represents a danger or an opportunity and whether or not the situation seems amenable to change (Mishel, 1988). If a situation seems to lend itself to change, an action-oriented, mobilizing approach involving information seeking, vigilance, and direct action tends to be used. On the other hand, when appraisal of the situation indicates that nothing can be done to change a harmful situation, a defensive emotional coping response is more likely to be used. This involves strategies of faith, disengagement, and cognitive support (Cohen and Lazarus, 1973; Mishel, 1988).

Psychophysiologic Responses to the Stress of the Diagnostic Phase

Fear and anxiety are common psychophysiologic responses to the stresses of the diagnostic phase of the cancer experience. The level of severity ranges from moderate to severe.

Fear

For patients undergoing diagnostic procedures, fear is heightened by anticipation of and participation in specific diagnostic procedures, such as exploratory surgery, biopsy, bronchoscopy, cystoscopy, colonoscopy, computed tomography (CT), and magnetic resonance imaging (MRI). There can also be fear of the post-test discomforts, and certainly of what the findings will be.

Anxiety

In addition to the fears attached to specific events, patients usually suffer from anxiety as they perceive a genuine threat to their ability to function, their appearance, and their lifestyle. Life itself appears to be threatened. While most people recognize that they will die some day, death is an abstract concept to them. Since cancer is commonly seen as life-threatening, suddenly death is no longer an abstraction. The abstract question, "What would I do if I discovered that I had cancer?" is replaced with the here and now question, "What will I do if it is cancer?"

For family members or companions who share the patient's daily living, moderate to severe anxiety also occurs. They experience concern over the threat to the patient. Additionally, they often experience a threat to their own way of life as they contemplate the need to provide care to the patient and dependent family members, an uncertain quality of life for the patient and themselves, changes in their relationships with the patient, and the possibility of having to live life without the patient.

Psychophysiologic Effects

The psychophysiologic responses to the stressors of events and dangerous uncertainties can result in:

Disorganized thinking

Easy distractibility

Decreased attention to cues in the external environment because attention is focused on internal matters, leading to:

A narrowed focus of attention on external cues

Attention only to the cues the person sees as most important

Loss of important new cues, resulting in decreased cognitive reappraisal of the situation

Decreased ability to remember, including:

Decreased memory for previously familiar activities and knowledge (e.g., phone numbers, location of items in the home, routes to the store or clinic, appointments)

Decreased capacity to link incoming information with previous experiences, plans, and values

Sleep disruption

Loss of desire to eat

Fatigue

Decreased social interaction, with withdrawal and apathy

Possible increased irritability, anger, and crying

Daily living goes on, but the capacities to meet its requirements are impaired and disrupted for the patient and those who share the experience.

Coping With Uncertainty That Has Negative Elements

When an individual experiences uncertainty for which the alternative is negative certainty (e.g., an unknown diagnosis versus a known diagnosis of metastatic cancer or a highly virulent cell type), the person may engage in behavior to *maintain uncertainty* (Mishel, 1988a). Only with uncertainty is hope possible. Strategies used to maintain uncertainty and hope include:

Creating illusions: Constructing beliefs out of uncertainty by emphasizing favorable aspects (Taylor, 1983)

Buffering: Blocking stimuli that might destroy the illusions and uncertainty. This is done by ignoring, minimizing, or misinterpreting communication that would give negative input about the situation and focusing only on the positive aspects and unpredictability (Mishel, 1988a).

A patient's need and behavior to maintain uncertainty rather than face an unpleasant confirmed diagnosis of cancer can interfere with acceptance of the diagnosis and the task of making an informed decision about treatment.

Another form of coping with the threats of the diagnostic phase is *intellectualizing*. These individuals adopt a highly rational approach that not only denies feelings but actually demeans them. A flat affect is maintained. An example of this approach would be the business person or professional who seeks information on the exact time duration of the tests, calculates the time needed for the tests plus transportation time, and then closely schedules work-related appointments around them. It is important to make a differential diagnosis between the person who is using intellectualizing as a coping response and the one who deals with the emotional elements of the situation, but prefers to do so privately.

While some patients and families avoid considering a serious outcome, others leap to an expectation of a fatal outcome. They give up on the basis of speculation or earlier experiences.

There is no ideal way of coping with the diagnostic phase, only the reality of variability. Each patient and family member tends to interpret information and respond in a personal way. Factors that can influence reactions during the diagnostic phase include:

Past experiences with cancer or other life-threatening situations—personally or among family and friends

Other concurrent stressors in their lives

Cultural variables

Religious beliefs

Other Factors Affecting Functioning and Management of Daily Living During the Diagnostic Phase

Other factors have been found to affect functioning and management of daily living during the diagnostic phase. Some of the important influences are education, social support, and the nature of the health care environment.

Education

Education can affect the person's and family's capacity to manage daily living during the diagnostic phase both indirectly and directly. Indirectly, the knowledge base acquired from earlier education sometimes can provide meaning and context to the experiences and events of the diagnostic phase (Mishel, 1988; Braden, 1986). In terms of direct impact, individuals having less than a high school education were found to see greater complexity in the health care activities and to have greater difficulty in understanding the health care system (Mishel, 1985). In each of these ways education can affect the nature of patient and family participation in daily living during the diagnostic phase.

Social Support

A functional social support system is important for the patient, the family, and care givers. A social support system that permits members to clarify the meaning of events through discussion and supportive interaction enables them to explore meanings, consider options, and plan responses in a safe environment.

A support group can also be a source of additional information. It can help to reduce disorganization and discomfort by providing input from others who have faced the same experience. It can serve as a network that provides predictable sources of physical assistance. Family members and significant others also can make the patient feel loved and cared about (Fitch and O'Brien-Pallas, 1990). The absence of such support networks or the inability to interact with them can add to the difficulties in managing the diagnostic phase.

Health Care Environment

Familiarity or unfamiliarity with the diagnostic environment, the people in it, and the procedures are important factors affecting functioning and daily living. Lack of familiarity with the environment and the equipment raises uncertainty and stress. So too does unfamiliarity with the roles required in the diagnostic phase—not knowing what to expect from others or what diagnostic personnel will expect. Even resourceful people can lose their sense of mastery when they are placed in situations in which they have no previous experience or knowledge on which to base their performance (Braden, 1986). On the other hand, familiarity with painful procedures can add to anticipatory stress.

Another challenge during the diagnostic phase is being shuttled from one diagnostic group to another. The patient and family often leave the comfort of their usual physician for one or more oncology specialists. Not only is the environment new, but each encounter brings a new group of health care providers who have their own specialized diagnostic focus, their own way of communicating, and their own set of expectations for patient behavior.

One patient outcome of this multidisciplinary approach to oncologic diagnosis is the requirement that the patient tell his "story" over and over as each new health care provider seeks a data base upon which to function. Most clinicians prefer to gather their own patient history rather than rely on one collected by another person or a member of another discipline. Having to repeat the symptoms and the history of the problem can be physically taxing for some patients who are ill, such as those who are admitted with an advanced state of cancer or whose cancer is characterized, even initially, by exhaustion (e.g., leukemias). Telling the story over and over can also be emotionally taxing. If there has been a delay in seeking health care, the discomfort of guilt may be increased with each telling, or the fear and anxiety generated by verbalizing the symptoms can be increased. There can also be some anxiety associated with the question of whether health care providers within the system communicate with each other, when each one seems to need the same information.

Usually there is no single individual designated as a case manager who will guide the patient and family through the various parts of the system, relating to and focusing on patient experiences and needs rather than on system-based needs. This lack of continuity can add to the sense of isolation and fear the patient is experiencing.

Informed Consent

Once all of the diagnostic activities have been completed, physicians decide on the options for treatment. Then the patient (and possibly the family) face the final task of the diagnostic phase—choosing what form of treatment (or nontreatment) to accept.

Informed consent involves both legal and moral dimensions. Consent that is not informed is invalid and does not give the physician the right to proceed with diagnostic activities or treatment (Schoene-Seifert and Childress, 1986).

The most stringent regulations for written informed consent are associated with treatment within federally supported investigative studies. These consent forms must provide information on the purpose of the study, treatment procedures, time of inpatient and outpatient treatment, side-effects, risks, assurance of confidentiality, responsibility for payment, and the right to withdraw from the study protocol at any time.

Oncologic treatments that do not involve government-sponsored investigative studies have much more latitude as to what constitutes informed consent. Here the physician, not the government, is the moral agent. A wide range of approaches is used by physicians in seeking informed consent. At one end of the continuum are physicians who are quite directive (e.g., "This is the treatment that is needed"). Such physicians may have a concern that emphasis on risks and side-effects might cause the patient and family to reject life-saving or life-prolonging treatment (Schoene-Seifert and Childress, 1986). Others offer a full disclosure of options for treatment and nontreatment, offering what reasonable individuals and families need to know in order to make sound decisions about treatment.

Informed consent deals with autonomy and self-determination in the use of one's body. Informed consent is an expression of the patient's right to decide where his or her interests lie, to choose among the medical treatment options proposed, to withdraw from treatment in progress, or to forego proposed medical treatment. Informed consent incorporates moral and value-related issues as well as risk–benefit and cost–benefit issues (Schoene-Seifert and Childress, 1986).

Implementation of informed consent involves obtaining written consent prior to treatment that is based on:

Competency: Determination as to whether the patient can understand this situation well enough to comprehend the information and variables involved, weigh the alternatives, and make valid choices

Voluntariness: Determination that the consent is given freely without subtle or overt coercion, and that each party (patient and physician) is taking into account the position of the other party in a mutual transaction. Voluntariness is seen to be particularly difficult for the cancer patient since special anxiety and vulnerability exist.

Disclosure: Provision of the necessary information on the patient's health situation, the treatment options, and all of the relevant benefits and risks of each treatment option (e.g., odds for survival, usual duration of survival, immediate treatment, long-term care issues, quality of life during and following treatment, type of personal assistance likely to be required, and costs of treatment—short-term and long-term)

Understanding: Provision of information in a language, vocabulary, and form that the patient can genuinely comprehend given the expected constraints on the patient's capacity to process information at this stressful time; use of body language and tone of voice that share the experience rather than intimidate; and allowance for sufficient time or multiple sessions to permit the patient (and family) to assimilate the information and its implications

(Chamorro and Appelbaum, 1988; Pellegrino, 1981; President's Commission for the Study of Ethical Problems in Medicine and Biomedical and Behavioral Research, 1982; Trandel-Korenchuk and Trandel-Korenchuk, 1986)

Deterrents to the patient's ability to give informed consent include high anxiety in the patient, with its associated impairment of taking in and processing information; lengthy medical instructions; consent forms written in technical language or in small, closely spaced print; the patient's lack of familiarity with medical knowledge and language; and the patient being elderly (over 65), seeing "only one way out," or asking the physician to make the decision as a means of avoiding awareness of possibly negative information (Cassileth et al, 1980; Chamorro and Appelbaum, 1988; Morrow and Hoagland, 1981).

Another issue in informed consent addresses the right of others (e.g., family members), to have the information or to decide for the patient. The guiding principle is a respect for the patient as a person. Competent patients have the right to know the information and make the decisions (Schoene-Seifert and Childress, 1986). They also have the right to determine who else will be given the information. There is no moral or legal warrant for disclosing information to the family without the competent patient's permission, nor for deferring to family wishes if the patient is competent and if this authority has not previously been delegated to the family (Schoene-Seifert and Childress, 1986).

Nursing Diagnosis and Treatment

Nursing diagnosis and treatment address problems in daily living and areas of dysfunction associated with issues and tasks of the diagnostic phase. Important data in the data base include:

Identification of the patient's key support figures, geographic distance from them during the diagnostic phase, relationships with them, and any patient wishes regarding how much others should know of the health situation

Critical roles the patient is attempting to maintain, difficulties in negotiating role adjustments to accommodate the demands of the diagnostic activities, and impaired capacities for managing role requirements during the diagnostic phase

Educational and ethnic background and language skills, as these influence understanding of the health situation, procedures, and information needed to make decisions

Previous experiences with persons who have had cancer, as these might affect expectations, worries, and uncertainties

Previous experiences with clinics, diagnostic equipment, and hospital facilities, as these affect the need for information and support during diagnostic activities

Diagnostic Targets

Persons to be considered for assessment, diagnosis, and treatment include the patient and, if the patient wishes others to be involved, key significant others designated by the patient.

Risk Factors

Patients at greatest risk of not managing daily living effectively during the diagnostic phase are those who:

Have premorbid depressions, anxiety states, a pessimistic orientation to life, psychosis, history of alcoholism or drug dependency, many past regrets

Have serious existential or religious concerns

Lack the personal resourcefulness to learn about the diagnostic experience and environment as a basis for maintaining a sense of competence in those areas that can be personally controlled

Lack the verbal skills or courage to make their needs and wishes known to health care providers

Are male (Fobair, 1981)

Live alone (Fobair, 1981)

Lack a comfortable, predictable support system with whom to share and process the experiences and feelings generated during the diagnostic phase

Lack people willing to give assistance with the physical demands of daily living as needed

Do not feel cared about (Fitch and O'Brien-Pallas, 1990)

Have concerns about major role responsibilities (employment, home, community) and difficulties in adjusting the role or finding surrogates to assume responsibilities

Have limited verbal and reading skills (this may be due to having English as one's second language)

Have been frightened by previous experiences involving individuals with cancer

Have financial concerns

Lack a case manager (nurse or personal physician) to lend continuity and assistance within the multidisciplinary activities of the diagnostic phase (Mishel, 1988a; Weisman and Worden, 1976; Worden, 1981)

Significant others sharing the diagnostic phase who may have difficulty managing daily living during the time the patient is undergoing diagnosis include those who:

Live with the patient or closely share daily living

Are dependent on the patient for physical or emotional well-being in daily living

Are depressed, highly anxious, or pessimistic

Have had previous negative or frightening experiences with cancer in themselves or others

Diagnostic Areas

PATIENT

Difficulty in implementing prescribed regimens or difficulty in participating effectively during the diagnostic tests related to (R/T):

Anxiety-based reduction in cognition leading to (L/T) reduced capacity to understand instructions

Limited vocabulary or nonfluency in English

Physical constraints (e.g., inability to lie perfectly still for extended periods for CT or MRI scans, claustrophobia in the MRI gantry, urinary frequency, coughing, pain)

Unfamiliarity with or fear of (specified) health care environment

Culturally based differences in expectations about health, illness, diagnostic procedures, hospitals, relationships with health care personnel

Difficulty in relinquishing control of self, daily living, privacy R/T:

Health care system's data collection strategies, documentation, or communication systems

Health care environment

Difficulty in making needs and desires known to health professionals R/T:

Lack of adequate communication skills

Lack of courage

Lack of knowledge about the system, how to make oneself heard, and what accommodations are possible

Difficulty in maintaining ongoing role obligations during the diagnostic phase R/T:

Anxiety-based distractedness, lack of ability to concentrate or attend to the external environment

Physical deficits (specify) associated with the diagnostic preparations, after-effects, or pathology

Inability to locate a surrogate or negotiate for others to give needed assistance

Difficulty in taking in reality-oriented information regarding the health situation R/T need to maintain uncertainty by ignoring, minimizing, or distorting any cues or input that would suggest negative possibilities, leading to (L/T):

Frustration in others seeking to break down these defense mechanisms

Unpreparedness for moving toward informed decision making

Loneliness R/T facing the stresses of the diagnostic phase physically or emotionally distant from one's support system

Difficulty in making an informed decision regarding the proposed treatment R/T:

Inability to "hear" or accept the diagnosis of cancer

Mental "shut down" after being told the diagnosis

Giving "ignorant consent" by waiving the right to full disclosure and knowledge and leaving the decision with the physician (Chamorro and Appelbaum, 1988; Nokes, 1987)

Difficulty in understanding the medical language (medispeak) used by the physician in explanations of the options (Chamorro and Appelbaum, 1988; Pellegrino, 1981; Reiser, 1980)

Limited ability to understand spoken or written English

Not knowing what questions to ask

Receiving little encouragement to consider any variables except those related to treatment of the tumor

Subtle or overt pressure from health care providers to take a certain course of action

Fear of alienating health care providers who will be needed to provide ongoing care during whatever treatment or nontreatment is chosen

Feeling there is only one viable treatment option

Feeling rushed to make a decision

Difficulties in decision making regarding telling others about the diagnostic activities and their possible significance or about the actual diagnosis of cancer R/T:

Fear of the difficulties or harm it may cause the person (e.g., ailing spouse, young children, aged parents)

Fear of an irreversible and undesired change in a relationship (e.g., possibility of distancing or abandonment) (Bergholz, 1988; Fisher, 1981; Kagan and Kagan, 1983)

Fear of losing status, influence, or position, or of being seen as unemployable (Hoffman, 1989; Mellette and Franco, 1987)

Lack of "scripts" or strategies for presenting the information to particular individuals or groups

FAMILY*

Difficulty in adjusting to changes in the patient's physical and emotional status or patterns in managing current daily living R/T not knowing what is occurring or why the patient is "not the same as usual"

Difficulty in relating to the patient R/T possessing accurate knowledge of the diagnostic activities and the possibility of cancer being found

Inability to share in the physical and emotional experiences of the patient during the diagnostic phase R/T:

Need to maintain illusion that "everything is OK" (Mishel, 1988a)

Preoccupation with their own role obligations

Geographic distances

Difficulty in relating to the patient's suffering R/T preoccupation with own fear and anticipatory grieving over possible loss of an important person or a way of life

Manifestations

PATIENT

The patient may report:

Being unable to function because of being distracted, unable to concentrate, not "hearing" what people say, forgetting, getting lost, just sitting and doing nothing (when this was not the usual pattern)

Crying, being sad, being more easily irritated than usual

Difficulties in sleeping

Loss of appetite

Fear of particular procedures, fear of experiencing claustrophobia with the CT or MRI equipment, fear of the findings

Fatigue

Worrying about how others will relate when they know about the tests and the possible diagnosis; worrying about who to tell and how to tell them

Not wanting to burden specific individuals with knowledge of the situation because the stress could cause physical or emotional harm to them

Feeling that others who do know are "acting different"

*See Chapter 2 on families. Family is "who the patient says it is."

Not understanding (e.g., "I don't know what questions to ask." "I don't really understand what they are telling me." "I'm afraid to ask for further explanation after they've told me once." "I don't know what to expect." "I don't know what I am supposed to do.") (Karani and Wiltshaw, 1986)

Feeling alone

Feeling that "everything will turn out all right" or "it's in the hands of the Almighty"

The nurse may observe in the patient:

Lack of attending to what is said (e.g., difficulty in following instructions, not responding appropriately, having a "glazed look")

Patterns of attending and information processing used to maintain "fragile optimism" (e.g., patient stresses similarities with others who are cancer free or doing well and ignores differences from them; minimizes new information by denial or misinterpretation; focuses only on the positive aspects of unpredictability) (Mishel, 1988a)

Episodes of forgetting

Sad facial expression or crying

Apathy, handing over of decision making to others, helplessness, or the reverse: aggressively seeking to control events and people

Easy irritability

No mention of family, unaccompanied by others, no visitors, no phone calls or mail, or the reverse: too many people involved for a patient who prefers privacy in this situation

FAMILY

If they have any contact with health care providers, the family may report:

Concern about the patient's situation or the patient's responses to the situation

Wondering about what is going on, or feeling that they know the situation but the patient doesn't

Worry about management of the patient's role responsibilities if the patient is dysfunctional for a period of time

Concern about how to interact with the patient, particularly in discussion of health status

The family may be observed to be:

Interacting comfortably with the patient—sharing the experiences and concerns

Overprotective, controlling, answering for the patient, making decisions for the patient

Superficial, avoiding health-related topics, physically avoiding the patient

Preoccupied with their own emotional discomforts and unable to deal with the patient's suffering

Prognostic Variables

Poor prognosis for managing daily living and functioning effectively during the diagnostic phase may be R/T:

Premorbid depression, a usual high level of anxiety, helplessness

Less than high school education, lack of command of oral or written English language

Lack of familiarity or comfort with the health care system and its personnel

Lack of trust in the capacity of science to deal with the pathology

Lack of or distance from a functional emotional and physical support system

Inadequate transportation resources

Complex and prolonged diagnostic procedures

Inability to take information provided by health care providers and integrate it with personal–family priorities and resources as a basis for making decisions about treatment

Lack of skill and confidence in communicating with medical and nursing personnel

Being given only part of the information needed for informed decision making, being given the information in unusable forms, or being pressured for an immediate decision

Preoccupation with costs and financing

Complications

Failure to manage daily living effectively during the diagnostic phase can further compromise the body's resources to deal with the cancer and the rigors of treatment. Failure to make a decision that is satisfactory to the patient, family, and health care providers can result in ongoing stress and disturbed interpersonal relationships at a time when the patient needs predictable, comfortable support. It can also result in failure to follow through on the planned treatment (Nokes, 1987).

Treatment Guidelines

Nursing treatment for the patient and others who are sharing the patient's experiences focuses on helping them to participate as effectively and comfortably as possible in the diagnostic activities and to manage daily living with the associated psychophysiologic responses. An ethical concern throughout relates to questions of the patient's right to control what information is given to others (e.g., family members) versus others' desire or need to know in order to manage their own daily living.

PATIENT   *Barriers to information processing R/T moderate to severe levels of anxiety*

Assess the level of anxiety.

Use short sentences, short words, and lay language, not medical–nursing jargon (unless the patient is a physician or nurse or is familiar with the language).

Where specific patient behavior is desired, make precise direct requests, not general suggestions.

Say important things first and stress important material.

Group ideas together (e.g., taking fluids and eating).

Repeat important information.

Ask the patient to recall or discuss important information or instructions with you.

Supplement verbal material with clearly written material† (if the patient is literate), video tapes, or audiotapes the patient can use in the institution or can take home (Molbo, 1986).

Provide phone numbers where additional information can be obtained (e.g., American Cancer Society, 1-800-ACS-2345; the National Cancer Institute, 1-800-4-CANCER).

Some nurses make their work and even their home phone numbers available to selected patients about whom they are concerned so that they can respond to questions as they occur.

Potential role incompetence and stress R/T unfamiliarity with upcoming diagnostic environments and experiences, and expectations for participation in them

Determine how much the patient knows and really wants to know versus what knowledge would only add to the stress (e.g., Would it be helpful or frightening to see the MRI equipment or the surgical recovery room beforehand?).

If the patient wishes to know what will happen (e.g., with bone marrow aspiration or a CT scan), describe what will be experienced in terms of sights, sounds, and sensations (or lack of them) in words that are neutral but specific. Link the upcoming sensations or experiences to something with which the patient is familiar (Chapman, 1988). (See Chapter 6, section on Pain Treatment Guidelines.)

†Written materials are available from all American Cancer Society offices and the National Cancer Institute.

Describe the behaviors or activities the patient will be asked to perform and any strategies other patients have suggested that make participation easier (e.g., deep breathing, shallow rapid breathing, counting, thinking of other things, positive self-talk).

Suggest prediagnostic activities that will make participating in the diagnostic procedure easier (e.g., emptying the bladder; asking for a cough suppressant; asking for an analgesic if this is not contraindicated; tying the big toes together before a bone scan, CT, or MRI to permit the patient to relax instead of expending energy to hold the feet together in an unmoving position).

Point out to the patient that it is not uncommon to be frightened or nervous and that health care providers want the patients to ask for help.

Following the procedure, help the patient to process the experience: In what ways did the patient feel relatively competent or incompetent? How was the experience congruent or incongruent with expectations? Are there any residual discomforts, emotional or physical, from the experience? What would the patient tell others to do as the best way of managing the experience? (This is less threatening than, "What would you do differently if the procedure were to be repeated?" Some painful procedures, such as bone marrow aspirations, may well be repeated.)

Prepare the patient for the interval of waiting for findings (e.g., indicate a range of time and the reasons the findings take this time—the need for the oncologist or team to put all the findings together in order to ensure the most accurate diagnosis). (Note: Some patients perceive the words cancer and tumor to mean different things. Make a decision on the provider team about which word is to be used with this patient, then take steps to assure that the terminology used is consistent.)

Concern about relinquishing control of self, of information about self, of daily living

Gather data on needs or desires for control, areas in which control is particularly important, and any discomfort with giving over some measure of control for a period of time in order to make a precise, individualized nursing diagnosis. This includes current wishes about who should be given information about possible diagnoses, tests, and findings.

Based on patient concerns, discuss areas in which it is possible to negotiate for maintaining control during this planned diagnostic phase, and rationale for relinquishing control in other areas in which health care providers or the system require control.

See also treatment guidelines on:

Patient decisions to share information about the health care situation with others

Negotiating with the system

Loneliness

Differentially diagnose between aloneness and loneliness (Carnevali, 1986).

Ascertain the reasons why person(s) the patient misses cannot be present.

Where possible, mobilize resources to permit a significant other to be with the patient.

Mobilize a former patient who has successfully managed the diagnostic phase to be a contact person or sounding board (often available through the American Cancer Society CanSurmount program) or, designate a primary nurse to provide continuity and a sense of caring in the fragmented, multidisciplinary diagnostic environment.

Difficulty in communicating one's needs, desires, or situation to health care providers

Differentially diagnose the basis for the difficulty (e.g., command of language, English as a second language, lack of courage, lack of knowledge of the system and strategies for making it accommodate one's needs, belief that making light of the symptoms will result in a better outcome).

Help the patient (or family member) determine what is to be communicated to given health care providers and what outcomes are desired.

If the person has the capacity to engage in the interaction, suggest strategies and scripts that could be used to communicate. When several have been developed that feel usable and comfortable to the person, role play the situation with the nurse (who knows the other party) assuming the usual behavior of the person the patient will be addressing. Consider several potential responses the other person might make in response to the patient's statements and plan for ways of responding to them. Ask the patient if the nurse's presence would be supportive or unneeded.

If the person indicates inability to undertake the interaction, offer to serve as advocate to present the situation, patient wishes, and goals.

If the patient or family wish to learn about the system in order to function in it more effectively, share information about the formal and informal networks and strategies for most effectively using the system to achieve desired outcomes.

Difficulty in managing requirements of daily living because of distractedness, inability to attend to cues, memory loss, or inability to concentrate

Suggest that these responses are not unusual, given the stresses of the diagnostic phase and that one manages them by adjusting the requirements of daily living to accommodate to these temporary dysfunctions.

Suggest that they might try to:

Avoid or delay critical tasks requiring sustained concentration, or break the tasks into smaller parts that can be dealt with in short blocks of time

Move from one task to another, doing physical tasks that don't require much concentration when distractedness is a particular problem

Carry social security numbers, important phone numbers, lists of tasks or shopping needs, and other important material in writing, in case of memory loss

Seek a companion or use written directions or maps to minimize getting lost

Concern about unusual emotional responses such as increased irritability, anger, crying, or being withdrawn

Indicate to patient (and to family if appropriate) that such emotional responses are quite common and might be expected, just as one expects coughing when a person has bronchitis, or pain when one sprains an ankle.

Explore with patient any "triggers" that escalate emotional responses, then explore with family the strategies they could undertake to avoid or minimize these trigger situations at this time.

To those who are sharing the daily living and experiencing the changed temperament of the patient, explain why *all* of the participants, and particularly the patient, are so vulnerable, and encourage them to take special care of each other and accept these unusual responses in themselves and others who are involved, putting them into the perspective of the unusual daily living of the diagnostic phase.

Difficulty in negotiating adjustments in role obligations during the diagnostic phase

See Chapter 6, section on Role, under Treatment Guidelines.

Need to maintain uncertainty by developing positive illusions and avoiding, minimizing, or distorting input that would lead toward a negative certainty (Mishel, 1988a)

Differentially diagnose between inability to process information associated with high anxiety levels versus behavior used to maintain uncertainty (i.e., ignoring, minimizing, or distorting cues that could be perceived as negative).

Support the person in acknowledging the stress of the situation. Realistically identify positive elements, actions taken, and behavior that shows wisdom and strength.

Use the same words the patient uses in describing perceptions of the situation, but be ready to sense and change when the patient seems ready to move on to other terminology.

Give honest answers to questions (when the physician has already given the information), using neutral words and simple language. (Be aware that if the diagnosis of cancer is confirmed, sudden, serious attempts could be made to substitute reality for the patient's illusion as a step toward gaining informed consent in treatment decisions.)

Offer a contact with someone who has gone through the diagnostic phase, as a source of expertise with whom to share the experience, if you sense that the patient is ready to listen to another person's experience and compare it to his own.

Lack of personal capacities to manage the activities of informed consent

Do not assume that people who have previously held strong positions and been active decision makers will automatically maintain this behavior when the area for decision making is cancer treatment (Pierce, 1985).

Help the patient draft a list of questions to take into the conference with the oncologist or a follow-up conference with an oncologic nurse specialist. Indicate that the list is like an insurance policy—it will not be needed if no problem is found. It is a way to be certain to get all the information needed in order to make satisfying decisions and plans that include daily living issues, problems, and values in this patient's situation. Point out that it sometimes is difficult to think of the questions to ask during the conference. To get the ideas started, ask the patient, "Would it be important to you to know . . . ?" (Select one of the questions below or one of your own choosing. Start with the least threatening areas.)

What areas of quality of life are altered during the treatment proposed? after each of the treatment options? if no treatment is undertaken?

What changes in functional capacities for managing my personal requirements of daily living will occur during the proposed treatments? after the treatment? What long-term or late functional changes may occur?

What kinds of assistance (if any) are likely to be needed with routine tasks of daily living such as shopping, food preparation, home maintenance, laundry, transportation?

What are the costs of immediate treatment? of ongoing follow-up? of prosthetics, cosmetic devices? of medications during treatment or after initial treatment?

Can I continue to work at my type of job? How much time away from the job is likely to be needed with each of the proposed treatments? If I have no treatment, about how long can I expect to continue to work?

(If applicable) How will the treatment affect sexual functioning? childbearing?

Do relationships with others tend to be affected by the results of this treatment? (e.g., after head and neck dissection, mastectomy, laryngectomy, colostomy, pelvic irradiation, prolonged immunosuppression)

What is the average or median life span with treatment? without treatment? (Note: This is a different question from one that addresses odds for survival. For example, a patient was told that his tumor had been growing for about 2 years and that he had a 50% chance for survival with treatment for his lung cancer with surgery, chemotherapy, and radiation but only a 20% chance without it. No mention was made that the average duration of survival with and without treatment is less than 2 years [Greenberg et al, 1988; Huhti et al, 1981]. The patient and his wife interpreted survival to mean cure and consented to the full treatment. Within 3 months of completion of an aggressive course of therapies he became seriously dysfunctional with brain and liver metastases.)

Suggest that the patient tape record the conference with the physician, so that there will be an opportunity to take in the information several times after the initial hearing. Have tape recorders for loan, and tape cassettes available (Cassileth et al, 1980).

Tell the patient that it is appropriate to ask to keep the consent document overnight or for several days in order to understand it more than is possible on one reading.

Offer to answer questions and explain any words that the patient cannot understand, or provide a glossary that translates into lay language the common "medispeak" words used in consent conferences. Indicate that there are no "dumb" questions. If something is of concern to the patient, it is important. Often it is managing the ordinary aspects in daily living that contributes to the effectiveness of the therapy.

Maintain a library of pamphlets in frequently used foreign languages that explain particular forms of therapy and their effects on the tumor, on body systems and functioning, and on the patient's and family's daily living. (In addition to translating the words, the information provided should take into account ethnic diets, common belief systems, and family or group relationships that will affect or be affected by their participation in the treatment.)

Desire to delegate decision making responsibilities to the physician (ignorant consent)

Note early in the diagnostic phase patient behavior that suggests a risk of or pattern of abdication of responsibility in decision making.

Introduce the idea that health care involves more than the treatment of a tumor or symptoms; it also involves managing daily living with the treatment for both the patient and family.

Indicate daily by words and behavior that patients are seen as *the* experts on their own daily living, their values and priorities, their resources, and their usual environment. The doctor is the expert on recognizing the pathology and its treatment. Both points of view are needed for a mutually satisfying decision.

In routine day-to-day interactions, gather data on the patient's lifestyle, priorities, strengths, and deficits in internal and external resources. Make the patient aware that you see these as important. Whenever possible, show how the elements of the patient's lifestyle link to health care activities in the institution and at home.

Point out that it has been generally established that patients who understand health care treatment and actively participate in the decision making tend to get along better (Chamorro and Appelbaum, 1988).

Risk that the patient will be unable to "stand his ground" in interaction with physicians

Observe for cues in patient and family behavior suggesting that they "don't know how to talk to doctors" or are intimidated by them.

Help the patient (and family if they are to be involved) to prepare for the diagnostic and treatment conference by describing the usual pattern of events (e.g., how their physician usually approaches these conferences).

Provide information on the options and rights patients have in making informed decisions—that informed decisions about medical treatment involve a negotiation between the patient's wishes and the expertise of the physician (Pellegrino, 1981).

Offer some scripts that have proven effective in other such conferences (e.g., "I can't make a decision right now. I need some time to think it over and discuss it with some others who are involved."). Use one or more of the questions provided earlier if they are appropriate.

Ask if there is any support the patient or family would like from the nurse in approaching the physician.

See Chapter 6, section on Role, under Treatment Guidelines.

Problems associated with decisions to share information about the situation with others

Gather data on the specific concerns about revealing the situation to particular individuals or groups.

Suggest that the patient think of three of the best things that could happen if the person were to be informed and two or three of the worst possible outcomes. Discuss with the patient possible strategies for avoiding or minimizing the worst contemplated consequences. Ask the patient to consider whether it is realistically possible to delay or conceal the situation from others.

If the patient decides not to tell others for the present, help (if needed) to develop "explanations" for the patterns of clinic visits or signs and symptoms that may raise questions.

If the patient desires help in planning for the encounter when the information is to be shared, help to:

Determine a "good" time for having the discussion

Develop possible scripts and plan what language to use. (Note: The approaches and language will vary with the age [e.g., children] and the relationship [e.g., spouse, children, parents, employers].)

Rehearse the scripts or role play them with a range of responses

Suggest that it is important to have at least one interested and understanding person with whom to share openly and comfortably the experiences of the diagnostic phase (Mishel, 1988a)

New distress R/T disagreement between the competent patient's wishes regarding treatment and those of family members

Indicate to the patient that, legally, the decision regarding treatment belongs to the patient, not to others. If the patient is willing, gather data on the rationale for the choice. Determine whether any assistance is desired in communicating with the family (e.g., assistance in developing possible scripts and strategies, the nurse being present when the patient talks to the family, or the nurse or doctor talking with the family).

Listen to the verbalized concerns of the family and the possible hidden agendas, fears, or tensions that use this issue as a release. If the family approaches treatment options from a logical point of view, point out to the family that the decision for treatment legally belongs to the competent patient, unless that responsibility has been delegated to another person. If the patient has given permission, indicate the basis for the patient's decision. If desired, put the family members in touch with other family members who have had similar experiences. Suggest that it is important to resolve their differences without creating additional stresses for the already stressed patient, who needs all available physical and emotional energy to manage the treatment and the disease at this point in time.

FAMILY

Concern about the patient and the situation when the possibilities or diagnosis are not known

Indicate to people who question or express concern that the physician is investigating some symptoms or findings and that no diagnosis has been made.

Acknowledge the legitimacy of their concern and the difficulty that uncertainty brings.

Suggest that they communicate their caring to the patient, but withhold questioning until more is known and the patient indicates a willingness to discuss the situation.

Concern about the patient and the situation when the serious possibilities or diagnosis are known by both patient and family

Acknowledge the discomfort being experienced. Explore their perceptions of the situation and the concerns and daily living implications it raises for them Discuss resources or strategies appropriate to the concerns expressed. Indicate your availability to answer questions, and suggest resources as the need for information and assistance arises.

Explore the usual ways in which the patient and family members relate to each other. Ask what they think the patient wants or needs from them at this time. Gather data on what the patient wants from the family at this time. Explore any difficulties they are having in meeting the patient's needs in the relationship. Mutually develop strategies that are feasible and relatively comfortable. Offer strategies the family members can use in relating to the patient, such as:

Verbalizing the discomfort they are experiencing in the relationship now that the cancer diagnosis is shared knowledge

Offering to listen and talk about the diagnosis, or not to talk about it, depending on the patient's wishes

Using the same words to describe the experience and feelings that the patient uses

Continuing to be with the patient in spirit as well as in physical presence (really be there for the patient)

Making physical contact in ways that are usual and are currently acceptable to the patient

Being open and sharing with the patient when the patterns of relating are not comfortable

Finding another person with whom to share the cancer experience from the family member's point of view and to consider strategies for continuing to meet the patient's needs

If family members of former patients are available to talk with family members of current patients, ask the family if it would be helpful to talk with someone who has managed daily living during the diagnostic phase. Arrange for the contact if desired.

Difficulty in relating to the patient when the family members know there is cancer or that a high probability of it exists and the patient maintains the illusion that "everything is OK"

Explore the feasibility, advantages, and disadvantages of the patient's maintaining the illusion for a longer period of time (e.g., if the doctor's recommendation is that curative treatment is not appropriate and only comfort measures be offered at this time).

Explore the possibility that the patient is maintaining a facade in order to protect the family from additional emotional burdens, or that overt cheerfulness is the patient's chosen way of dealing with the situation in relating to others.

Point out the importance of following the patient's lead: using the words the patient does in describing the illness and daily living experiences with it, and being perceptive about changing the words as the patient does.

Evaluation

Evaluation of responses to nursing treatment focuses on the degree of effectiveness, comfort, and satisfaction the patient and family achieve in daily living during the diagnostic phase. Areas for evaluation are based on the diagnoses made. These can include:

Effectiveness of the patient in carrying out the preparatory regimens for diagnostic tests

Willingness to ask questions of nurses in areas of concern or knowledge deficits

Cues indicating level of understanding of information given

Degree of understanding and acceptance of emotional and behavioral responses to stress; strategies for accommodating or compensating for deficits in memory, inability to concentrate, easy distractibility, emotional responses that are not usual; or unmanaged difficulties in daily living occurring because of these deficits

Appropriateness of or difficulties associated with maintaining uncertainty and illusions in the presenting situation

Preparedness for participating in the diagnostic conference

Strengths or deficits in participating in the diagnostic conference. Degree of satisfaction with physician's and own behavior and with the interaction

Degree of satisfaction with personal decision for treatment option or for nontreatment

Status of patient's repertoire of scripts for discussing the health situation; status of family's repertoire of scripts in interacting with the patient in health-related areas

Congruence of patient and family wishes regarding therapy or effective strategies for managing the differences

Comfort and effectiveness of patient and family in making individual needs and desires known to each other and to health care providers

Status of current resolution of decisions to inform specific individuals or groups about the patient's health status

Bibliography

Bergholz E. Under the shadow of cancer. New York Times Magazine, p 73. December 11, 1988.

Braden CJ. Self-help as a learned response to chronic illness experience: a test of four alternative theories. Ph.D. dissertation, University of Arizona, 1986.

Campbell L. Hopelessness and uncertainty as predictors of psychosocial adjustment for newly diagnosed cancer patients and their significant others. Ph.D. dissertation, University of Texas at Austin, 1986.

Carnevali D. Loneliness. In: Carnevali D, Patrick M, eds. Nursing management for the elderly. 2nd ed. Philadelphia: JB Lippincott, 1986.

Cassileth BP, Zupkis RV, Sutton-Smith K, March V: Informed consent: why are its goals imperfectly realized? N Engl J Med 1980;302:896.

Chamorro T, Appelbaum J: Informed consent: nursing issues and ethical dilemmas. Oncology Nursing Forum 1988;15:803.

Chapman CR. Pain related to cancer treatment. Journal of Pain and Symptom Management 1988;3:188.

Cohen F, Lazarus RS: Active coping processes, coping dispositions and recovery from surgery. Psychosom Med 1973;35:375.

D'Angio GJ; Ross JW. The cured cancer patient: a new problem in attitudes and communication. In: Proceedings of the American Cancer Society Third National Conference on Human Values and Cancer. Washington, DC, April 23–25, 1981.

Fisher R. A patient's perspective on the human side of cancer. In: Proceedings of the American Cancer Society Third National Conference on Human Values and Cancer. Washington, DC, April 23–25, 1981.

Fitch MI, O'Brien-Pallas LL. Defensive coping. In: McFarland G, Thomas M, eds. Psychiatric mental health nursing: application of the nursing process. Philadelphia: JB Lippincott, 1990.

Fobair P. Program planning for cancer patients. In: Proceedings of the American Cancer Society Third National Conference on Human Values and Cancer. Washington, DC, April 23–25, 1981.

Folkman S, Lazarus RS. An analysis of coping in a middle-aged community sample. J Health Soc Behav 1980;21:219.

Greenberg ER, Chute CG, Stukel JA et al. Social and economic factors in the choice of lung cancer treatment: a population-based study in two rural states. N Engl J Med 1988;318:612.

Hoffman B. Cancer survivors at work: job problems and illegal discrimination. Oncology Nursing Forum 1989;16:39.

Huhti E, Sultinen S, Saloheim M. Survival among patients with lung cancer: an epidemiological study. Am Rev Respir Dis 1981;124:13.

Kagan AR, Kagan JD. The quality of which life? Am J Clin Oncol 1983;6:117.

Karani D, Wiltshaw E. How well informed? Cancer Nurs 1986;9:238.

Lynn J. Choices of curative and palliative care for cancer patients. CA 1986;36:100.

Mandler G. Thought processes, consciousness and stress. In: Hamilton V, Warburton DM, eds. Human stress and cognition: an information processing approach. New York: John Wiley & Sons, 1979.

Mellette SJ, Franco PC. Psychosocial barriers to employment of the cancer survivor. Journal of Psychosocial Oncology 1987;5:97.

Mishel MH. Perceived uncertainty and stress in illness. Res Nurs Health 1984;7:163.

Mishel MH. The nature of uncertainty in women with gynecological cancer. Presented at the National Symposium of Nursing Research. San Francisco, CA, November, 1985.

Mishel MH. Coping with uncertainty in illness. In: Proceedings of the University of Rochester and Sigma Theta Tau International Epsilon Xi Chapter Conference on Stress, Coping Processes and Health Outcomes. Rochester, NY, April 14–15, 1988, p 51.

Mishel MH. Uncertainty in illness. Image 1988a;20:225.

Molbo D. Cancer. In: Carnevali D, Patrick M, eds. Nursing management for the elderly. 2nd ed. Philadelphia: JB Lippincott, 1986.

Morrow GR, Hoagland AC. Physician–patient communications in cancer treatment. In: Proceedings of the American Cancer Society Third National Conference on Human Values and Cancer. Washington, DC, April 23–25, 1981.

Mullan F. Seasons of survival: reflections of a physician with cancer. N Engl J Med 1985;313:270.

Nokes K. Letter in "Practice corner." Oncology Nursing Forum 1987;14:91.

Pellegrino ED. The moral foundations for valid consent. In: Proceedings of the American Cancer Society Third National Conference on Human Values and Cancer. Washington, DC, April 23–25, 1981, p 171.

Pierce P. Decision-making by women recently diagnosed as having breast cancer. Ph.D. dissertation, University of Michigan, 1985.

President's Commission for the Study of Ethical Problems in Medicine and Biomedical and Behavioral Research. Making health care decisions. Washington, DC: US Government Printing Office, 1982.

Reiser SJ. Words as scalpels: transmitting evidence in the clinical dialogue. Ann Intern Med 1980;92:837.

Schoene-Seifert B, Childress JF. How much should the cancer patient know and decide? CA 1986;36:85.

Scott DW, Oberst MT, Bookbinder MI. Stress-coping response to genitourinary carcinoma in men. Nurs Res 1984;33:325.

Taylor SE. Adjustment to threatening events: a theory of cognitive adaptation. Am Psychol 1983;38:1161.

Trandel-Korenchuk D, Trandel-Korenchuk K: Disclosure of information in nursing. Nursing Administration Quarterly 1986;10:69.

Weisman AD, Worden JW. The existential plight in cancer: significance of the first 100 days. Psychiatry in Medicine 1976;7:1.

Worden JW: Teaching adaptive coping to cancer patients. In: Proceedings of the American Cancer Society Third National Conference on Human Values and Cancer. Washington, DC, April 23–25, 1981.

6

Managing Daily Living During Initial Medical Treatment of Cancer

Medical treatment of cancer can be undertaken at various times during the course of the disease. However, patients and families face the initial medical treatment differently from later therapy. These differences affect both patients' and families' approaches to the management of problems in daily living associated with the disease and its treatment.

With the initial diagnosis and treatment there is the emotional shock of the new diagnosis or confirmation of suspicions, and the sense of threat to life that the word "cancer" brings. But there is also hope for control of the disease that brings with it an energy for managing the problems in daily living that arise from the treatment. Both the newness of the diagnosis and treatment experiences and the hope are variables that nurses will factor into the diagnoses and treatment plans.

The challenges to daily living that can appear during the initial active treatment stage of the cancer experience are not limited to this stage. The dysfunctions and impairments and the changes in daily living that occur in this stage are often found in the post-treatment period and again later if the cancer reemerges as a chronic or end-stage disease. Thus, the diagnostic areas addressed in this chapter may reappear in subsequent chapters. In the context of this chapter, the dysfunctions and challenges to daily living tend to be "new." There is little past experience of success or failure in managing them. This inexperience can be both an advantage and a disadvantage, but in either case it is a reality that is incorporated into both the nursing diagnosis and the treatment plans at this stage.

Medical treatment may begin at any stage of neoplastic growth, depending on the point at which the cancer was diagnosed. Nursing's data base incorporates the reality that this is an initial medical treatment effort and takes note of the predicted course of events and outcomes associated with the pathology, findings, and staging. These variables help to shape nursing's perspective as to which problems in daily living and functioning can or cannot be prevented or cured. The medical data are also considered in diagnosing the problems in daily living in which prevention and cure are not possible and in which palliative and supportive care is the required nursing treatment (see Chapter 10).

In this chapter, some of the common phenomena associated with problems in managing daily living effectively during the initial active treatment stage are discussed. [*] Each problem area is approached as a distinct phenomenon with associated diagnostic areas and treatment options appropriate to that particular problem. This may suggest that one problem in daily living occurs in isolation from the other problems; of course, this is rarely the case. In the initial active treatment stage, more often than not, there are several concurrent problems affecting one another. Anorexia, fatigue, vulnerability to infection, or mechanical difficulties in eating are not experienced in isolation. Each dysfunction and its associated problems of daily living casts its shadow over each of the others, and tends to compound the difficulties in managing them. Daily living is managed in the face of the composite of concurrent dysfunctions and problems. However, in terms of knowledge, because each is a distinguishable phenomenon and requires separate consideration, the problem areas are discussed separately.

In clinical practice there is no question that nursing diagnoses and treatments must integrate the problem areas. The clinician is expected to adapt knowledge about the specific phenomena to the individual patient based on data related to the patient's pathology, stage of disease, signs and symptoms, medical treatment, initial and modified functional status, daily living patterns and requirements, and external resources. The ideas in this chapter, then, are a springboard for the precise and integrative thinking that must emerge in the individual patient situation.

Living With Role Alterations Associated With Cancer and Its Treatment

Change in roles is a requirement in daily living that occurs during the initial treatment stage, not only for the person experiencing cancer, but also for those who share that experience. The changes involve both the addition of new roles and adjustments in usual roles and role relationships. These changes and adjustments may be taken for granted by oncologic health care personnel who daily encounter patients and families facing these challenges. However, failure of nurses to diagnose and treat problems in effective role management in daily living can diminish patient and family well-being and may well complicate the response to the cancer treatment.

Being given a confirmed diagnosis of cancer has been likened to entering a special place that one person called "the land of the sick people" (Trillin, 1981). She found it to be a rather ordinary place where the rules of life had not changed. However, others who still lived in the land of the well people behaved as if there were a distance and boundary between these two lands. Persons from the land of the well people could visit the land of the sick people, but always returned to the land of the well, a place where the individual diagnosed as having cancer could no longer go.

Persons who are known to have cancer come to be seen as different from who and

---

[*] Oncologic emergencies can occur at any point in the cancer experience. They are discussed only once in the book, however, in Chapter 10.

what they were before the diagnostic label was applied to them. Role relationships change and are marked by a new separateness. This may be a means for others to preserve the illusion of their own immortality when it is threatened by the uncertainty of life in another (Trillin, 1981). Sometimes that new separation is marked by added concern, solicitude, and kindness; sometimes by avoidance and actual physical distancing in the work place, in children's play, or in social activities. This change in relationships presents new requirements for insights and skills, an additional burden in daily living to be managed by the person experiencing the cancer and its treatment.

In addition to the changes in interpersonal relationships associated with the diagnostic label of cancer, the disease and medical treatments produce other conditions that alter role relationships. The treatment itself and the geographic location of the treatment center can physically isolate the person from others during treatment. The transient iatrogenic effects and long-term sequelae of the treatment can also create or necessitate changes in previous role relationships and role responsibilities.

With entry to the health care system, new roles are added. These include the *sick role*, as well as variations of the *patient role* encountered in the multiple diagnostic and treatment settings involved in the provision of oncology care.

Many factors come into play to change the patient's usual role constellation. New roles are added, there is an altered capacity to fulfill usual roles and role responsibilities, and there are changes in the way others are prepared to function in their usual role relationships to the patient.

Initial treatment usually occurs shortly after a diagnosis has been confirmed. Thus, the person experiencing confirmation of the cancer diagnosis is making significant treatment decisions, signing informed consent sheets, taking in new knowledge, and moving into the patient roles associated with the various treatments while adjusting to intrapersonal changes.

At the same time, family members, employers, co-workers, and colleagues who may be affected are adjusting their own daily activities, thoughts, feelings, and role expectations in relationship to the patient. They are dealing with their own issues of mortality and the threat of loss. They are shifting the patient into somewhat different roles or changing their expectation of the patient's capacities for fulfilling usual roles for a period of time.

The loss of role comfort and stability for patients and those close to them can present pervasive challenges in daily living. There are decisions to make and subtle or overt interpersonal problems to address, quite aside from the psychologic and physiologic strains of the disease and treatment.

Nature of Role Alterations

As the person moves into initial cancer treatment several role alterations occur. These include not only the various new or altered roles the patient must occupy, but also difficulties in being competent and comfortable in them.

Illness Role

The illness role is generated and developed by the person who is experiencing the signs and symptoms. It is the set of behaviors the individual undertakes as a result of the perceived signs and symptoms and the associated interpretation of their importance.

Classically, this has been linked to health care seeking behavior (Kasl and Cobb, 1966). It can be conceived more broadly to incorporate the moods, activities, and behaviors linked to the illness experience that the person sees as appropriate and acceptable in assuming a personal version of the illness role. For example, the illness role of one person with iatrogenic nausea and vomiting may be to continue usual role obligations by limiting activities only on days of peak dysfunction and resuming normal activities on the "good" days. For another person with the same pattern of iatrogenic nausea and vomiting, the illness role may be seen as legitimately withdrawing from as many usual role responsibilities as possible for the duration of the treatment cycle and symptoms.

Sick Role

The sick role is assigned by others when a person is seen as being incapable of maintaining normal role or task performance, including both physical and interpersonal tasks, because of a health problem (Parsons, 1958). Societal role expectations associated with the sick role include the sick person's (Parsons, 1958):

Not being held responsible for the incapacities being experienced

Release in varying degrees from normal role obligations

Obligation to recognize that illness is undesirable and to express a desire to get well

Obligation to seek competent help, cooperate with treatment, and accept the decisions of health care providers

There can be conflicts between the illness role an individual experiencing cancer adopts and the sick role those around assign. Further, there may be incongruence in assigning the sick role to the patient among the various groups involved with the person (e.g., health care providers, employers, co-workers, and the family). The possibilities of role conflict and role ambiguity are high.

Initial medical treatments, which frequently include surgery, radiation, and repeated chemotherapy cycles, can cause the individual to be intermittently functional and dysfunctional for months—sometimes in unpredictable patterns. Thus, the adoption of the illness role and the assignment of the sick role can fluctuate over prolonged periods of time. This cyclic pattern of iatrogenic dysfunction offers additional opportunities for role incongruence and confusion among the participating parties.

Role Incompetence

Role incompetence may occur when the patient faces new requirements and expectations while participating in unfamiliar oncologic treatment activities and prescribed institutional or home-based regimens. It may be compounded by constantly changing health care personnel, who may have different role expectations or who communicate them in unfamiliar ways. The patient's own care givers may be overwhelmed in their new care-taking roles by the technology, frightened by the symptoms, or frustrated by the inability to meet the patient's dietary needs or to control symptoms. Spouses or family members who are uncomfortable with or frightened by any illness may feel incompetent in relating to the patient.

Role Ambiguity

Role ambiguity may be associated with transitions into and out of the illness or sick roles. It may also occur when the patient and others attempt to adjust role relationships and responsibilities to the ups and downs of patient functioning during cycles of treatment or post-treatment sequelae.

Role Conflict

Role conflict may occur for patients and others. The patient's priorities for working or giving care to children or dependent others may conflict with the oncologists' expectations for participation in treatment protocols or adherence to dietary or other health care behaviors. The oncologists may expect the patient to accept them in the authority and expert physician role and thus to unquestioningly accept their treatment recommendations. However, the patient may maintain a highly autonomous version of the patient role and make decisions that conflict with the recommendations. Expectations of friends, family, and social or religious groups as to the appropriate treatment for cancer can strongly conflict with the approach the patient and family have chosen.

Care givers and family members who have other concurrent role responsibilities experience role conflict as they try to balance perceived role obligations to meet the patient's need for care with other important and valued roles. Employers may experience conflict between the need to remain cost-effective and to be a compassionate supporter of the patient. Co-workers may feel conflict due to the extra role responsibilities that must be assumed in taking up the patient's share of work while maintaining control over the quantity and quality of their own usual work load.

Summary

Role-related phenomena are areas of nursing concern in the pretreatment phase, during hospitalization, in preparation for returning home, during out-patient treatment, and in follow-up. It is not enough to consider only the patient's role problems. Family members and others in the patient's role constellation also need attention, since management of their role problems can be crucial to the patient's well-being.

Underlying Mechanisms

Pathophysiologic and Iatrogenic Factors

Tumor-Related Factors   Knowledge of a confirmed diagnosis of cancer plus information or preconceived ideas about the prognosis can cause the patient or others to alter role relationships.

Fear of death or threat of loss of a loved one generated by the patient's possibly life-threatening illness may initiate construction of defense mechanisms involving denial or subtle or overt separation behavior. These can create role stresses for the patient.

Tumor pathology or pathophysiology can change both the appearance of the individual and specific areas of functional capacity. Depending on the nature of these changes and the roles occupied by the individual, alterations in specific role relationships and functions may occur or require negotiation.

Surgery

Surgery to remove or reduce the tumor mass often involves disfiguration, and may alter functioning in ways that change role relationships and role competence. For example, prostatic resection, a mastectomy, or a colostomy can affect sexual roles; head and neck surgery alters appearance and can affect family, social, sexual, and business roles; altered eating ability can affect family and social roles.

Radiation

Radiation to certain parts of the body can alter appearance (e.g., alopecia or changes in breast texture). It can also change functional capacity, both during and after the treatment. During treatment profound fatigue, loss of appetite, difficulty in eating, diarrhea, or pain can seriously affect role performance and role relationships (see specific sections in this chapter). Long-term sequelae (e.g., loss of taste, dry mouth, chronic diarrhea, vaginal scarring, or impotence) can affect performance in a variety of roles. Post-radiation seizure activity and its control with anticonvulsant drugs alters the capacity to fulfill many roles. Role performance can be affected both during and after radiation treatment.

Chemotherapy

Chemotherapy has many side-effects during the actual course of treatment (e.g., fatigue, neuropathy, gastrointestinal symptoms, and leukopenia) that intermittently interfere with role performance. There may be long-term effects. For example, ovarian and testicular function can be impaired for several years, resulting in sterility or impaired gonadal function and the potential for genetic defects in offspring (Murinson, 1981).

Daily Living Factors

Activities in Daily Living

Role performance and role relationships are involved in most activities in daily living. Where cancer and its treatment are concerned, the role-related activities involved will be determined by the match between the role requirements in daily living and the patient's areas of dysfunction.

Role negotiation and renegotiation are a prominent and recurring activity in daily living as the patient's status or desires change during the course of treatment and as others who are linked to the patient's daily living seek to alter their own roles.

Events in Daily Living

As in activities, the events of concern for the patient are determined by the patient's role obligations in relation to mental and physical status and the desires and expectations of others for the patient's participation. Medical treatments are events that have associated new roles or that alter the capability for fulfilling usual role obligations. Other events are of a personal nature (e.g., social events, travel, or business events).

Roles and role skills developed in past events (medical or social) can be factors that determine role competence in present events.

Preparation for roles and role competence in predicted medical or other *future events* is also of concern in nursing diagnosis and treatment.

Demands in Daily Living

Self-expectations of role fulfillment, role obligations, and priorities in roles are important considerations. The patient can also be anticipated to have role expectations for others—health care providers, individual family members, other care givers, friends, employers, and co-workers—that may or may not be congruent with reality.

Equally important are the nature and strength of role expectations others have for themselves and for the patient.

The punishing and rewarding behaviors engaged in when demands are met or not met by the patient or others are important elements in understanding the dynamics of role relationships and in prescribing treatment.

Environment for Daily Living

Environmental features in daily living can either enhance or create barriers for those involved in trying to fulfill their role obligations to each other. Physical barriers (e.g., masks, gowns, gloves, lead or plastic walls, warning signs, or geographic distances) limit the physical closeness in a role relationship. Access to toilet facilities can limit one's competence in maintaining fecal or urinary continence. A one-bedroom apartment with only a double bed can cause sleep deprivation for the partner and limit that person's capacity to function in the role of care giver or employee. Cooking facilities and eating environments that permit control of odors can enhance the patient's ability to eat. Good, convenient laundry and washing facilities in the environment can facilitate effective management of daily living in the immunosuppressed, who face infection risks, or in those with incontinence problems.

Values and Beliefs

The values individuals and groups assign to their own roles and the roles of others create important dynamics in daily living for the person with cancer and those who share the experience. There are many opportunities for the daily living of each party to be enhanced when there is congruence in role values and expectations. By contrast, it is equally possible for daily living to be made miserable by conflicting values. For example, the medical team may value the patient's role of total compliance with the treatment protocol, while the patient may value the role of single-parent child care giver over the role of compliant patient; the patient with acquired immunodeficiency syndrome (AIDS) believes in the right to continue in the role of employee, while co-workers believe they are threatened by the presence of a person with AIDS-related Kaposi's sarcoma.

The belief systems and stereotypes that many people hold about cancer create stigmatization wherein the person who has cancer, or even a history of cancer, can be assigned the role of victim or outcast.

Functional Health Status

Strength and Endurance

Physical and emotional strength and endurance are important considerations in determining the patient's ability to carry out role obligations associated with initial treatment for cancer. They are often important for the care giver as well if the patient becomes dependent.

Cognition

The cognitive capacities needed to deal with role requirements during the treatment phase include the capacity to:

Learn new roles (e.g., the patient role in various treatment and monitoring settings)

Recognize and understand the role changes in self and others as a basis for participating in the roles and negotiating for needed or desired changes

Anxiety and fears associated with the cancer diagnosis and movement into initial cancer treatments may be severe enough to limit rational thinking or the capacity to learn new roles or make role adjustments at this point in time.

Egocentricity associated with the stress can limit the capacity to receive or act on input from persons in reciprocal roles (e.g., patient–nurse, husband–wife, parent–child).

Once treatment is underway and environments and body responses become more familiar, the capacity to receive and process information can be expected to improve for the patient and those who are close to the patient. At this point, consideration of ongoing role responsibilities and relationships can more productively be addressed.

Communication

Many of the roles, role relationships, and obligations an individual manages in daily living have built up over time in unspoken ways. Thus it may be difficulty to verbally negotiate them.

The special role of the "person with cancer" can add difficulties to communication with persons who do not have cancer (Trillin, 1981). Assistance may be needed in developing the vocabulary, concepts, and communication skills of negotiation in order to do effective problem solving in role negotiations with the family, care giver, employer, co-workers, and even some health care providers.

Nursing Diagnosis and Treatment

Nursing diagnosis and treatment regarding alterations in role can be concerned with several areas:

Congruence of roles and role responsibilities with physical, mental, and emotional resources to carry out those role activities

Implications of the patient's reduced capacity to maintain role performance for daily living of the patient and others

Role competence and capacity for taking on new roles or adjustments in usual roles

Desire and skills of those in reciprocal roles to negotiate for changes in role relationships or responsibilities

Patient's role ambiguity or confusion related to differing role expectations of differing oncologic teams and settings

Capacity to manage role conflicts arising at home or work or in social or health care settings

Diagnostic Targets	Diagnostic targets include the patient, family members, care givers, health care providers, employers, co-workers, and close associates.
Risk Factors	Individuals who may have difficulty in managing daily living in the face of altered roles are those who:

Have never thought much about the roles they occupy

Have few alternatives for changing roles or role obligations

Have those in reciprocal roles (e.g., spouses, companions, children, parents, employers, co-workers, care givers, doctors, nurses, radiation technicians) who are unable or unwilling to negotiate for changes in role relationships and obligations with the patient

Have pathophysiology and symptoms severe enough to interfere with fulfilling role requirements or engaging in role negotiations

Have alternating periods of being functional and dysfunctional during the course of treatment

Have limited verbal or negotiating skills

Feel powerless to introduce change or negotiate

Must engage in role negotiations with others whose stereotypes and beliefs about cancer and cancer treatment create major barriers

Diagnostic Areas

The diagnostic areas described are major categories that will need to be greatly refined by the synthesis of data from the specific situation of the individuals and groups involved in the role and role relationship. (Note that diagnoses may apply to the patient or to others.)

Disruptions in role relationships (specify) related to (R/T) dysfunction(s)†

Lack of competence in the role of *_____ (* e.g., patient, care giver, employee, sexual partner) R/T:

Unfamiliarity with role expectations

Lack of (specified) skills

Lack of desire to learn the role

Lack of cognitive or physical ability to learn the role or gain the skills

Dissatisfaction with perceived (specified) changes in role relationships with *_____ (* e.g., child, spouse, friend, employer) R/T that person's use of defense mechanisms of denial, distancing, or depersonalization

Unsatisfying or dysfunctional role relationships R/T:

Lack of negotiating skills on part of participant(s)

Patient or care giver's sense of powerlessness to negotiate with *_____ (* e.g., husband, doctor, children, patient)

Being placed in victim or outcast role by *_____ (* specify the person or group)

Decreased effectiveness in role or role relationships R/T an environmental barrier (specify) (e.g., isolation precautions, radiation precautions, geographic distances)

Role conflict between patient and *_____ (* e.g., spouse, care givers, specific health care provider, children, employer, coworkers, other family members) R/T differing priorities, differing expectations of role obligations, distancing, or failure to communicate or negotiate

Manifestations

PATIENT

Reported:

Uncertainty about how to function in treatment settings, with self-care procedures, or with particular health care providers

Unhappiness, anger, or depression R/T perception of emotional or physical distancing by significant other(s)

---

† In a working diagnosis, the nature of the reduced capacity, dysfunction, and disruptions in daily living is identified specifically, based on current data from the patient situation. The specific role of the patient or other person should also be used in the diagnostic statement.

Not knowing how to talk to someone about desired changes in their relationship or role responsibilities

Uncertainty about whether or how to give information about one's cancer diagnosis and treatment because of concern over how it will affect the relationship

Feeling torn between responsibility for self and for others

Feeling guilty because behavior or response is not what another person wants

Concern about risks of alienating those upon whom the patient must depend for medical treatment or personal care

Observed:

Uncertainty, hesitancy, or ineffective actions associated with treatment-related activities or with interaction with certain (specified) or all health care personnel

Lack of skill in self-care activities related to (specific aspects of) oncologic treatment regimen or technology

Evidence of fatigue, pain, anorexia, nausea, or vomiting that would be predicted to interfere with the known requirements of the patient's current roles in daily living

Changes in attitude or behavior that reflect negative feelings, sadness, or anger during interaction with family or friends

Passiveness or air of resignation in interactions in which decisions are made regarding role and role responsibilities, even when the outcomes do not seem to be in patient's best interests

Aggressive, controlling behavior in negotiations regarding role that generates defensive responses and anger in others

OTHERS   Family members' or care givers' reported:

Lack of usual comfort and ease in relating to the patient—not knowing what to talk about or how to talk with patient about health status

Concern about how they will manage to provide care or support, given their own physical status or other role obligations

Feeling torn, angry, or guilty about trying to meet the obligations to the patient together with other role responsibilities

Previous unsatisfactory role relationships (e.g., child or spouse abuse) that make it difficult to be genuinely supportive to the patient (Copstead and Patterson, 1986)

Fear of or the actual experience of being incompetent in role of care giver because of the technology or the patient's symptoms

Utter frustration with the patient's failure to respond in a positive way to care giving efforts of family or care giver; wanting to give up on care giver/supporter role

Observed:

Failure to visit the patient; failure to come with the patient to out-patient treatments or care conferences; missing appointments with the nurse to learn patient care skills

Maintenance of a physical distance from patient, not touching the patient

Maintenance of a consistently superficial conversation or being predominantly silent

Procrastination in learning patient care skills and management of technology that will be used in home care

Attempts to take over and control patient roles and role responsibilities where patient wishes to or can engage in self-care

Ineffectiveness in patient care skills or activities evidenced in patient status

Specific physical conditions in the care giver that interfere with assisting the patient in necessary areas

Ineffective communication with health care personnel regarding role relationships with the health care system or the patient

Prognostic Variables

Poor prognosis for managing roles and role relationships in daily living is associated with:

Severity of symptoms sufficient to interfere with functioning in current roles or learning of new roles

Previously poor role relationships between patient and family, care givers, or other support figures

Having demanding roles that do not easily accommodate change

Lack of negotiating skills

Having severe symptoms that interfere with attention to role relationships

Feeling powerless

Having those in reciprocal roles who will not accommodate the patient's changing role capacities or will not negotiate for changes

Complications

Failure to effectively manage role alterations during active treatment can result in frustration with role relationships, depression, or giving up by the patient or care givers; the patient feeling isolated and alone; the family or care givers feeling angry or guilty; lack of adequate care for the patient with resultant loss of well-being and possibly a negative outlook for the disease; loss of job and income; loss of valued roles, status, or identity.

Treatment Guidelines

Role performance impairment R/T health status or daily living situation

Gather data on the specific role tasks in daily living that are impaired and the health-related factors that contribute to the problems.

Explore options for changing the role responsibilities by modifying, postponing, or reducing the tasks, or recruiting some assistance in fulfilling role responsibilities.

Help the patient and others involved, if needed, to structure a plan that is acceptable and feasible for accomplishing tasks and maintaining satisfying relationships.

Provide opportunities for feedback on the course of events and satisfactions, problems with the implementation of the plan, and needs for adjustments.

Role incompetence R/T unfamiliarity with role expectations or skills

Gather data on any past personal or vicarious experience with the role that may affect current role expectations.

Gather data on any cognitive, emotional, or physical factors that may impede the person's learning of the role or role-related skills.

Provide information regarding the nature of the role and role responsibilities in the clinical setting where they will be used (e.g., the amount of variation in behavior that is tolerated, the accepted limits on deviating from role expectations, the nature of feedback that will be offered for role guidance, or the skills involved in implementing the medical regimen). This information can be given in writing (unless the patient is illiterate) and supplemented by discussions and exposure to the environment and equipment.

Rehearse role behaviors and skills in a safe environment or give participants ideas about how they may engage in such role rehearsal on their own. Where the behavior or skills must be transferred from one setting or situation to another, address the specific changes or adjustments that will need to be made for each situation. If there is a possibility that the learner may not retain the information, make an audiotape of the interaction that can then be replayed as often as needed and under less stressful conditions.

Reward successful elements of role performance specifically, generously, and genuinely.

Help the person(s) to correct and improve role behaviors that are not yet effective in ways that will be perceived as useful, not embarrassing or derogatory.

Arrange for feedback on progress, problems, need for adjustments, questions, and status of satisfaction with the role and role competence.

Dissatisfaction with role relationships associated with the health care situation—role strains, role conflicts. (Treatment may be offered to patient, family member(s), care giver, or health care provider.)

Gather data on the role relationship that is not satisfying: What was the relationship like in the past and how has it changed (if it is not a new relationship)? What does the person want the relationship to be like? What factors does the person believe might explain the change in the relationship or the unsatisfactory nature of a new relationship (e.g., an encounter with a radiologist, oncologist, or nurse)?

Explore what the person is willing or feels able to do to try to change the relationship and what the other person could do to improve the relationship.

Provide objective information about factors that might normally affect relationships during this type of a health situation and some of the ways others have managed them.

Discuss the strategy for role negotiations. For example, the person desiring the role change may change his or her own behavior in order to modify the response of the other person—without discussing it explicitly; or, explicit negotiations may be used to try to initiate desired role changes. Help the person to choose the strategy that seems most useful or comfortable in the presenting situation.

If the person decides to try to change his or her own behavior as a basis for changing the other person's response, help in planning the behavior to be used in particular circumstances and the adjustments to be made if the other person's response is not the desired one. Propose that the person develop and rehearse scripts (planned verbal approaches) or behaviors for particular situations; assist if needed. Suggest that the patient take note of the other person's response as a basis for determining what action to take next.

Assess whether the person feels capable of carrying on the negotiations alone or needs help. If the person needs help:

Confer about when is a "good" time for the parties to discuss their roles and role relationships. Is there a particularly good place for the discussion to take place?

If needed, help to plan a script to introduce the role negotiation. For example, "Doing _____ is very difficult for me at this time. It would be helpful (or, it is critical) for us to consider some changes that would be workable for, and acceptable to, each of us."

Offer general guidelines for role negotiation (Bartos, 1970):

Determine how their views of the role and relationship differ. The person seeking change can gather data on the other person's view and desires and share information on his or her own view and desires—the difficulties being experienced, the values involved, and the goals.

Work to find the "payoffs" and exchanges that will be "fair" for each party under the circumstances as a basis for coming to a workable agreement.

Remind the person that functional capacities may fluctuate during the treatment phase, so that ongoing negotiations are likely to be necessary; therefore, setting a pattern for this can be important.

Sense of powerlessness interfering with role relationships

Gather data on the basis for feelings of powerlessness and determine whether this is a new or long-standing perception.

Where the health status of the individual does not permit use of empowering strategies, offer to serve as an advocate in role negotiations.

Where health status is such that the individual can participate in empowering activities:

Encourage the patient or family to describe themselves as people (not patients) in terms of their personal strengths, goals, priorities, values, and beliefs.

Legitimize the right to make decisions regarding health care and roles.

Identify areas for negotiation within the system. For example, "You don't have to put up with that." "You are paying for this health care, you can. . . . "

Alert them to consequences that may result from specified negotiations. "By contracting with the children to set the table and clean up after dinner, you can make them feel that they are making a contribution and at the same time you can get a bit more rest at a time when you have been having greater fatigue."

Alert them to consequences of failure to negotiate for particular role behaviors. For example, "Dr K.'s pattern with patients is to give them information they specifically request, so if you want to know, you will have tell him how much information you want and ask questions."

Offer the degree of nurse support or action in the role negotiations that the person desires; for example:

Patient takes total responsibility.

Nurse teaches the patient how to negotiate in the specific situation.

Nurse is present to support, as pre-planned or as needed.

Nurse negotiates for the patient.

Prepare others to participate in role negotiations the patient wants to undertake in order to support the patient's power.

Assist the patient to use the critical words needed in negotiations with people in the health care disciplines or bureaucracies, or translate for the patient.

Offer strategies for gaining verbal or written contracts of goals and role responsibilities.

Support the patient's belief about his capacity to make sound judgments when he has adequate information and has considered the options.

Environmental barriers to effective role relationships and role performance

Gather data on the specific nature of perceived role difficulties and environmental factors contributing to them (e.g., lack of convenient laundry facilities, lack of a kitchen, too many people needing to use one bathroom, a single bedroom with a double bed for patient and partner, no place for privacy for patient or others, no telephone, substandard housing (dirt, vermin), no close public transportation).

Mobilize resources to reduce the barriers, if possible.

Work with those who occupy the same housing to develop schedules and behaviors that will accommodate the patient's current needs.

Evaluation

Response to nursing treatment of role alterations and dissatisfactions can be evaluated in terms of:

Effectiveness in performance of observed roles in the health care system (e.g., patient interactions with physicians in the various oncologic specialty areas, interactions with nurses, participation in the treatment regimen and self-care activities, care giver effectiveness in providing care to patient; family member's comfort and effectiveness in maintaining degree of mutually desired closeness with the patient)

Reports of status of satisfaction with role relationships or outcomes of role negotiations by one or more participants

Evidence of patterns of renegotiation of roles and role obligations as patient status or care giver status changes

Evidence of reduction in environmental barriers or mobilization of other support systems

---

Living With Loss of Desire to Eat

Loss of desire for food can be one of the first symptoms of cancer, an ongoing problem in the cancer experience, and the first evidence of recurrence or progression. Many factors associated with both the disease and its treatment alter the desire to eat, including the psychologic impact of the diagnosed disease and the local and systemic effects of the neoplasia itself. Appetite may be affected by each form of cancer therapy. Thus, loss of the desire for food can be an early and persistent problem.

Medical Perspective

The medical perspective on anorexia most frequently addresses the anorexia in terms of potential clinical malnutrition. The malnutrition may, in turn, influence the effectiveness of the therapy.

Nursing Perspective

The nursing perspective concerns the disrupted eating patterns and the associated discomfort, as well as problems in daily living experienced by the patient and others closely involved in food- and eating-related activities. These problems in daily living, if improperly diagnosed and treated, can compound the patient's malnutrition and further reduce well-being.

Description of Loss of Desire to Eat

Several psychophysiologic phenomena are associated with the desire or lack of desire to eat.

Hunger is a physiologically based craving for food, an urge to eat to fulfill the body's requirement for food.

Appetite is a positive attitude toward eating food and often involves preferences for particular foods or nutrients.

Satiety is the feeling of having consumed sufficient food and a desire not to eat more.

Anorexia is an active disinterest in food and a lack of desire to ingest food.

Food aversion is a distaste or dislike for a particular food. It may be long-standing or a recent conditioned response, for example, related to association of a particular food to nausea and vomiting (iatrogenic or other). Food aversion may also result from taste changes.

People with cancer often experience anorexia and develop food aversions. Additionally, many experience early satiety.

Loss of desire to eat has an impact on daily living. Eating and food preparation tend to have prominent and regular places in daily living. They involve well-developed patterns affected by culture, social customs, established role relationships, emotions, memories, and physical environmental factors.

It is hard to escape regular visual and auditory stimuli about eating. Wherever the person is or goes there are billboards, newspapers and magazines, radios and televisions, restaurants, supermarkets, and smaller specialty food shops, all with reminders about food and eating. Social interactions often involve food and eating. Role relationships within families include behaviors associated with food preparation and eating. These relationships and interactions can be disrupted when either food preparation or eating are disturbed by changed eating patterns in the person who has cancer. Thus, a complex psychosocial, cultural, and physical set of variables interact to create problems in daily living, not only for the person with cancer whose eating is disturbed, but also for those who share in the eating and food preparation activities.

Underlying Mechanisms

Pathophysiologic and Iatrogenic Factors

The physiologic basis for anorexia is complex and, as yet, poorly understood (Behnke, 1986; Williams, 1986). For the person with cancer there may be both physiologic and psychophysiologic factors at work.

Tumor-Related Factors

The following tumor-related factors can be linked to anorexia:

Tumor growth alone can cause anorexia, depending on the site and extent of disease (e.g., oral, pharyngeal, gastrointestinal, hepatic, pancreatic, and gallbladder cancers).

Side-effects of the cancer such as ascites, dyspnea, and pain are related to anorexia.

Metabolic changes (e.g., decreased insulin sensitivity associated with changes in metabolism of glucose and triglycerides, and imbalances of specific plasma amino acids) that are associated with neoplasia can be linked to a false sense of satiety (De Wys, 1982; Theologides, 1981).

Neurotransmitter production changes (e.g., changes in serotonin levels) may cause changes in appetite by acting on appetite centers in the brain (Chance, 1983; Theologides, 1981; Wurtman, 1984).

Encroachment on or obstruction of gastrointestinal space occurs with cancers growing within that tract. Cancers growing near the gastrointestinal tract (e.g., hepatic, pancreatic, ovarian, renal, or uterine tumors and intra-abdominal metastatic lesions) create pressures on it and also narrow the lumen. Ascites creates broad, generalized pressure on intra-abdominal structures.

Dyspnea from a variety of tumor-related factors can decrease the desire to eat.

Taste changes associated with cancer include increased sensitivity to bitterness, aversion to meat (possibly related to the amino acids, polypeptides, and purines in meat, which in pure form taste bitter), decreased sensitivity to sweetness, and decreased salt recognition in patients with colon resections followed by antimetabolite chemotherapy. The mechanisms of taste changes are not well understood, but zinc deficits may be implicated. Taste changes affect the desire to eat.

Noxious odors due to necrosis, infection, urine, feces, fetid breath, and jaundiced skin, which are associated with neoplasia or artificial body portals, can cause anorexia.

Surgery

Immediate side-effects of anesthesia and surgical procedures (e.g., pain, decreased peristalsis) and narcotics usually decrease appetite temporarily.

Surgical alterations including permanent reduction of space for food (e.g., gastric resections) may have the long-term effect of decreasing appetite and increasing early satiety; short bowel syndrome secondary to removal of segments of the bowel may also affect appetite.

**Chemo-
therapy***

Nausea and vomiting related to emetic properties in certain chemotherapeutic agents is thought to be caused primarily by the effect on the vomiting center in the brain of stimulation of the chemoreceptor trigger zone. Stimulation of peripheral vagal impulses, resulting in gastric irritation, may also be a factor. Anorexia tends to be present with nausea or vomiting. Higher cognitive centers can affect appetite. Certain stimuli (sights or smells) associated with chemotherapy or recall of the experience can induce anorexia, actual nausea and vomiting, or learned aversion to food eaten in the time periods near the treatments (Coons et al, 1987). Stomatitis, mucositis, and xerostomia create pain or mechanical difficulties that decrease the desire to ingest food.

Radiation

The effect of radiation on appetite depends primarily on site, but dosage also has some effect. Radiation to the head and neck can destroy taste buds and production of saliva. Radiotherapy to the mediastinum, esophagus, and stomach causes nausea, dyspepsia, and pylorospasm, with high dosages causing dysphagia, anorexia, nausea, and vomiting. Where the radiation field affects the intestines, there are major effects on the crypt cells, shortening of villi, and denuding of intestinal mucosa. When this occurs in the small intestine, it results in nausea and vomiting. Pelvic irradiation results in anorexia, diarrhea, and

* The actual presence of anorexia or its severity will vary with the individual, with the site and stage of the disease, and with the treatment regimen.

cramping (Hilderly, 1987). All of these can decrease the desire for food.

Biologic Response Modifiers

Anorexia and weight loss (an average of 4%) are common with treatment involving biologic response modifiers (Mayer et al, 1984).

Infection-Related Factors

Given patients' increased vulnerability, infections are a relatively common complication associated with cancer and its treatment. Systemic reactions to infections usually include a decrease in appetite. Additionally, some specific infections, such as hepatitis and pancreatitis, particularly affect appetite. Herpes simplex, herpes zoster, and candidiasis create local pain and secondarily decrease the desire to eat.

Emotional Factors

Emotional responses of anxiety, depression, and fear tend to be either ongoing or recurring features of daily living with cancer, its diagnosis, and treatment. These psychophysiologic responses, transmitted by the autonomic system (sympathetic and parasympathetic) as well as hormonal responses, can negatively affect appetite. Persistent hopelessness creates anorexia even in healthy individuals (Holland et al, 1977). People who have head and neck surgery may be ostracized or may isolate themselves because of their appearance. Such negative experiences depress the desire to eat. It is important to differentiate between depression (disinterest in all aspects of life) and anorexia (disinterest in eating) because of the difference in treatment (Behnke, 1986).

The behavior of others in relationship to the patient's appetite and eating can also have an effect. Undue attention, whether oversolicitousness, criticism, or nagging, can also have a negative impact on the desire to eat.

Diet

The diet itself, whether the texture, the foods themselves, or the monotony of the limited foods or textures can contribute to loss of desire to eat.

Fatigue

Fatigue, a frequent concomitant aspect of cancer and its treatment, can have a depressing effect on appetite (McCorkle, 1973).

Daily Living Factors

Activities in Daily Living

Food preparation: Food procurement, preparation, and presentation may suffer in two ways. The patient may be the food preparer for self and others and may experience tremendous difficulties with shopping and with the sights and smells involved in food preparation. A care giver or family member may be the one who prepares the food and can experience intense frustration, anger, and often guilt when the patient is intolerant of odors involved in food preparation or refuses to eat what is prepared or what he may have requested or formerly tolerated. Frustration can also occur with the monotony of preparing only the one food the patient will eat—day after day after day.

Social interaction: Companionship at meals can become a negative influence when the behavior of the patient's meal companions is changed by alterations in the patient's appearance or participation in the mealtime experience. Meal companions may send verbal or nonverbal messages to the patient that he is disturbing their own eating or they may urge food on the patient that he is unwilling or unable to ingest. This, in turn, may create further emotional distress for the patient. Some of the patient-based elements that can have impact on mealtime interaction include:

The need to have a different diet (e.g., pureed or liquid foods)

The inability to tolerate the sights and smells of foods eaten by others at the table

Lack of appetite and unwillingness to "try to eat" when part of the recognized therapy is maintenance of adequate nutrition

Changes in the patient's appearance

Decreases in stamina that prevent the patient's remaining at the table for a whole meal

A negative prevailing mood or the patient's need to talk about his condition and treatment

Offensive sounds in swallowing, or choking and coughing when eating

The presence of noxious odors

As a result of discomfort between the patient and meal companions, the patient may suffer many blows to his self-concept and may experience psychologic or physical isolation in the activity of eating, whether self-created or mandated by others. Eating in public places may be similarly affected.

Events in Daily Living

Medical diagnostic and treatment-related events can decrease desire for food, as can fear or anxiety associated with medical and treatment events and findings (diagnoses and prognoses). The emotional impact of nonhealth-related events that either increase or decrease anxiety, depression, and tension also affects desire to eat.

Social events in which eating is an element can cause difficulties when the desire not to eat is strong.

Demands in Daily Living

Self-expectations: The patient may have self-expectations of:

Obligations related to preparing food, or the right to be excused from such responsibilities

Eating what has been prepared or feeling free to eat only as desired

Participating in activities involving eating or avoiding such activities

Eating in order to survive or not eating in order to shorten life

Expectations of others: These include expectations that the patient either will or need not:

Maintain role of food preparer

Eat according to others' prescription or expectations (institutional and noninstitutional)

Participate in eating related to work or social activities

Eat because it will affect survival

Environment for Daily Living

The nature of the physical environment (institutional and home) that can affect desire to eat includes:

Architecture that does not permit avoidance of cooking odors

The aesthetics of eating areas

Environmental barriers to food procurement and preparation when the patient is the food preparer or the food preparer also has physical limitations

Values and Beliefs

Cultural and social values and beliefs associated with food and eating patterns, particularly in relationship to health and cancer, include:

Valuing the roles associated with food and eating

Valuing the quality of life and survival—this valuing affects participation in dietary aspects of the treatment regimen

Beliefs in the effects of food on health and illness

Family or care giver beliefs that feeding is loving and that eating what is prepared is also an expression of love and appreciation

Functional Health Status

Cognition

Cognition associated with the desire to eat involves the capacity to:

Understand how nutrition is, and is not, related to health status and response to treatment in the presenting circumstances (e.g., taking megavitamins instead of taking in calories and protein can have a nontherapeutic outcome)

Understand the reasons for loss of appetite, taste changes, and food aversions as a basis for managing these factors

Learn about options for managing difficulties in daily living related to eating, food odors, food shopping and preparation, and eating-related social or work situations

Acquire or retain organizational skills for managing food preparation and eating-related tasks in the presence of anorexia

Strength and Endurance	Strength and endurance involve the capacities to feed oneself, chew, procure and prepare food, or even be interested in food.
Mobility	Mobility involves the capacity to move about in food procurement and preparation and to chew and swallow food and fluids.
Mood	The patient's usual outlook and mood (e.g., optimism, cheerfulness, and enthusiasm versus depression, pessimism, moodiness, and anxiety) can affect appetite.
	Emotional response to presenting situations can also have a transient affect on the desire to eat.
Communication	Communication capacity related to loss of desire to eat involves the ability to describe personal experiences (verbally or in logs), wishes, needs, or problems related to food preparation roles and eating experiences, and the capacity to negotiate for needed changes in daily living associated with food preparation and eating.

Nursing Diagnosis and Treatment

Prevention

Nurses can predict the loss of appetite, early satiety, and food aversions for individual patients based on their knowledge of the diagnosed neoplasia and projected treatment. They know the areas of high risk in daily living associated with these eating problems. As they gather data about the patterns of daily living in the high risk areas for individual patients and their families, it is possible to predict problems that may arise and take early action to prevent some problems, minimize others, or enable patients and families to take action to deal more effectively with problems as they occur.

Once a diagnosis of a possible problem is made, treatment is directed toward:

Promoting successful eating experiences

Preventing or minimizing predicted eating problems

Planning ahead for predicted problems in food preparation, either by the patient or other care givers

Preparing patient and meal companions for any problems in communal eating or eating in public places

The risk factors listed below can be used to help the nurse focus observations and data collection to include or rule out problems that lend themselves to prevention. Many of the diagnoses listed under Diagnostic Areas could be viewed in terms of prevention. Many of the treatments described under Treatment Guidelines in this section can be beneficial if introduced prior to the experience of anorexia or disruption of food preparation and eating elements in daily living.

Diagnostic Targets	Individuals who can be the focus of diagnosis and treatment when the patient experiences loss of desire to eat during antineoplastic treatment include the patient, care givers (including family members, lay persons, nurses, and other health care personnel), food preparers, those who eat with the patient, and food servers in cafeterias frequently serving patients receiving radiation therapy or chemotherapy.
Risk Factors	Patients who may have difficulty in managing daily living with loss of desire to eat include those who:†

Have given food an important place in past patterns of daily living

Have little or no knowledge of nutrition, appetite, and factors that affect them

Have taste changes and xerostomia

Live alone or eat alone

Are depressed

Have inadequate financial resources to purchase appropriate food and supplements

Need but do not have a consistently available, caring primary care giver to shop and prepare food

Have primary responsibility for food preparation for others in the family

Have a care giver who believes that loving is feeding and that eating food offered is returning that love

Live with people who emotionally or physically distance themselves

Are intolerant of institutional food

Find the required texture or food substances monotonous and unappealing

Use decreased eating as a means of withdrawal from living

---

† Many of these risk factors can be adjusted to diagnose potential problems for care givers as a basis for early treatment and prevention.

Have care givers who lack time, knowledge, skill, interest, or physical capability to prepare foods the patient accepts

Have a lack of support and assistance (for the patient who must serve in the role of food preparer)

)iagnostic
Areas
PATIENT‡

Anxiety, ineffective food preparation, or impaired eating behavior R/T lack of understanding of the underlying mechanisms of changes in appetite, taste, or development of food aversions

Fear of eating or exploring new approaches to food or eating R/T current problems with eating

Ineffective management of food preparation and serving R/T lack of knowledge of options and creativity for managing nutrition, given the loss of appetite, monotony of diet, or food aversions

Decreased interest in eating R/T monotony of foods or food textures that patient perceives as being possible to eat and retain

Decreased desire to eat R/T inability to escape from distasteful food odors in the environment

Guilt, anger, fatigue, or ineffective role behavior of patient as food preparer R/T lack of an understanding, functional support system

Difficulty in managing interactions with others in eating situations (institutional, social, or work situations) R/T failure to develop and rehearse usable scripts or plans for handling these encounters

Decreased incentive to eat R/T ostracizing or distancing behavior of eating companions

Purposeful decrease in food and fluid intake R/T desire to escape from the current and predicted quality of life

FOOD PREPARER

Frustration and anger when food preparing efforts are continually rejected by the patient

Frustration with the monotony of preparing only the one form of food the patient is willing to eat R/T lack of knowledge and skills in providing usable options

Decreased incentive to eat R/T having to see and hear distasteful sights and sounds from the patient

Difficulties in scheduling and arranging for meals R/T times of treatment, limiting intake to minimize nausea and vomiting, lack of food services in clinic, or waits for transportation

‡Many of these nursing diagnoses may also apply to those involved in care giving, food preparation, or sharing ating experiences.

Manifestations	Pattern of ongoing weight loss
PATIENT	Expressed fear of trying to eat after unsuccessful eating experiences
	Apathy in food choices and decisions about eating
	Failure to eat usual amounts and foods
	Neutrality in responses to questions about appetite or eating: "Oh, I eat pretty well—small amounts, but frequently"; "I eat when I feel like it"; "Food isn't as important as it once was." This may mask serious anorexia.
	Requesting special foods and then not wanting them
	Refusal of medications to reduce nausea or improve appetite
	Rejection of all food
	Attitude of increasing withdrawal or resignation
	Perception that others would rather that the patient not be present at mealtimes or that the patient is being required to eat alone
	Failure to eat on treatment days
	Reports of or behavior indicating deteriorating self-concept
CARE GIVER	Reports frustration with inability to satisfy the patient or prepare foods the patient will eat: "Nothing I fix appeals to her"; "He won't even eat his favorite foods anymore."
	Reports difficulty in cooking because of patient's aversion to food odors
	Reports anger or guilt over inability to prepare foods the patient needs to maintain nutrition and will accept
	Threatens to "give up" in trying to please patient
	Reports not understanding why the patient "refuses to eat normally"
	Reports that the patient "isn't even trying"
	Reports discomfort or distancing behavior of meal companions R/T patient symptoms, mood, or behavior
Prognostic Variables	Poor prognosis for managing daily living to improve eating in the presence of loss of desire to eat is associated with:
	Hopelessness, depression, or a weak will to survive
	Lack of desire or skills to find strategies for managing the problem
	Minimal knowledge of nutritional options
	Iatrogenic effects of aggressive oncologic therapy (nausea, vomiting, pain, fatigue)

Lack of predictable, caring, competent, care givers and food preparers and lack of support systems for the care givers

Distancing behavior in people who have been a source of support to the patient

Complications   Failure to manage daily living effectively in the areas of eating or food preparation can result in:

Malnutrition

Diminished physiologic resources for building tumor resistance and desired response to the treatment regimen

Establishment of a downward spiral: not eating leads to even less desire to eat, which leads to fatigue and malnutrition

Depression secondary to malnutrition and electrolyte imbalance

Loss of will to live, withdrawal from the treatment protocol

Burnout in the food preparer

Treatment Guidelines   One option for gathering data on eating patterns, preferences, aversions, and actual food consumed is the use of an eating log. A sample is shown in Figure 6-1. This can give a baseline prior to medical treatment effects and show any change that occurs in association with the disease–treatment trajectory and nursing intervention.

The following treatment guidelines are intended for either institutional or home settings.

Lack of understanding of loss of desire to eat in present situation

Provide information on factors that can affect desire to eat based on the *specific* nursing diagnosis (i.e., pertinent to the individual patient's physiologic, emotional, social, and daily living situation). Use informal discussions in ongoing contacts, more scheduled teaching sessions, reading materials (if patient and care giver are literate), and audio cassettes. Use language, sentence structure, drawings, etc. that are appropriate to the person's language, education, and cultural background. Consider also the effect of anxiety on the capacity to learn.§

Lack of awareness of options or skills for managing food preparation and eating in the presence of lack of desire to eat

Explore acceptable and feasible modifications in daily living that can improve eating patterns. Recommend the following strategies to the patient. To combat:

§ See US Department of Health and Human Services. Pretesting in health communications: methods, examples and resources for improving health messages and materials. Bethesda, MD: US Department of Health and Human Services, NIH Publication 84-1493, 1984.

Appetite and Eating Log

Name _____   Date _____

Day of week (*circle*)   S   M   T   W   Th   F   S

Record as accurately as you can your appetite, the foods and amounts you actually ate, plus any comments such as food aversions, sensations after eating, successes in eating, and any problems. You and your nurse can use this information to plan for more comfort and good nutrition.

Time	Appetite Code	Names of Food or Fluid Ingested	Amount Ingested	Comments

Appetite Code
+2 very hunger
+1 somewhat hungry
 0 no desire for food
−1 nauseated
−2 vomiting

Guide for Recording Amount Eaten or Drunk (numbers of)
T: tablespoons
t: teaspoons
B: bites taken (eg, meat, bread)
C: cup (8 oz) or portion eg, ¼, ½
#: number of, eg, chips, nuts, grapes, cherries, cookies, crackers

Figure 6-1.   Sample appetite and eating log.

Anxiety at having to eat when there is no desire to eat: Engage in systematic relaxation prior to major meals to counteract the effects of anxiety on appetite; plan to eat larger amounts during the "best" time of day. Note: Gastric emptying of solid meals ingested in the evening has been found to be 53.6% longer than in the morning; liquids showed a similar pattern (Goo et al, 1987).

Fatigue: Try to plan for a 30-minute rest before meals (Mc-Corkle, 1973); use prepared foods that don't require much effort in preparation; prepare and freeze meals on the "good" days for use on the "bad" days; accept or ask for help from friends, being specific about foods that can and cannot be eaten (US Department of Health and Human Services, 1986).

Pain: Take pain medications so that there is maximum analgesia at eating times; for mouth–throat pain suck ice chips and place ice packs on throat; use food temperatures that are most comfortable to the patient.

Odors: Try to get someone else to do the cooking or use frozen entrees that can be warmed at a low temperature or microwaved; avoid frying foods; avoid brewing aromatic beverages; go for a walk or stay in another room with the door closed while food is cooking (US Department of Health and Human Services, 1986).

Nausea: Take antiemetic medications 30 to 60 minutes before eating; serve smaller portions; use foods low in fat; eat salty foods and avoid sweet foods (particularly after a period of vomiting); do not eat especially enjoyed foods near times of predictable nausea and vomiting; take clear, cool liquids through a straw in small, slow sips 30 to 60 minutes before meals rather than during meals; avoid lying flat or engaging in activity for 2 hours after eating; wear loose clothing (US Department of Health and Human Services, 1986).

Early satiety: Eat smaller meals more often; keep nutritious snacks available; do not eat too slowly (try to ingest more food before the satiety signal is sent); limit fatty foods; drink nutritious liquids but limit the quantity taken during meals (US Department of Health and Human Services, 1986).

Altered taste: Eat poultry or fish in place of meat; cook on a barbecue if possible; add bacon bits, ham strips, or pieces of onion to vegetables; try tart foods or herbs to enhance flavor if there are no mouth and throat problems; try adding wines, beer, or mayonnaise to soups or sauces for flavoring; marinate meats, fish, and chicken and add herbs to marinades; try temperature change in serving food—cold or room temperature; alter the taste in the mouth by drinking more liquids or eating foods that leave a taste of their own (e.g., fresh fruits, hard candies) (US Department of Health and Human Services, 1986). Head and neck radiation increases a "burnt" taste—avoid deep roasted coffees, use cream in coffee, don't deeply brown or roast meats. Cisplatin makes meat taste "metallic"—use small amounts of meat in sauces that disguise the meat taste.

Patient's difficulties regarding obligations as food preparer for others

Help the patient to find ways to increase awareness of usual patterns in food preparation and explore ways that current symptoms require a change in these patterns. Explore possible acceptable alterations: What are the hours or days that the patient feels the most energy and least symptoms? Could foods be prepared at this time in larger amounts and stored for the "bad days"? Are there others in the family who could do the shopping or help with meal preparation? Are there family or friends who could bring in some meals or help with shopping or other food-related tasks? Could medications be taken on a schedule to reduce symptoms during meal preparation and eating?

Explore patient expectations versus the options that are available in the presenting situation.

Identify elements of the tasks that are creating or will create difficulties.

Help the patient, as needed, to write a plan and schedule a definite trial period of alternate approaches that will be reevaluated at a designated nurse–patient contact (personal or telephone). Modify or continue plan based on its effectiveness.

Help the patient or family to set up a "cardiac kitchen" with stools of appropriate height for sitting while preparing foods and frequently used utensils and staples at convenient heights.

Where nausea or fatigue preclude completing all food preparations, propose hanging on the refrigerator the menu, the location of remaining items to be set on the table, and any instructions for final preparation so that others can take over and the patient may have the energy to eat.

Patient's, care giver's, or family's values and beliefs that create barriers to effective management of daily living with anorexia

Explore values and beliefs associated with food preparation, eating, and food-related behavior and interaction as these affect the presenting situation.

Determine the relative strengths of the values—they may range from "needs permission to change" to "totally resistant to any change."

Explore what the person thinks is the worst and the best that could happen if specific changes were to be undertaken.

Explore acceptable strategies and occasions for introducing changes.

Assist person to develop a script or repertoire of behaviors to use in responding to others' reactions to change(s).

Care giver's or food preparer's difficulties in participating in food preparation and eating activities in light of the patient's loss of desire to eat

Gather data on food preparer's or care giver's understanding of the difficulties the patient is experiencing in eating and the critical nutritional needs.

Gather data on the food preparer's knowledge, skill, and available time as these relate to food shopping, cooking, and serving. Propose resources that will address identified problems.

Seek to detect the presence of "to love is to feed" belief and any pressures or difficulties this may be having on eating interactions.

Meet with food preparer–care giver alone and assure confidentiality. Explore any difficulties the person is experiencing (lack of knowledge, time, or skill; negative emotional responses; burnout; or conflicts due to cultural factors).

Serve as a resource to the person in considering acceptable and feasible options or strategies that will cause either the patient to eat more or the care provider to be more comfortable with the eating situation. Refer to other patients or care givers who have experienced or are experiencing similar challenges. Legitimize the emotional responses of frustration, anger, or guilt or feelings of being "used." Explore options for respite or outlets for emotions.

Propose negotiating with friends who wish to contribute food for either patient or food preparer about what foods are currently palatable and usable, the need to prepare in single-size servings for refrigeration or freezing for the patient, and appropriate serving sizes for food preparer or family.

Isolation of patient or distancing behavior during mealtimes

Arrange for or suggest arranging for companionship at mealtimes (in institutional or home setting).

Explore with eating companions the elements in the patient's condition or behavior that create difficulties for them in eating with the patient.

Explore acceptable options for minimizing these negative stimuli or altering their responses (e.g., develop a pattern of suctioning tracheostomies before each meal and having a clean cravat over the stoma, have clean dressings applied prior to meals).

Explore practical options for altering the eating situation in ways that will not create alienation or distancing behavior between patient and eating companions (e.g., arrange for the patient to join the family for only the latter part of the meal; plan a dessert that the patient can easily eat).

Follow up on outcomes of any changes introduced in mealtime activities and behavior. Stress the importance of avoiding pity.

Presence of environmental factors that are a deterrent to eating when anorexia is present

Help the patient and care givers understand that the environment for eating and the aesthetics of food presentation are important.

Offer the following strategies to care givers:

Try a change of the patient's position or location for meals (e.g., bed to chair; living room to eating room).

Experiment with serving the portions for everyone at the table, rather than serving "family style."

Offer smaller portions of food on smaller plates. Avoid presenting food that looks like "sick person's food"—that is, bland and colorless. Use garnishes or colorful plates for eye appeal.

Consider having a glass of wine or beer before meals if this is seen as a usual pattern or a treat (with physician approval).

Try to make the eating environment aesthetically pleasing. Use flowers or a candle on the table or tray. Play music that is enjoyable or turn on a favorite TV show. Recruit someone to talk with the patient who leads the conversation into areas of interest and diversion to the patient. Any or all of these strategies may provide an environment to help a waning desire for food.

Encourage the patient to prepare for the "event" of eating—freshen up, use mouth wash, change clothing for evening "meal" or a meal with companions or the family.

Difficulties in scheduling eating times on treatment days

Gather data on current patterns of eating on treatment days and the symptoms that dictate this schedule (e.g., anticipatory nausea and vomiting, motion sickness on the ride to the treatment site, post-treatment nausea, vomiting, pain, diarrhea, or having to wait around the treatment area for laboratory tests or for transportation home).

Using the data, plan for the most nutritious and acceptable eating schedule and menu for these days.

When the anorexic patient must eat in the hospital cafeteria on treatment days, specifically plan strategies for obtaining food in order to minimize fatigue, indecision, and exposure to food odors.

Deliberate reduction in caloric intake as a means of withdrawing from life itself or seeking an escape from conflicts over eating

Observe for signs of resignation or "giving up." (Note: In advanced cancer, failure to eat may be a signal that the patient is moving into the terminal phase of the illness. Since the cancer may be well-advanced at the time of the initial treatment, it is wise to be aware of this possibility.)

Explore the patient's expectations and goals in the situation. Help the patient to consider alternatives.

Evaluation

Patient or care giver response to nursing treatment may be evidenced by collecting and evaluating data in the following ways.

PATIENT

Observe pattern of weight. Obtain and evaluate food diaries to determine appetite and intake patterns.

Obtain data on status of taste and its effect on appetite.

Obtain feedback on strategies used to manage food preparation and eating, relationship with food preparer, and sense of skills and control in food-related social situations. Ascertain any elements in environment or food presentation that make eating easier or more difficult; ascertain satisfaction or dissatisfaction with any changes introduced; and collect data on responses of others.

Observe for cues indicating discouragement or negative changes in self-concept and sense of control over daily living and relationships. Note: Progress is often slow, so help patient and care giver to look for small signs of returning desire to eat.

If the patient has been hopeless or seeking a way out of the situation, seek data on any change in his or her perception and consideration of options.

CARE GIVER

Obtain feedback on planned strategies that have been attempted and the outcomes.

Obtain data on status of emotions (e.g., discouragement, endurance, sense of control, respite).

Seek data on current self-expectations in present food-related situations.

Determine status of care giver's other responsibilities and how these affect activities associated with patient's eating.

Look for patterns in food diaries.

Gather data on status of support actually being used in assisting with food preparation and care giver's comfort with it.

Living With Difficulties in Eating

During the course of the active treatment phase, one of the problems in managing daily living involves actual mechanical and pain-related difficulties in taking in, masticating, and swallowing food and liquids. While these can co-exist with and contribute to loss of desire to eat, they form a distinct problem area and require different approaches to nursing diagnosis and treatment. Side-effects of treatment are the predominant causes for difficulty in eating; however, advanced tumors of the mouth, throat, and esophagus may play a role.

Medical Perspective

The medical perspective in this phenomenon tends to be concerned with:

The observed status of the tumor and surrounding tissue

Maintaining nutrition and fluid and electrolyte balance to promote wound healing and reduce infection risks

Preventing associated complications

Determining whether the iatrogenic response requires any modification in the treatment protocol or palliation in order to permit the patient to continue in the protocol

Nursing Perspective

Nursing diagnosis and treatment is concerned with preventing and managing daily living problems associated with difficulties in eating. Areas of concern include:

Interference of eating difficulties with nutrition and hydration

Implications of increased vulnerability to infection for food preparation and mouth care

Problems of self-esteem and grieving over losses associated with deficits in eating competence

Strains on role relationships and social or work situations created by the patient's eating difficulties

Description of Difficulties in Eating

Difficulties in ingesting food and fluids during the active stage of treatment tend to involve mechanical deterrents, pain, or both.

Mechanical deterrents to eating include:

Obstruction of the passage of the bolus of food to the stomach

Inability to prevent escapement of food or fluids from the oral cavity to the outside in the process of eating or drinking

Difficulties in chewing

Difficulties in moving the bolus of food from the front of the mouth to the throat and down the esophagus

Lack of normal quantity and quality of saliva for mastication

Presence of thick ropey saliva that prevents normal preparation of the bolus of food for swallowing and is in and of itself difficult to swallow or spit out

Pain as a deterrent to eating involves:

Oral, pharyngeal, and esophageal pain of an intensity that makes masticating and swallowing of food and fluids difficult if not impossible

Loss of eating competence includes:

Changes in eating competence, and appearance and sounds while eating that can erode self-concept and disrupt former patterns of companionship at mealtimes. It may also alter the capacity to fulfill former role responsibilities that include eating with others. The patient may be grieving over the loss of former eating competence, food patterns, and eating-related relationships.

Monotony of diet involves:

Limitations in capacity to masticate and swallow that restrict both textures and kinds of foods to a narrow range, resulting in a monotonous diet that creates decreasing interest in eating

Underlying Mechanisms

Pathophysiologic and Iatrogenic Factors

Tumor-Related Factors   Oral and pharyngeal tumors tend to spread to neighboring structures and to extend into underlying structures. However, they are not usually painful in early stages, and thus do not interfere mechanically with eating until they are advanced. Difficulty in swallowing usually indicates extension of the tumor.

Neoplastic ulcer formation may cause pain that deters eating.

Surgery   Surgical treatment can create difficulties in eating in several ways, depending on the location and the nature of the surgery.

Areas of Resection/ Type of Treatment	Effect on Eating
Lips, cheeks	Food escapement Difficulty in holding food in the mouth
Mandible/maxilla	Difficulty in chewing and in holding food in the mouth
Tongue	Difficulty in moving food bolus for chewing and swallowing Loss of taste
Palate, floor of mouth	Difficulty in moving the bolus to point of swallowing Food escapement
Neck dissection	Possible removal of neck muscles and nerves associated with swallowing, leading to paralysis of the tongue, which interferes with ability to move the bolus of food for mastication and swallowing Loss of involuntary propulsion movements of the esophagus, leading to food remaining in esophagus rather than moving on to the stomach (also increasing the risk of aspiration)
Immediate postoperative trauma	Postoperative swelling of oral and throat structures Postoperative pain Excessive secretions and difficulty in swallowing or managing them

Chemotherapy	Selected antimetabolites and antitumor antibiotics may cause damage to basal layers of oral mucosa. This inhibits replacement of superficial layers and leads to ulceration (stomatitis). The pain of ulceration may preclude eating.
	There is a high risk of pain-producing oral infections with chemotherapy, due to immunosuppression and denuded membranes (e.g., candidiasis, herpes simplex), and dyspnea that does not permit normal patterns of chewing and swallowing.
Radiation	Radiation to the head and neck may produce:

Stomatitis and oropharyngeal mucositis (patchy white membranes that become confluent and can bleed if disturbed), which are painful

Dental caries, which may interfere with chewing and cause pain

Rarely, trismus (continued tonic contraction of jaw muscles), which interferes with normal opening of the mouth and chewing

Radiation of the salivary glands may produce xerostomia, which may be temporary or permanent, depending on the dosage and the extent of the glands radiated. The mouth and lips become dry, and the normal washing action of the saliva does not take place, resulting in greater risk of infection and dental caries. Dentures no longer fit tightly. Speech becomes difficult. Saliva becomes thick and ropey, making it hard to swallow or spit out; this causes gagging. Mastication of food is difficult.

Radiation of the mediastinum may cause:

Esophagitis with edema and dysphagia

Substernal pain, perhaps severe

Globus—a sensation of a "lump in the throat, only deeper" and a sensation that food "catches" in the esophagus

Daily Living Factors

Many of the same problems in daily living that were cited in the Loss of Desire to Eat section apply to difficulties in ingesting food and fluids. In reality, anorexia and mechanical or pain-related problems in eating often coexist. However, disruptions in daily living may be more severe and can involve different areas when serious mechanical problems in eating occur. Medical therapy has often changed patient appearance and created problems in the person's capacity to manage the control of food and fluids in the mouth and throat. The sights and sounds of food escaping from the mouth, the choking and gagging, or behavior to manage the food or ropey saliva can repel both the patient and any eating companions. Social isolation and damaged body image and self-concept are at risk.

The types and consistencies of foods that the patients feel they can control and swallow may be more restricted than in anorexia. Thus the problems cited in the previous section relating to the food preparer also may be more extreme.

Many of the iatrogenic, mechanical problems that disrupt eating are of limited duration. Iatrogenic effects of radiation and chemotherapy tend to decrease and disappear within weeks of discontinuation of the therapy, although xerostomia, taste changes, and dental caries can be long-lasting. Plastic surgery and repairs of surgically created defects can improve appearance and functioning, but there is a time lag of 6 to 12 months. With mechanical difficulties in eating, the demands on financial and human resources are heavy.

The acts of eating, shopping, food preparation, and socialization around eating are all affected when the person with cancer experiences mechanical difficulties or discomfort with eating. These activities involve not only the patient, but also food preparers and eating companions.

Activities in Daily Living	One or more of the following new activities may become a part of daily living. The duration (temporary or permanent) and nature of these activities will vary, depending on the kind of eating difficulties encountered and their etiology.
PATIENT	Incorporating into daily living activities to manage pain and permit the greatest degree of comfort while ingesting food
	Learning strategies to prevent escapement of food and fluids from the oral cavity
	Managing the changing fit of dental prostheses
	Learning new strategies for masticating and swallowing food with the presenting impairments

Negotiating with others (nurses, food preparers, or hostesses) for foods that are acceptable and are of a consistency and temperature that can be masticated and swallowed, given the specific eating difficulties

Managing the ropey, tenacious saliva that often cannot be swallowed, is difficult to spit out, and can cause gagging

Managing the grief work associated with temporary or permanent losses in competence and lifestyle due to eating dysfunction

Discovering and gaining skill in strategies for managing to eat with others (family, friends, and in public places) in spite of eating impairments

Developing and gaining skill in using plans and scripts for meeting difficult situations associated with eating impairments

Trying to communicate with altered oral and throat structures, edema, ulcers, dry mouth and lips, inflammation, surgical alterations, and pain

CARE GIVER OR PATIENT AS OWN FOOD PREPARER

Discovering ways of dealing satisfactorily with the need to prepare foods that tend to be visually unappealing (e.g., pureed meats and vegetables and a range of food options that is very narrow)

Developing strategies for providing the most nutritious and appealing "meals" possible under the circumstances

CARE GIVER

Developing strategies and resources for handling one's own stress and feelings in such a way as to maintain personal mental health and to promote that of the patient, given patient appearance and eating difficulties

FAMILY, COMPANIONS

Developing strategies for dealing in a satisfying manner with the patient's changed appearance and functioning during eating situations (e.g., making plans and engaging in behavior that are acceptable to all and that do not add to the patient's stress, loss of self-esteem, loneliness, or loss of will to live)

Events in Daily Living

Events in daily living associated with eating difficulties include:

First awareness of the reality of eating impairments or subsequent episodes of exacerbation

Success in overcoming one or more eating difficulties, or failure in an attempt to manage eating difficulties in a particular situation

Realization that eating difficulties are abating or that they are becoming a chronic problem

Demands in Daily Living

The following are possible expectations or demands that may present with the problem of eating difficulties.

Self-expectations

Expectations of how one is to appear or sound in the process of eating

Expectations regarding self-care in management of eating difficulties or ropey saliva

Level of competence expected in self-care involving tube feedings, use of blenders, hyperalimentation, and related technical equipment

Expectations about experiencing pain and its control

Role expectations regarding participation in eating with family members and others

Expectations regarding maintaining former role obligations associated with food procurement and preparation

Others'
Expectations
CARE GIVER

Status of expectations regarding the obligation of the patient to consume food based on previous patterns or prescribed diet

Possible perception that patient failure to eat or to "try hard to eat" regardless of the discomfort or dysfunction represents "failure" on the part of the care giver

FAMILY

Status of expectations that patient will continue previous role functions as food preparer

EATING
COMPANIONS

Possible expectations that the patient "would know enough" to restrict his appearances during shared meals if his dysfunction or eating management strategies are offensive to others

Environment
for Daily
Living

Environmental factors that will affect management of difficulties in eating include:

Options for privacy while learning how to manage the new difficulties in eating (in the hospital, at home)

Options for socialization during the nonthreatening, nonembarrassing aspects of eating

Availability of "safe" environments in which to practice one's skills of eating in public facilities or in social situations

Access to needed adaptive devices, supplies, and equipment

Values and
Beliefs

A variety of values and beliefs can affect patient and family responses when patient eating difficulties occur. These include:

Ingrained values regarding acceptable and unacceptable eating behavior as they have impact on the presenting situation

The degree of deviance from these established standards that is tolerable

The nature of sanctioning behavior in the presenting situation

The degree of acceptability of allowing the person to be in the sick role and the duration of the sick role that is acceptable, given the specific forms of medical treatment

- The belief that the patient is obliged to try to get better (eat) as an aspect of the acceptable sick role, and the behavior others engage in to support this belief

Beliefs about acceptable levels of pain and pain control

Ethnic beliefs related to the need to create a balance between the "hot" and "cold" effects on the body of the pathology, treatment, and diet (Harwood, 1971). Note that the concept of hot and cold may involve different words or ideations in various ethnic groups, but the concept of taking action—for example, adjustment of the diet to maintain balance between these forces—remains central in many major ethnic groups (e.g., Asians, Hispanics, Indians, and Middle Easterners).

Beliefs about what constitutes food, including texture (e.g., the "meat and potatoes person" who does not see pureed or finely ground meat as constituting food because of the change in texture)

Previous values associated with eating a low cholesterol and low fat diet and conflict with a concentrated high calorie diet containing high fat

Values related to vitamin supplementation

Beliefs that food is medicine—part of the healing prescription that permits the patient to participate in the treatment of his cancer

Functional Health Status

Several areas of functional capacity are involved in managing the requirements of daily living with physically impaired eating ability. They include physical strength and endurance, motivation, cognition, emotional responses, and communication ability.

Strength   Strength is involved in the ability to chew and swallow. These tasks are affected by disruption in bone, muscle, and nerve function and pain.

Endurance   Endurance is a consideration in the length of time and the consistency of food one is able to chew and swallow in the face of dyspnea, pain, muscle weakness, difficulty in moving food to the throat, or xerostomia.

Motivation   Motivation is characterized by the status of willingness to keep on trying, use new strategies, and try different foods, different quantities, different eating environments, or different adaptive devices.

Cognition	Cognition affects:

The capacity to understand how the particular treatment produces the side-effects of eating difficulties; what the patterns of emergence, abatement, or chronicity of symptoms are; and what the disabilities and structural changes are in the course of treatment, and the capacity to incorporate this understanding into plans for managing daily living to cope with the dysfunction and maintain nutrition

The ability to perceive applicability of adaptations and equipment that are available to manage specific presenting eating difficulties and lifestyle

The capacity to develop a repertoire of behaviors and scripts to manage encounters with others involving one's eating difficulties

Emotions	Patient, care givers, and family will have emotional responses to the current eating difficulties and the projected course of events.
Communication	Iatrogenic or tumor-based speech dysfunction and limitations in expression may hinder communication about the nature of the experience and the problems in daily living associated with the eating difficulties.

Nursing Diagnosis and Treatment

Nursing diagnosis and treatment of mechanical eating difficulties during the active treatment stage concern themselves primarily with the specific barriers to effective eating and nutrition. Another focus is the impact altered eating behavior has on the psychosocial aspects of daily living.

Prevention

The specific mechanical difficulties in eating that are associated with the various forms of treatment tend to be predictable, although patients having the same treatment can vary widely in the amount of dysfunction encountered. Nursing's perspective in prevention is to prevent, minimize, or delay high-risk problems in daily living that result from pathologic or iatrogenic dysfunctions.

In the process of giving informed consent, the patient and family have usually been introduced to information about the side-effects of the treatment. Nurses can at this point indicate that there are adaptive equipment and strategies to help in managing the dysfunction and the problems in daily living. However, patient and family anxiety regarding the threat inherent in the diagnosis of cancer and its treatment often makes it impossible for them to take in information at this time. Further, talking about the dysfunction rarely prepares the person for the actuality. On the other hand, some patients never experience expected dysfunctions.

Based on a patient–family data base collected in the pretreatment period, nurses can make tentative diagnoses regarding issues in daily living associated with mechanical eating problems that are likely to be difficult for them to manage. They then can assess the status of internal and external resources for managing the anticipated problem areas.

Nursing treatment to anticipate and minimize the difficulties in daily living for both the patient and the care givers begins as soon as the patient and care giver are emotionally and physically able to participate. The participation may be passive initially, as the nurse provides the care and information. However, given the short hospital stays, active participation in learning the specifics of problem prevention and management in daily living in the face of the presenting dysfunctions and health care requirements must be begun at an early stage. Preparing patients and care givers for what to expect tends not to result in their experiencing additional symptoms, but rather to give a greater sense of control. Consider two examples:

> Patients can learn that effective and regular oral hygiene can reduce the risks of oral infections and the additional pain and eating difficulties infections bring. This can give a sense of control over some aspect of daily living when so much seems to be out of their control.

> Care givers can learn that it is not uncommon for food preparers to experience frustration and possibly anger or guilt in the course of trying to promote good nutrition for the patient on a day-to-day basis. The nurse can then identify strategies or resources for managing these experiences.

Advance preparation can provide a sense of normalcy or legitimacy for the potential experiences as well as knowledge of strategies for managing them.

Prevention associated with mechanical or pain-related eating difficulties involves the nurse in helping patients, care givers, and meal companions to become aware of the challenges that the specific dysfunctions can pose in their particular patterns of daily living. The treatment plan involves the offering of options and resources to minimize or manage the difficulties. Many of the problems identified in the following section under Diagnostic Areas and Treatment Guidelines can be considered prospectively rather than waiting for the problem to arise.

Diagnostic Targets	With eating difficulties the targets for diagnosis include the patient, care givers (those who prepare and serve the food or who are concerned with nutritional intake, including nurses, dietitians, and physicians), and companions who share eating experiences.

Risk Factors
PATIENT

Persons at greater risk for not managing daily living effectively are those who:

Live alone and have no one to:

Assist in swallowing emergencies

Procure and prepare food

Help in developing better eating strategies

Share in failures and successes

Are easily discouraged by adversity and who give up

Receive aggressive medical therapy that particularly disrupts the oral cavity, throat, and esophagus

Wear dentures

Have limited resources for obtaining food supplements and adaptive equipment

Do not discontinue their use of tobacco and alcohol (both cause irritation and dryness to mucous membranes)

Are accustomed to a diet that includes "hot" spices (curry, chili powder), hot peppers, tart fruits, or coarse foods (whole grains, raw vegetables, potato chips)

Are mouth breathers

Have care givers that:

Lack time, interest, knowledge, or skill in using the technology, or lack patience

Equate their own success with the patient's eating according to care giver expectations

Are unable to understand the mechanisms of patient eating difficulties or the relationship of symptoms associated with the treatment. (Care givers and companions with this characteristic are also at greater risk.)

CARE GIVER

Care givers at greater risk for not managing daily living effectively are those who:

Have health or emotional problems of their own in addition to the care giving responsibilities

Lack their own support system to allow them to debrief, explore options, and experience respite

Are highly anxious and frightened by the appearance and dysfunction of the patient or their perception of the patient's prognosis

Diagnostic Areas
PATIENT

Reluctance or refusal to eat R/T:

Anticipation of pain; oral, pharyngeal, or esophageal dysphagia; choking; or other difficulty in eating

Unsuccessful past attempts to manage choking, escapement of food, swallowing, or pain

Ongoing oral tissue trauma R/T difficulty in avoiding cigarettes, alcohol, spicy foods, or substances that irritate the mucous membranes

Difficulties in coordinating chewing and swallowing with breathing R/T severe dyspnea

Reduced food intake or "giving up" R/T difficulties in eating associated with xerostomia, denervation, pain, stomatitis, esophagitis, alteration in musculoskeletal structures, ulcerations, or edema

Ineffective management of (specified) eating impairment(s) R/T lack of understanding of the particular mechanical difficulty

Reduced eating R/T boredom with the monotony of the food options

Chewing difficulties and potential for infection R/T ill-fitting dentures

Reduced food and fluid ingestion in the presence of oral, pharyngeal, or esophageal pain R/T:

Lack of knowledge about effective use of analgesia

Belief system negating pain relief

Grief R/T loss of:

Preferred meals and foods

Normal eating competence and behavior

Being able to eat with others

Being able to eat in public

Reduced self-esteem R/T manifestations of own or others' distaste at perceived eating difficulties

Ineffective management of eating R/T lack of:

Availability of equipment

Skills in using equipment

Money or insurance coverage to obtain equipment

Difficulty in managing social eating situations R/T failure to develop adaptive strategies that are usable or acceptable in social situations

Social isolation (of patient or companions) R/T unwillingness to be seen by others in eating situations

CARE GIVER   Depression R/T lack of positive feedback in the form of patient success in eating or being thanked for food preparation efforts

Frustration R/T the narrow range of foods the patient will accept and eating patterns the patient will tolerate

Anxiety or frustration R/T sense of inability to control the course of events and outcomes in eating activities

Manifestations   *Signs and symptoms of mechanical impairments*

PATIENT   Complaints of oral, pharyngeal, or substernal pain

Dyspnea and increased respiratory rate severe enough to interfere with normal chewing and swallowing

Edematous mouth or lips

Oral, labial, pharyngeal, or esophageal ulcerations

Signs of oral or labial infections

Discontinuation of wearing dentures or dental prostheses

Decreased clarity in enunciation

Dry, cracked lips, dry-appearing mouth

Mouth breathing

Gagging or choking (observed or reported)

Escapement of food and fluids from mouth

Grimacing or unusual muscular effort during swallowing

A greater than 10-second delay in rising of the cricoid cartilage after food or liquid is taken into the mouth

Signs and symptoms of difficulties in managing daily living with mechanical eating difficulties

Refusal to try to eat

Taking one or two bites and giving up

Pattern of postponing eating

Ineffective use of analgesia in relation to eating

Report of ineffective pain control

Narrowing of range of foods or fluids ingested or limiting of consistency of food ingested

Nonuse of adaptive devices

Reported lack of success in use of adaptive strategies to control dysfunctions

Weight loss, dehydration

Reported discouragement: "If only I had known, I never would have started the treatment."

Missing of treatment appointments or discontinuation of the treatment

Increasing social isolation, apathy, depression

CARE GIVER See Manifestations in section on Loss of Desire to Eat

Prognostic Poor prognosis is associated with:
Variables

The severity and duration of symptoms and dysfunction

Depression

Lack of success in managing eating dysfunctions

Loss of cherished social activities

Loss of self-esteem

Deficits in external resources and personal support systems

A care giver who has difficulty accepting the changes in the person's eating ability

A care giver who is perceived by the patient to nag about eating or be oversolicitous

Lack of knowledge and skills in managing eating difficulties on the part of either patient or care giver

Complications
PATIENT

Failure to manage daily living with difficulties in eating can result in:

Giving up on trying to eat or to manage daily living with the dysfunction

Malnutrition, fluid and electrolyte imbalance

Infection

Pain

Social isolation

Depression

CARE GIVER

Failure to manage daily living effectively for care givers can result in:

Discouragement and burnout

Social isolation

Overcompensating in care giving efforts related to the sense of helplessness to change the patient's situation

Overemphasis on food and eating, creating a patient back-lash and increased resistance to eating

Treatment Guidelines
PATIENT

Reluctance to try to eat R/T anticipation or experience of specific problems, dysfunctions, or discomfort associated with eating

Pain

Arrange for medical orders for analgesia at a level and frequency option that controls pain associated with eating attempts and using a route that is compatible with the swallowing dysfunction (e.g., rectal suppositories, local anesthetics). If nausea occurs as a result of narcotic analgesics, obtain an order for an antiemetic drug.

Give medications or teach patient or family to schedule medications so that peak action occurs at time of eating.

For pain related to stomatitis and mucositis, use one of the available medications containing a local anesthetic, an antacid, and an antihistamine to coat, soothe, and relieve. Offer 5 to 10 ml of the mixture and instruct the patient to swish it around the mouth, holding it in the mouth for a few minutes before spitting it out. Use ad lib unless the patient shows a pattern of swallowing the rinse; if so, discontinue its use. Before meals, apply with cotton-tipped applicator to oral areas, avoiding the tongue (to minimize loss of taste) (Goodman and Stoner, 1985).

Maintain oral hygiene:

Prestomatitis: Schedule oral care before and after meals and at bedtime. Proper care involves gentle tooth brushing with a soft toothbrush (e.g., Oral B, Sulcus, or Right Kind) using a fluoridated type of toothpaste, and gentle flossing with unwaxed dental floss. Rinsing or irrigating the mouth at least four times per day with a solution of ½ teaspoon of baking soda and ¼ teaspoon of salt in 1 pint of water will not only cleanse, but will raise the pH level and help to prevent overgrowth of aciduric organisms, particularly *Candida albicans* (Bersani and Carl, 1983; Carl, 1983). Instruct the patient not to use a water pick unless it has been regularly used previously. If used, the pressure should be low and the stream directed horizontally to avoid lacerating the mucosa and floor of the mouth (Carl, 1983). Water-soluble gel should be put on the lips after oral care.

If stomatitis occurs: Schedule oral care every 2 hours during the day and every 6 hours at night (Dauffler, 1981; Strohl, 1985). Apply cold to the painful area for a short time before attempting to eat (e.g., suck ice chips, apply ice pack to throat). Suggest use of antacids, milk, or milk products (e.g., yogurt, sour cream, cottage cheese) to promote coating and comfort—unless mucus is copious. Adjust temperature of food to cause the least discomfort (usually a tepid temperature is more comfortable than hot or cold). Avoid spicy, tart, salty, or briny foods. Prepare the food in a consistency that causes the least discomfort and trauma in mastication and swallowing.

Escapement of food or fluid from the mouth

Instruct the patient to do the following:

Experiment with the use of cups with longer spouts (for lip resections) and use long-handled spoons to place the food well back in the mouth and on the opposite side from the defect.

Use scrupulously clean aseptic syringes or "basters" to place fluids in the back of the mouth. Introduce fluids *slowly* in small amounts—no faster than can be swallowed (to prevent aspiration).

Tilt the head away from the area of leakage.

Place the hand not being used in feeding over the area of escapement to support it and minimize leakage.

Difficulty in chewing

Discuss with the patient the foods he enjoys that are in the liquid or "soft" category (e.g., well-cooked vegetables and fruits, pasta, mashed potatoes, pudding, ice cream, and fish, poultry, and meats that are finely ground and well cooked). Propose use of a blender if even soft foods cannot be managed. Help patient and food provider to explore how they can adapt their preferred or usual menus to the currently required textures, and discuss the best ways to fit the adapted dishes into patient and family eating patterns. Identify ways to present food and liquids attractively, using attractive small glasses, bowls, or plates, and variations in presentation as well as in food flavors and colors.

Dentures or dental prostheses that don't fit

Remind patient that dentures may no longer fit as tissues in the mouth are affected by treatment.

Strongly recommend a dental visit before treatment. If fit becomes a problem, recommend a dental visit to get a relining of dentures or adjustment of partials. If finances or transportation are problems, seek resources for patient.

If it is not possible to get a good fit with the dentures, recommend that the patient wear them only when eating and modify the diet to minimize gum trauma.

Ropey saliva

Ropey saliva is usually a problem that is resolved before the patient leaves institutional care. Suctioning the patient and teaching him how to suction himself is the usual method of control. A salt and baking soda mouthwash is helpful in dissolving the viscous mucus that makes swallowing difficult (Bersani and Carl, 1983).

Dry mouth (xerostomia)—may be temporary or permanent

Recommend frequent sips of water during day and night to keep mouth moist while oral tissues are too sensitive for artificial saliva.

When oral tissues tolerate it, recommend use of artificial saliva in spray form (e.g., Moi-Stir, Salivart, Ora-lub) (Bersani and Carl, 1983). Its effect is transient, so it needs to be used frequently.

Recommend careful oral hygiene before and after meals: rinse with saline–bicarbonate solution, floss, then brush.

Instruct patient to avoid smoking and alcohol because they dry as well as irritate the mouth.

Difficulty in moving bolus of food to back of throat for swallowing

Instruct patient to:

Use thinly pureed foods.

Place the food in the back of the mouth with a long-handled spoon or a catheter-tipped syringe or baster.

Recline upper body to 45 degrees. Allow gravity to move the food. Do not hyperextend the neck (McNally, 1982).

Choking (indication of food or fluid entering trachea)

Work to prevent choking episodes that in turn may create high anxiety and less control over eating skills.

Show diagrams and describe to the patient the phases of swallowing and those activities that the patient can control. Encourage the patient to ask questions during teaching and later when he has had time to think and to practice.

Swallowing sequence: The entire tongue is lifted as the bolus of food moves toward the soft palate, then the base of tongue is elevated. The food then enters the pharynx. The *larynx is elevated against the base of the tongue* (this is the most important mechanism for preventing aspiration), the vocal cords close, and the base of the tongue is forced against the posterior pharyngeal wall. The contraction of pharyngeal constrictors creates a stripping wave to empty the pharynx (Goodman, 1987).

Help the patient build up swallowing skills and strategies while the feeding tube is still in place. Use the following sequence: ice chips, then nectar, then Jello.

Instruct patient to (1) inhale, (2) place small amount of food in mouth, (3) swallow, (4) exhale and cough as needed, and (5) wait a short time before taking the next bite (Grady et al, 1985).

Remind the patient to cut solid foods into small portions and to take small sips of liquids.

Encourage the patient to concentrate on the act of swallowing—not to take it for granted as an automatic process. Note that this need to concentrate can affect conversation. Conversation that is distracting may make it more difficult to concentrate on voluntary swallowing (Axelsson et al, 1989).

See section on dry mouth for suggestions on eating with inadequate saliva, as it contributes to swallowing difficulties.

Esophageal edema and inflammation

See the Treatment Guidelines for Pain, above. Note that analgesic mouthwash would need to be swallowed to provide relief of esophageal pain.

Advise use of high-calorie, high-protein, high-carbohydrate liquids or soft food (e.g., milkshakes, or commercial liquid supplements). Other foods can also be used when put in the blender if swallowing thicker substances is possible. Strain particles out of liquids (e.g., soups) if these are felt to "catch" or "stick" in the esophagus.

Reassure the patient and care giver that the dysfunction and discomfort will abate within a few days to a few weeks of the completion of radiation therapy.

Arrange for medications to be given in liquid or suppository form rather than in tablets.

Ineffective food preparation

Instruct patient and care giver to:

Use favorite foods, but prepare them in a manner to make them *softer and moister* (e.g., by cooking with water or broth, or using gravies, sauces, soups, or fruit juices).

Use a blender or food processor. If the food is to be cooked, blend after cooking for better flavor.

Choose soft foods such as mashed potatoes (made a little moister than usual), yogurt, custards, cottage cheese, gelatins, pasta (well cooked), and creamy cereals.

Soak and soften dry foods (e.g., toast, dry cereals, cookies) in coffee, tea, milk, or cocoa.

Avoid tart, acidic, or salty foods (e.g., substitute fruit nectar for orange juice).

Avoid "hot" spices; try using more delicate herbs instead.

Adjust food temperature for comfort. Patients who find cold foods soothing may want to add ice or ice cream to milk or make milkshakes; make and chill high-calorie, high-protein drinks; use frozen yogurt or ice cream; and chill watermelon or other melons. For patients who find tepid foods more comfortable, liquids should be brought to room temperature and foods normally served hot should be heated only to tepid. It is important to refrigerate foods appropriately and to bring them to the desired temperature just before eating rather than to allow them to sit at room temperature.

Seek as much variety as possible among acceptable foods, in type, texture, and appearance (e.g., try various types of melons; different flavorings can be used in high-calorie drinks; vegetables, chicken, shellfish, and other fish can be used in cream soups; sauces can be varied with different seasonings and herbs).

Eat several small meals rather than fewer large meals.

Sip on fluids (cold or lukewarm) frequently to maintain hydration and keep the mouth comfortable.

Reluctance to try to eat R/T previously unsuccessful attempts

Gather data on specific problems associated with unsuccessful eating experiences.

Propose other adaptive devices or strategies to minimize dysfunction or discomfort (see above).

Actually go through the eating task with the patient (and care giver, if this is appropriate), using the suggested equipment or approaches to test their effectiveness for this patient and to give added suggestions and support.

Check back by phone to determine what subsequent eating experiences were.

Grief R/T loss of eating competence, preferred foods, social or business encounters involving eating

Determine the nature of the specific loss(es) this patient is experiencing. Make a clinical judgment as to the anticipated duration of the losses.

With long-term deficits, determine the degree to which the patient can find satisfying goals related to eating that are less than a total restitution of previous lifestyle and skills.

If the duration of the dysfunction is limited, emphasize the time-limited nature of the loss (e.g., by marking days off on a calendar).

Indicate the normalcy of the grief being experienced and the legitimacy of grieving behavior: "Of course you are angry (or depressed)—you've had a big loss." Point out that awareness of the normalcy of grief and its stages does not permit escape or minimize the suffering associated with it.

Where losses in eating competence or preferred foods can be improved, offer assistance or resources when the person is able and willing to try them.

Explore the nature of social encounters that are lost or avoided and discuss possibly acceptable alternatives.

Can the person manage to eat dessert in a group setting?

Are there foods that cause less problems, so that a menu could be developed that is "safe"?

When new skills of eating have been learned, accompany patient to a "safe"area in the hospital cafeteria or other public place to try out public eating.

Help the patient develop plans and scripts for setting the stage for eating with others or for dealing with any problems that may arise. These should include preparing others for the patient's eating difficulties and offering options (e.g., "I'd like very much to come over for dinner, if you don't mind my bringing my own food—I'm still having difficulty swallowing, so I'm rather limited" or "My eating still isn't very skillful; you may want to wait till I get better at it" or "I couldn't manage a whole meal out, but I'd like very much to join you for dessert" or "My breathing tube (tracheostomy) still makes some noises and I do have to cough at times. I may have to leave the table occasionally so that I won't bother the others. If this is all right with you, I'd enjoy coming.") Some scripts should be developed for the occurrence of sights and sounds that are not usual during social situations (e.g., the sounds or odors from an ostomy, difficulty with food leakage).

Teach the person how to order "safe" foods from a menu or a cafeteria selection, then rehearse. It may be possible to have a supply of typical menus for different types of restaurants available on the unit or in the clinic for this teaching experience.

Explore with the patient who among family and friends are low risk for early practice at eating with others.

Make arrangements for feedback after experiences. Be generous and genuine with praise. Accept difficult experiences as unfortunate, but not unexpected. Diagnose the exact difficulties and help the patient develop alternative strategies and scripts.

Loss of self-esteem related to eating competence and altered options for eating companionship

Model acceptance of the patient. Find accomplishments or aspects of the person that are genuinely praiseworthy and be both specific and generous in offering praise. Do not become "professionally busy" in the presence of the patient—make necessary activities secondary to relating to the patient. Make contacts with the patient even when no signal or task would make them necessary.

Gather data on situations the patient will face in which there are risks of being stared at or avoided. Work through strategies that the patient feels will enable him to manage with some degree of comfort or control.

Give examples of scripts that can be used (e.g., the "advanced warning script": "I'd like to accept that cup of coffee, but I have to warn you that I do make slurping noises when I drink these days." Ask the patient to modify the scripts so that they are personally usable and comfortable. Ask the patient to give samples of others that might be needed and the situations where they might prove useful.

Teach patient to negotiate with prospective meal companion or host about what to expect in terms of what can be eaten and appearance or sounds to anticipate. The patient determines whether this is acceptable, and if so what strategies would be most comfortable for hosts and guests. (See previous section under treatment strategies for grief regarding eating loss for additional examples.) Ask patient to give other situations and options for action. Make specific arrangements for feedback after experiences (e.g., telephone contact, next visit).

Acknowledge and reinforce specifically areas you see that are going well. Help the patient to "process" the situations that did not go well.

Suggest that the patient identify one representative among his meal or social companions who could assume responsibility for preparing others to accept the patient's eating difficulties. Ask the patient to identify to this person the nature and pattern of the difficulties; explore the anticipated responses of eating and social companions; identify alternative responses that are both feasible for them and are most likely to be helpful to the patient at varying stages of the dysfunction; and request companions to use these responses.

Lack of equipment

Provide the patient (and care provider, if needed) with opportunities in the hospital and clinics to gain skill in using the equipment that will be used later in the home (e.g., long-handled spoons, cups with spouts, syringes with or without tubing, drinking straws, feeding tubes, enteral nutrition formula bags, pumps, obdurators). Make specific arrangements for linkage to telephone or personal support system if problems or questions arise at home.

Determine the patient's resources for obtaining the needed equipment. Mobilize resources to make equipment available if there is a resource deficit.

Gather data on environmental factors that will affect the use of the equipment in the noninstitutional settings and plan with the patient how to function effectively within those environments.

Arrange for specific feedback sessions in which patient can discuss experiences and issues in daily living with the equipment.

CARE GIVER   *Dissatisfaction with the lack of any positive feedback from the situation*

Talk over status of:

Patient's limitations in giving positive feedback (e.g., egocentricity during illness and suffering, the body's energy conservation mechanisms and the priority for self-healing, patient anxiety and discomfort)

Patient's strengths or resources for giving positive feedback (e.g., past patterns, warmth of relationship, possibility that patient might be willing to offer more positive cues or words of appreciation to the care giver if it were suggested)

Explore the importance of setting *small* goals.

Identify the normalcy and legitimacy of the feelings the care giver is experiencing and some of the "safe" options for discharging them.

Arrange for opportunities for the care giver(s) to debrief on their experiences and reactions and seek new options (e.g., have they tried sharing their feelings with the person who is ill in order to gain comfort from the commonality of suffering?).

Identify and arrange for opportunities for contacts with other care providers who have gone through similar experiences.

Sense of loss of control over patient situation and personal daily living

Help the care giver anticipate that there may be times when feelings of helplessness arise, and assure person that many care givers experience this.

Explore areas in which care giver does and does not have control. Ascertain the level of control in each that would offer an acceptable degree of satisfaction and comfort to the care giver.

Consider strategies for taking control in areas that are accessible, or creating a sense of control. Show the care giver how to *reframe* the situation by looking at the patient's problem as a basis for the behavioral symptoms the patient is presenting rather than only looking at the symptoms. This sometimes gives a sense of control over what cannot be changed or offers insight into the possible sequence of symptoms. For example, the patient is grieving over the unexpected severity of the difficulty in eating and is expressing that grief with anger and depression. Instead of focusing on the angry behavior as a personal attack, suggest that it be seen as an expected symptom, just as the coughing is a symptom of secretions in the bronchi. Help the care giver plan behavioral responses and scripts to use in the most troublesome areas.

Suggest participation in cancer family support groups. Offer to be available to receive feedback and give further ideas as needed. Be generous and genuine in giving specific praise when care giver has managed the situations to reduce feelings of frustration.

Discouragement and feeling of wanting to give up

Discuss the need for the care giver to maintain physical and emotional endurance in order to continue to give patient care in a situation that may be slow to change.

Suggest that care giver arrange for respite periods away from the home and the patient. These should be regularly scheduled and of long enough duration to give some genuine respite.

Explore with the patient and care giver the development of a schedule of surrogate care givers (family, friends, or home health care personnel) who will offer security and peace of mind to both patient and care giver during the regular care giver's absence.

If needed, help the care giver plan for the most satisfying and effective use of respite periods. One option during this time is participation in a support group meeting.

Address the issue of preventing or minimizing any guilt feelings that the care giver might have about enjoying himself or herself while the patient is suffering. Remind the care giver that the patient is dependent on the care giver's physical and emotional strength and well-being, so that maintaining that well-being is crucial to the patient. Explore what would happen to the patient if the care giver "burned out" and became unable to give the needed care.

Arrange for feedback on respite experiences and the status of care giver's feelings of renewal.

Frustration with the monotony of preparing the same foods in the same way day after day

Ask care giver to identify foods, textures, and food temperatures the patient will accept, then explore other foods with similar tastes, textures, temperatures, and seasonings that might be tried.

Review patient's possible fear of producing additional discomfort or lack of success in eating to prepare care giver for possible patient reluctance to accept deviations from current diet and eating patterns.

Work out scripts that the care giver can use that encourage but do not appear to "nag" (e.g., "You've had pretty good success with (name the food). I've made some (name the food) that is almost the same, but would give you a little variety. You could try a small bite to see how it goes for you, and if it feels OK you can try a bit more.")

Evaluation   Nursing treatment can be evaluated in terms of the following factors.

Patient   Status of success in preventing food escapement and in chewing and swallowing

Status of comfort in eating

Status of actual social interaction versus that desired

Degree of satisfaction with adjustments and adaptations in daily living

Status of availability and effectiveness in using adaptive equipment

CARE GIVER   Status of care giver's stresses and resources for providing acceptable food and positive eating experiences to the patient

Status of care giver's respite schedule and activities

COMPANIONS   Status of family's and companions' responses to the patient in eating situations and their satisfactions and dissatisfactions

---

Living With Nausea, Vomiting, and Retching

Nausea, vomiting, and retching, separately or together, occur in individuals with some forms of cancer. They are also common at various times in many of the cancer therapies. These body responses, together with associated emotional distress, affect daily living. For some people nausea or vomiting causes daily living to become totally disrupted. Others are able to take some initiative to try to control or work around the symptoms and manage daily living in a reasonably acceptable form in spite of the symptoms.

Medical Perspective

Medicine looks on nausea and vomiting as pathophysiologic responses accompanying certain tumors and tumor locations and as unavoidable side-effects in some forms of therapy. Medical treatment involves prescribing antiemetics and sedation to reduce symptom occurrence or emotional distress, and managing any associated nutritional deficits or fluid and electrolyte imbalances.

Nursing Perspective

Nursing's perspective addresses the prevention or minimizing of nausea and vomiting through alterations in approaches to daily living. It also involves helping the patient and family members to manage the requirements of daily living as effectively and comfortably as possible where nausea, vomiting, retching and associated emotional distress are present.

Description of Nausea, Vomiting, and Retching

While nausea, vomiting, and retching often occur together, each can occur in distinctive patterns in the cancer experience (Rhodes et al, 1985; Rhodes et al, 1987). The emotional distress an individual experiences in the presence of nausea and vomiting can be congruent or at variance with the actual symptom occurrence (i.e., minimal symptoms can produce great emotional response, or modest emotional responses may accompany intense symptoms) (Rhodes et al, 1987). Nausea and vomiting can occur as physiologic responses to tumor or treatment, but may also appear as conditioned responses, as in anticipatory nausea and vomiting (Duigon, 1986).

Nausea is a vague but distinctly disagreeable queasy feeling in the stomach and a tightening sensation in the throat accompanied by a strong revulsion toward food and eating. It is usually preceded by anorexia. The anorectic person can become frankly nauseated when confronted with food. Nausea, like anorexia, is accompanied by decreased gastric motility. It may also be accompanied by signs of diffuse autonomic activity, including profuse watery salivation, sweating, and increased heart rate. Acid secretion in the stomach is decreased, so food remains undigested and fails to move on to the duodenum (Blacklow, 1983).

Vomiting is a sudden, powerful oral expulsion of stomach contents. It is usually, but not always, accompanied by nausea. The "true" or integrative vomiting center, in the medulla, is located near and linked to the chemoreceptor trigger zone. Input may come directly to the integrative vomiting center from the vestibular system, a peripheral system made up of the pharynx and gastrointestinal tract, and from higher cortical and brain stem structures (Billings, 1985). The chemoreceptor trigger zone can be stimulated by various agents, including certain toxic chemicals. It, in turn, transmits impulses to the vomiting center, with the resultant vomiting.

Vomiting has a psychosocial component. It is considered repulsive in many societies, to the point that seeing a person vomiting may cause the observer to gag or actually vomit. Vomiting and retching also represent a loss of control over body functions, and thus can create increased anxiety (Norris, 1982).

Retching is the violent, spasmodic movement of respiratory muscles of the chest wall and the diaphragm, accompanied by opposing expiratory contractions of the abdominal muscles and a closing of the mouth and glottis. The heart rate slows and respirations cease during the act of retching. Retching precedes vomiting, but it may also occur without any expulsion of stomach contents; this is known as "dry heaves." Painful soreness of chest and abdominal muscles, lasting for several days, occurs with the repeated severe retching experienced in some forms of chemotherapy with high emetic activity.

Underlying Mechanisms

Pathophysiologic and Iatrogenic Factors

Tumors themselves, systemic neoplastic effects (e.g., hypercalcemia), and many forms of cancer therapy can produce nausea or vomiting. However, the responses can vary. Given the same treatment, some patients will vomit, while others will not (Rhodes et al, 1986). Both physiologic and psychologic factors can play a role.

Tumor-Related Factors	Certain tumors tend to cause nausea and vomiting. These include brain tumors, meningeal carcinomatosis, advanced stage gastric tumors, late stage liver tumors, obstructing intestinal tumors, and those causing hypercalcemia (e.g., parathyroid, lung, kidney, ovary, and colon tumors and metastatic breast tumors).

Surgery   Vomiting may occur in the immediate postoperative period associated with the nature of the surgical procedure itself (e.g., gastric surgery or adrenal insufficiency related to adrenalectomy).

Anesthetic agents and other medications given in the perioperative period may contribute to nausea and vomiting.

Narcotic analgesia can cause nausea and vomiting through either direct vestibular effect or effect on the chemoreceptor trigger zone.

Chemotherapy   Many of the antineoplastic drugs have an emetic side-effect, although individual patients vary in their emetic responses. See Table 6-1 for a listing of some antineoplastic drugs, the strength of their emetic properties, and onset and duration of effect. Chemical stimuli reach the chemoreceptor trigger zone through the blood and spinal fluid. The exact mechanism is not known, but it may be by direct action of the drug, production of other substances such as intermediate metabolites from tissue damage, or stimulation of activity of neurotransmitters such as dopamine and acetylcholine (Harris, 1982; Kennedy et al, 1981). Sources of stimuli directly to the integrative vomiting center from chemotherapy include gastrointestinal irritation and distention.

Radiation   Radiation directed to the whole abdomen or portions of it, large pelvic fields, the hypochondrium, epigastrium, or para-aortic areas will create some degree of nausea and vomiting. Dosage is also a factor. Whole brain irradiation or wide mediastinal fields may cause some degree of nausea. In the gastrointestinal tract the mucous membranes and glandular tissues swell, causing partial obstruction of the ducts. Secretions in the involved organs are inhibited due to damage to the acini (Hilderly, 1987). Such changes contribute to nausea and vomiting.

Psychologic Factors

Brain stem and higher cortical centers can influence nausea, vomiting, and retching. Preoperative anxiety has been linked to postoperative vomiting (Dumas and Leonard, 1963). Overall attitude or morale can affect nausea in cisplatin therapy (Ash, 1981). Trait anxiety (usual levels of anxiety) has been linked to post-chemotherapy retching. State anxiety (anxiety associated with a presenting situation) following the second and third cycles of chemotherapy has been linked to increased vomiting (Rhodes et al, 1986).

Anticipatory nausea and vomiting is a conditioned response in which the sights (e.g. needles, the building, room, nurses, or doctors), smells (e.g., rubbing alcohol), or sounds (e.g., the nurse's voice on the telephone) associated with the chemotherapy experience evoke responses of gagging, nausea, or vomiting. Recall of previous chemotherapy or anticipation of the next cycle can also produce anticipatory nausea and vomiting (Duigon, 1986).

Table 6-1. Chemotherapy-Induced Nausea and Vomiting*

Drug	Incidence	Onset†	Severity	Duration (hours)
Amsacrine	Low		Mild	
Asparaginase	30%–60%		Mild	
Azactidine	30%–60%	1.5–3	Moderate	
Bleomycin sulfate	10%–30%		Mild	12
Carmustine	60%–90%	2–6	Severe	4–24
Chlorambucil (Leukeran)	Low		Mild	
Chlorozotocin			Mild	
Cisplatin	90%	1	Severe	24+
Cyclophosphamide (Cytoxan)	60%–90%	4–6	Moderate	8–10
Cytarabine	10%–30% 90% (high dose)		Moderate	
Dacarbazine (DTIC-Dome)	90%	1–3	Severe	24–48
Dactinomycin (Cosmegen)	60%–90%		Severe	
Daunorubicin hydrochloride	Common		Moderate–severe	
Doxorubicin (Adriamycin RDF)	30%–60%		Mild–moderate	12
Etoposide	10%–30%	2–6	Mild	
Floxuridine (FUDR)			Mild	
Fluorouracil	30%–60%		Mild	
Hexamethylmelamine	30%–60%		Moderate	
Hydroxyurea (Hydrea)	10%–30%		Mild	
Mechlorethamine hydrochloride (Mustargen)	90%	1–3	Severe	8
Melphalan (Alkeran)			Mild	
Methotrexate sodium injection (Mexate)	10%–30% 60%–90% (high dose)		Mild	12
Mitomycin (Mutamycin)	30%–60%	1–2	Mild	
Mitotane	Common		Severe	
Mitoxantrone			Mild	
Micamycin (Mithracin)	Common		Moderate–severe	24
Procarbazine hydrochloride	60%–90% early, then subsides		Moderate	
Streptozocin	90%	1–4	Moderate–severe	
Tamoxifen citrate	20%		Mild	
Thioguanine	<10%		Mild	
Thiotepa	10%–30%		Mild	
Vinblastine sulfate (Velban)	10%–30%		Mild	24
Vincristine sulfate (Oncovin)	<10%		Mild	

*Information on the incidence, onset, severity and duration is given where this could be found in the literature. *The emetic response to chemotherapeutic agents is quite variable, depending on the dosage, the health of the patient, and the pattern of use of antiemetics.*

†Hours after administration of the drug.

Daily Living Factors

Activities in Daily Living

Several areas of activity in daily living are affected by the presence of nausea and vomiting. They include:

Preparing food and fluids in ways that are acceptable and do not evoke further nausea or vomiting (e.g., avoiding foods with strong or disliked odors; avoiding high fat or calorie-rich foods that prolong stomach-emptying time and further inhibit food intake by afferent pathway stimulation [Koretz and Meyer, 1980]; serving cold foods that may stimulate stomach emptying [Bateman, 1982])

Changing eating patterns so that food is eaten in amounts and at times that minimize nausea and vomiting; avoiding eating immediately prior to or after radiation or chemotherapy sessions; adjusting liquid and food intake during vomiting episodes so as not to exacerbate vomiting

Stocking food supplies for menus and snacks so that food is available that makes every bite count nutritionally during periods when nausea and vomiting are in abatement

Managing transportation to avoid public transit systems during predictable vomiting episodes; planning ahead to have a kit of receptacles and towels available should vomiting occur en route

Scheduling self-care and essential tasks around times of peak nausea or vomiting

Planning strategies for managing social encounters in the presence of nausea or vomiting

Planning for diversion that is effective in distracting from the symptoms

Events in Daily Living

Medical and personal events in daily living that must be managed include:

Treatment days and the post-treatment period when symptoms are most pronounced

Growing dread associated with subsequent treatment cycle as treatment continues

Obligatory work, social events, or meetings with visitors who may have come some distance

Demands in Daily Living

Demands in daily living with respect to managing nausea and vomiting include:

Demands from self or others for maintenance of optimum nutritional intake versus self-perceived constraints on ingesting or retaining needed nutrients and fluids

Self-expectations that one take life in stride (including iatrogenic nausea or vomiting), or self-expectations that nausea and vomiting legitimize movement into an illness role for the duration of its predicted course

Expectations of health care providers that the patient will continue in treatment protocols despite severe nausea and vomiting and discouragement

Expectations of companions (perhaps not verbalized) that patient will manage symptoms in such a way that it does not make others uncomfortable or burden them with unwanted responsibilities

Environment for Daily Living

Elements in daily living related to the environment that require special attention in the presence of nausea and vomiting involve avoidance of some stimuli and planning for others. These include:

Avoidance of sights, sounds, and smells that are similar to those encountered in the chemotherapy experience that evoke nausea or vomiting responses

Availability of environments that are quiet and neutral or pleasantly distracting during periods in which episodes of nausea or vomiting are occurring

Availability of pleasant eating environments, with some distractions and a minimum of cooking odors

Avoidance of the vicinity of the chemotherapy treatments when driving or walking, to minimize anticipatory nausea and vomiting

Values and Beliefs

Value placed on self-control may be jeopardized by the act of vomiting or the uncertainty of when vomiting may occur.

Value placed on surviving can influence motivation to maintain nutrition and continue treatment in spite of nausea, vomiting, and symptom distress.

Societal values that make vomiting an unacceptable public activity can create serious stresses for patients whose situation requires them to remain active in work and social situations during treatment.

Possible confusion or conflict in societal values associated with assignment of the sick role during chemotherapy cycles, in which the patient experiences intermittent nausea and vomiting, can cause functional capacities to fluctuate markedly from week to week for 5 to 6 months.

Functional Health Status

Strength

Strength in the presence of these symptoms involves the status of physical strength to manage tasks of daily living and go to treatment; emotional strength to maintain motivation, hope, and interpersonal relationships in the face of symptoms; and intellectual strength to plan effective modifications in daily living and engage in tasks associated with work, school, or home life that make cognitive demands.

Endurance

Physical endurance to complete specific requirements in daily living can be compromised, as can psychologic endurance to stay with treatment and other demands in daily living in the face of current and predictable patterns of nausea or vomiting. Initiative to continue making adaptations in daily living in the face of presenting symptoms can become increasingly difficult if nausea or vomiting persist over extended periods.

Cognition

Where nausea or vomiting are predicted to occur, cognitive tasks in daily living involve the capacities to understand:

> The basis for the nausea or vomiting and the pattern that is expected or common with a given therapy
>
> Linkages between symptoms and planning for adjustments needed in daily living
>
> How to use antiemetic therapy most effectively
>
> How best to adjust food and fluid intake in the presence of nausea or vomiting

Cognition also involves the ability to put words to the symptoms being experienced and the activities undertaken.

Emotions

The emotional resources involved include:

> Overall morale and attitude toward therapy (Ash, 1981)
>
> Usual levels of anxiety (Rhodes et al, 1986)
>
> Anxiety at particular points in therapy (e.g., later cycles in chemotherapy [Rhodes et al, 1986])
>
> Status of "Symptom Distress" (Rhodes et al, 1987)
>
> Level of assertiveness in seeking to maintain control over daily living

Motivation

When patients are experiencing nausea or vomiting, there is a lessened capacity to accommodate elements of the health care system that do not seem to meet their needs or desires. This can lead to a loss of motivation to participate in the prescribed treatment that is creating such discomfort.

Motivation may also be affected by strength of will to survive and the desire or capacity to control life events.

*Communi-
cation*

Capacity to communicate accurately may involve the ability to convey information in such a way as to have credibility and receive appropriate attention related to:

The patterns of nausea, vomiting, retching, and related symptoms

The impact of symptoms and symptom distress on eating, drinking, sleeping, work, relationships, and other significant aspects of daily living

Personal daily living requirements and supports and their influence on the presenting situation

Nursing Diagnosis and Treatment

The experiences of nausea, vomiting, or retching added to the altered daily living of the patient and family during the initial treatment phase create new problems and complicate others. They can negatively affect eating, sleeping, control over activities, energy, and role relationships for the patients, and often for those who share their daily living. Individuals and families vary widely in their effectiveness in managing daily living in the presence these symptoms, and it is not always the severity of the symptoms that distinguishes those who manage and those who do not. Effective management of daily living during periods when nausea, vomiting, or retching are occurring presents a challenge to nurses in terms of diagnosis and therapeutic intervention.

Diagnostic Targets   Individuals who require diagnosis may include the patient, persons who share the patient's living space (e.g., care givers and family), and others who will be affected by the sights and sounds of the patient's symptoms, symptom distress, and changes in mood and lifestyle.

Risk Factors   Persons with increased risk of not managing daily living effectively in the face of nausea, vomiting, or retching include those who have:

Medical treatment causing severe iatrogenic nausea, retching, and vomiting

Tumors or tumor side-effects produce ongoing nausea and emetic effects

Concurrent symptoms of pain, fatigue, dyspnea, and so on that further reduce coping ability

Previous response patterns involving a tendency toward nausea and vomiting

Inappropriate expectations derived from past experiences or hearsay reports about the severity of the nausea or vomiting and lack of pharmacologic control

Low morale, depression, a negative attitude, and passivity

High levels of trait or state anxiety

Lack of a predictable, caring, skilled care giver or companion

Limitations on availability of preferred food (e.g., ethnic diets in the hospital)

Financial restrictions for obtaining appropriate food or food supplements

Lack of suitable transportation to and from the treatment site

Deficit in desire or ability to gather accurate data on symptoms and factors in daily living that relieve or exacerbate symptoms and to use the data as a basis for discovering relationships or patterns and making therapeutic changes in daily living

Diagnostic Areas

PATIENT

Inappropriate expectations of nausea and vomiting R/T lack of correct information about the incidence of iatrogenic nausea and vomiting and pharmacologic control

Ineffective use of antiemetics R/T lack of understanding of the best strategies for using them

Ineffective eating R/T lack of understanding of the best strategies for timing and food substances to cope with nausea and vomiting

Increasing restrictions in eating R/T to food aversions developing from associating a growing list of foods with subsequent vomiting episodes

Ineffective ability to manage the symptoms of nausea and vomiting in daily living R/T knowledge deficit of strategies for distraction, clinical relaxation, or hypnosis

Loss of will to "try" R/T past patterns of coping, severity of symptoms, or response to perception of stressors in daily life

Social isolation R/T nausea or fear of retching or vomiting in front of others

Ineffectiveness or failure to try to modify daily living in such a way as to minimize symptoms or to work around them R/T lack of knowledge, communication capacity, or support

Inability to obtain nutrients in a usable form R/T lack of financial resources or transportation

CARE GIVERS, COMPANIONS

Uncertainty about management of the environment, food preparation, feeding activities, or interpersonal strategies R/T knowledge deficit about the dynamics of the patient's specific presenting situation with regard to nausea, vomiting, retching, or symptom distress

Distancing behavior R/T personal revulsion with patient's activities of retching and vomiting

Discomfort in relationship with patient R/T uncertainty about how to interact with someone who is nauseated or vomiting

Manifestations
PATIENT

Signs and symptoms that the patient is not managing daily living effectively with the symptoms include:

Weight loss, observed or reported failure to eat and take in fluids, loss of skin turgor

Increasing abnormalities in laboratory values related to fluid and electrolytes

Reports of food intake that indicate inadequate nutrients, fluids, or electrolytes even on days when nausea and vomiting are reduced or not present

Belief that all patients who have radiation or chemotherapy experience severe nausea and vomiting

Increasing signs of depression and apathy

Reports on timing, frequency, duration, or amount of nausea, vomiting, or retching that are vague

Reports on patterns of taking antiemetic drugs that show that they are taken irregularly, infrequently, or ineffectively in relationship to the requirements of the presenting situation

Reports of major changes in patterns of daily living involving self-neglect, inappropriately reduced activity, sleep changes, and altered work or social relationships

No evidence of efforts to link data on symptoms and activities to effective modifications in daily living

CARE GIVER

Indications that the caregiver is not managing daily living effectively may be seen in reports of:

Anxiety, fear, frustration, or discouragement over patient's situation

Uncertainty or lack of knowledge about how to best help the patient with the symptoms of nausea, vomiting, or retching

Distaste or revulsion at having to be present or in the vicinity of the patient's retching or vomiting

Prognostic Variables

Poor prognosis for managing daily living effectively in the presence of nausea, vomiting, or retching episodes include intractable nausea and vomiting, presence of other symptoms that diminish adaptive resources, ineffective use of antiemetics, lack of a competent and reliable support system, personal coping style of passivity, lack of a strong will to survive, and lack of resources for appropriate food, fluids, and medications.

Complications

Failure to effectively manage daily living, particularly ingestion of food and fluids, can result in a cycle wherein malnutrition further promotes the symptoms and debility with a downward spiral in internal resources and response to treatment.

Health care workers can demobilize patient and family efforts to effectively manage daily living if they fail to offer hope, encouragement, and realistic positive information about the occurrence and management of nausea, vomiting, or retching.

Treatment Guidelines

PATIENT

Incorrect stereotypes about the occurrence and management of nausea, vomiting, and retching

Give realistic information about:

The emetic effects of treatment, including usual incidence and patterns of nausea and vomiting in the particular form of therapy (e.g., "with your type of chemotherapy, vomiting is not usual. If it should occur, it would not last beyond _____ hours after your treatment. You may feel somewhat nauseated beyond that time. Patients vary widely in the amount and severity of nausea or vomiting experienced with the tumor or with the different forms of treatment. Many have minimal difficulties"). (See Table 6-1 for occurrence and patterns of nausea and vomiting with some chemotherapeutic agents.)

New drugs and the therapy available to them to decrease nausea and vomiting and produce amnesia of the treatment experience

Gather data on patient expectations and clarify misconceptions:

Patients and families may equate the responses of nausea and vomiting to the efficacy of the treatment. Some may believe that the treatment isn't working unless the symptoms are present; others may see the symptoms as signs of treatment failure.

In dealing with patients and relatives, separate the kind of information that is required for the informed consent procedure ("Nausea and vomiting can be a side-effect") from that which will be used to prepare patients to manage their treatment experiences ("Quite a few of our patients have minimal problems with nausea and vomiting" or "We have many better drugs to help to control nausea and vomiting these days—so you are quite likely not to have the same experience as your mother did 10 years ago") (Rhodes et al, 1987).

Ineffective antiemetic use

Recommend that, for best control, the prescribed antiemetic medication regimen begin 1 to 12 hours prior to chemotherapy treatment and continue every 4 to 6 hours as prescribed for at least 12 to 24 hours. Continue as long as nausea and vomiting persist (Hogan, 1986). Inform the person that the drugs are not addictive and that consistent blood levels need to be established for effectiveness. Give specific information about duration and peak of drug action as well as dosage not to be exceeded. Suggest that a record be kept of when the antiemetic drugs are taken and the degree of relief obtained. (See Table 6-2 for onset and duration of antiemetic drug effects taken orally.)

Identify side-effects of antiemetic medication and their impact on daily living activities. Identify for the patient any precautions to be taken with antiemetic use (Grant, 1987).

Ineffective timing of eating in relationship to nausea and vomiting

Advise patient that many patients find it useful to avoid eating for several hours immediately preceding and following radiation or chemotherapy treatments and to eat less during the 1 to 3 days of nausea following chemotherapy.

Suggest rinsing the mouth to alleviate dryness and taking liquids in small sips during periods of vomiting.

Suggest that the person experiment and eat what works best for him when vomiting abates. A variety of strategies have been reported as effective for returning to more normal eating patterns. Some limit themselves to carbonated beverages, dry toast, crackers, dry popcorn, and baked or boiled potatoes—safe foods. Others report eating according to cravings, even pizza, with good results (Scogna, 1981).

Advise patient that in the presence of nausea, frequent smaller feedings (e.g., every 2 to 3 hours) seem to be better tolerated than three large meals per day.

Table 6-2. Common Antiemetic Medications Taken Orally: Peak Action and Half-Life

Drug	Peak Action	Half-Life
Ativan tablets (lorazepam)	60–90 min	16 hours
Benadryl-25 capsules (diphenhydramine hydrochloride)	60 min	4–6 hours
Cannabinoids (THC)	2–3 hours	4–5 hours
Compazine (prochlorperazine)	30–60 min	3–4 hours
Decadron (dexamethasone)	30–60 min	6 hours*
Inapsine (droperidol)	30 min	2–4 hours†
Marinol capsules (dronabinol)	2–3 hours	4 hours†
Reglan (metoclopramide hydrochloride)	1–2 hours	5–6 hours
Torecan (thiethylperazine)	30–60 min	3–4 hours
Valium tablets (diazepam)	30–60 min	4–6 hours†

Note: This information should help the nurse in administering the medication or in helping patients to schedule their antiemetic therapy to control nausea and vomiting most effectively.

*These numbers indicate the interval between doses. The half-life is long and there can be cumulative effects.
†Alterations in consciousness can occur for up to 12 hours.

Food aversions

Recognize that food aversions can develop when the person becomes aware that vomiting occurred after eating a particular food.

Recommend that favorite foods not be eaten before chemotherapy or at times when vomiting is likely to occur, but be reserved for times when vomiting is not likely.

Advise person that some patients have discovered that certain foods increase their vomiting while others decrease it. Suggest that the person pay attention to possible relationships between foods and vomiting patterns (Tiedemann, 1981).

Knowledge deficits about self-care options for managing daily living with nausea and vomiting

Be aware that in addition to antiemetics, other strategies may offer some degree of comfort. Their application and usefulness may depend on the degree of nausea being experienced.

Provide information or resources to develop necessary skills in progressive relaxation techniques as a means of reducing vomiting (Cotanch and Strum, 1987; Scott et al, 1983).

Explain strategies for resting (with or without relaxation activities) before meals so that fatigue does not affect eating.

Advise patient that deep breathing and fresh air may be helpful.

Advise patient to avoid major activity after eating.

If the person wishes to rest, suggest not lying flat for at least 2 hours after eating. Sitting, lying in a recliner, or lying in bed with 4-inch blocks under the head of the bed are more effective positions.

Explore available and usable options for distraction—radio, television, phone conversations, reading, visits, companions at meals. Recommend trying taste distractions such as tart hard candies or chewing gum, and varying the flavors among those that are acceptable.

Explore stimuli in the environment that create additional difficulties (e.g., music or TV played by others, the playing of children, behavior of others in the environment—whether hospital or home). Suggest strategies to reduce these stimuli.

Recommend trying liquids (e.g., food supplements) served in small amounts in small, attractive glasses (not cans) at the temperature the patient prefers; alter the flavors.

Recommend that the patient avoid clothing that is tight around the waist and abdomen.

Contract with patients to seek their own approaches; note what they tried and what their responses were as a means of gaining some sense of control. Encourage the setting of concrete, small goals.

Plan with the patient for specific contacts (phone or personal) in which feedback is given on the strategies tried and the outcomes.

Identify and communicate personal, warm pleasure in their successes, however limited.

Loss of will to continue treatment or to make any special effort to manage difficulties in daily living

Understand that, at times, the stresses of treatment, feeling miserable, and a bleaker-than-usual outlook make it difficult to mobilize one's resources to try to cope with daily living. The nurse as the constant on the treatment team can be a significant consistent support figure.

Emphasize the time-limited nature of nausea and vomiting associated with the particular therapy. Give a range of time rather than a specific time (e.g., the nausea tapers off within 1 to 2 weeks after the treatment is completed).

Listen to the patient's reports of patterns of nausea and vomiting—help to find the words as needed. Be empathic with the discomfort while assuring the patient that the symptoms are the expected ones under the presenting circumstances.

Help the patient to set small achievable goals in terms of managing daily living (e.g., using distraction, developing an eating schedule around symptom occurrence, adding a new food or texture, finding a successful strategy for improving the environment for eating, gaining a sense of control over some additional element in life associated with the symptoms or their management).

Offer warm encouragement. Identify and help the patient to identify successes. Offer specific praise. Where strategies haven't worked, negotiate for some alternatives to be tried during the next time period.

Social isolation R/T fear of vomiting in the presence of others

Recognize that the sights and sounds of retching and vomiting create problems for others as well as the patient. Cleaning up of an emesis can add to the embarrassment and difficulties. Even travelling to and from the treatment site may pose a problem because of anticipatory nausea and vomiting or post-treatment vomiting.

Offer as a strategy the possibility of determining the periods of highest risk for vomiting and where possible planning work and other activities around them.

Suggest that the patient keep a record of episodes of nausea, vomiting, and retching to determine patterns, then use the findings to schedule activities.

Suggest that private vehicles used in travel (e.g., to and from chemotherapy treatments) be stocked with a kit containing one or more receptacles with lids for emesis, moist wipes, clean cloths or towels, a bottle of water or other solution for rinsing the mouth, and a packet of breath mints.

For those who don't have personal private transportation, put them in touch with the local American Cancer Society for volunteer transportation (e.g., "Road to Recovery," also sometimes affectionately called "the buddy and bucket brigade"). Usually these volunteers have supplies to care for vomiting, but it might be wise for the patient to check ahead.

Difficulty in renegotiating usual roles to adjust to current patterns of nausea and vomiting

Help patient understand that:

It may be difficult for others (children, spouses, employers, co-workers) to adjust their role expectations for the person who is undergoing cancer treatment, particularly radiation or chemotherapy. These treatments are less tangible than the more visible surgical treatment and may seem more mysterious and frightening. With chemotherapy the iatrogenic symptoms often are cyclical. Thus the person's capability of fulfilling usual role responsibilities may wax and wane with each cycle of treatment. Others may wonder: Is the person placed in the sick role or not? One of the greetings reportedly disliked by patients is "How ARE you?" A more neutral "How are things going?" seems to be the form preferred by patients.

Accommodations to patient disability tend to be made by others for about 2 weeks; then they taper off. It is difficult to sustain an unequal relationship, except in the professional care roles.

Specific difficulties in negotiating for changes in usual role obligations will vary with the setting and situation (e.g., home versus work, mother with preschool children versus mother with adolescent or adult children, patient-spouse with responsibility for care of an ailing partner).

If the patient is predicted to experience major problems with nausea or vomiting, or is experiencing one or both, help patient consider:

The areas in daily living where periods of nausea or vomiting pose problems in terms of role obligations

The types of changes that need to be made and the persons who are affected by the proposed changes (e.g., children, spouse, employer, co-workers, and others)

What information would need to be shared

The possible impact of sharing the information—advantages and disadvantages (e.g., the employer or supervisor may—in kindness—take away more job responsibilities than the patient wishes to lose)

Help patient explore the issues and ramifications in his own specific situations as a basis for making informed decisions about sharing information with others. In work situations, given some prevailing myths or stereotypes about cancer (e.g., that it is contagious or that the person who has it is automatically dying), individuals in active treatment may be reluctant to reveal to others that they have the diagnosis and that they wish to renegotiate the job requirements or hours of work for a period of time.

Once the patient has made the decisions, be supportive in following up on outcomes and the periodic renegotiations as needed (e.g., increasing or decreasing role responsibilities).

(See section on Role for additional considerations)

Inability to obtain nutrients in a usable form R/T lack of money or transportation

Obtain data on any financial or transportation restrictions that may make it difficult to obtain dietary supplements, special dietary substances, or hyperalimentation equipment or formula.

Provide information on sources of assistance, if the person or family seem able to seek this help on their own. Negotiate for the resources if there is reason to believe that they cannot or may not do so (note that some persons who are perfectly competent in most areas have difficulty asking for help).

CARE GIVERS, *Ineffective management of patient's diet and symptoms R/T lack of knowledge*
COMPANIONS

Provide specific information about the reason for the patient's nausea or vomiting and the pattern that is to be anticipated.

Provide information verbally and in writing (if they are literate) about:

The kinds of foods and fluids that are often tolerated and helpful

The importance of a pleasant environment during eating (e.g., small portions of food served attractively using small plates and glasses; distraction in the form of music, interesting conversation, or television; and control of odors that the patient cannot tolerate).

Encourage care giver to:

Plan on several small "meals" rather than the usual three-meal schedule, but ensure the opportunity to eat some of the small meals with the family, if this is normal

Offer food, but not urge it (no nagging!)

Offer specific food options, rather than ask "What do you want to eat?"

Take the opportunity to provide more nutrients during times when nausea and vomiting are in abatement

Promote periods of rest and relaxation before and after eating

Check with the patient periodically to determine that the patterns being used in eating, foods, companionship, environmental stimuli, etc. are as comforting as is possible under the circumstances, and not to take for granted that current patterns are helpful

Avoidance or distancing behavior related to discomfort with the possibility of the patient's vomiting

If the patient requires assistance during vomiting, determine which care givers are available to help. Gather data on the difficulties they are having or anticipate having in being with the patient during vomiting episodes. Legitimize their responses as being normal. Offer care givers strategies for overcoming their own difficulties, such as:

Negotiate with the patient as to what actions he prefers the care giver to take during episodes of vomiting

Focus on the person and his needs, not on the emesis

Swallow hard if gagging occurs

Have a cloth or paper available to cover the emesis receptacle when carrying it for disposal, or use a receptacle with a lid

Have available water or dilute mouthwash for the patient to rinse his mouth and a damp cloth for wiping his face

Use aerosol or burn matches to dispel the odors associated with the emesis. (Check to see that the aromas from aerosol or matches are tolerable to the patient.)

When the patient does not require assistance, but family or visitors are afraid of having to witness vomiting, help the patient broach the subject, using the following nursing interventions:

Explore with patient any concerns about how family members or friends may respond to the risks of his vomiting when they are in his residence. Determine whether the patient is comfortable dealing with these persons directly or whether an intermediary would be preferable.

Explore whether it is possible to take a matter-of-fact approach when discussing these personally uncomfortable symptoms with others. Help the patient to rehearse scripts and tone of voice.

Suggest gathering data on vomiting patterns. (Many patients with iatrogenic vomiting have recognizable, predictable patterns of vomiting [Tiedemann, 1981].)

Suggest arranging for visits with family and friends during times when the patient is not likely to vomit. Inform them directly or through an intermediary that this is a "safe" time for a visit.

Suggest that, where family members or others are, of necessity, present during bouts of vomiting, the patient propose the use of sound barriers (doors) or masking noises (raising the volume on the radio or TV) to limit the sounds associated with vomiting.

Note that these interventions are dependent on the emotional and physical status of the patient. Concern for others' discomfort may be beyond the capacity of the patient if the patient is also experiencing other symptoms, such as severe pain, fatigue, and depression.

Evaluation   Evaluation of response to nursing treatment will address one or more of the following areas:

Status of understanding of the basis for nausea, vomiting, and retching and the patterns that are normal and expected with the particular tumor or treatment protocols

Status of understanding regarding the effective use of antiemetics for this presenting situation and the side-effects that need to be worked around or reported

Status of understanding about effective strategies for eating and drinking in the presence of symptoms of nausea or vomiting

Status of understanding regarding activities and environment that can reduce the symptoms or make them more tolerable

Status of understanding of how food aversions develop

Status of knowledge of supplies to be carried to manage emesis when a bathroom is not immediately available

Status of activities and behavior in daily living that actually put understandings into practice—from patient and family reports

Status of satisfaction or discouragement with alterations in daily living to manage the discomforts and disruptions caused by nausea and vomiting

Status of comfort and skills in relating to others in areas of interaction or role responsibilities affected by nausea and vomiting

Status of outcomes of these negotiations and satisfaction with them

Status of external resources—money, transportation to obtain needed nutrients, supplies, and equipment; use of the available resources

Status of care givers', food preparers', or companions' level of comfort and satisfaction in their relationships with the patient and with their own lifestyles in the presence of the patient's patterns of nausea and vomiting

Living With Constipation

Constipation can be a problem for some individuals during the initial treatment stage. Both neoplastic and iatrogenic factors can contribute to its occurrence.

Medical Perspective

The medical perspective addresses the pathogenesis of the condition and, most frequently, the prescription of diet and medications to relieve it. Surgical treatment may be needed when constipation is precipitated by intestinal obstruction or painful rectal conditions such as an abscess.

Nursing Perspective

Nursing diagnosis and treatment focuses on patterns in daily living associated with effective elimination. These include eating, fluid intake, mobility and exercise, laxative use, and toileting habits.

The basis for diagnosis will be specific data gathered by the nurse on the frequency, amounts, and stool consistency of bowel movements; any symptoms that are interfering with defecation; discomforts, concerns, and disruptions in daily living associated with the constipation; usual actions taken when constipation occurred in the past; and what, to the patient, constitutes the range of "normal" in expections of elimination patterns. Relief should be obtained, where possible, using strategies that the patient has previously found successful unless these are contraindicated in the present circumstances. Once the initial constipation is relieved, the underlying causes and associated issues in daily living can be diagnosed and treated.

Nature of Constipation

Usual bowel patterns can vary widely among individuals, as can interpretation of what constitutes constipation. As a basis for diagnosing the existence of constipation, specific information is needed on usual frequency, amounts, and consistency of bowel movements.

Constipation is defined as an undue delay in fecal evacuation (usually less then three times per week). Stool consistency tends to be harder and dryer than usual, with the possibility of a covering of mucus when there has been an inordinate number of days since the previous bowel movement. Evacuation is more difficult than normal and involves use of voluntary abdominal muscles (Peterson, 1983).

Patterns in daily living associated with diet, fluid intake, exercise, and promptness of response to the urge to defecate can influence the occurrence of constipation. However, it can also be an outcome of oncology treatment and tumor location or growth. Self-expectations about what constitutes "normal" or "desirable" patterns of bowel evacuations in patterns of daily living tend to be idiosyncratic. These data form the baseline for determination of what changes in bowel movement patterns constitute "constipation" for a given individual.

Underlying Mechanisms

Pathophysiologic and Iatrogenic Factors

The underlying mechanisms for constipation when cancer is present can include factors related to both the tumor and the treatment—specifically, treatment with surgery and chemotherapy. Other forms of cancer therapy are more likely to cause diarrhea than constipation.

Tumor-Related Factors
Tumors may have the following constipation-causing effects: Spinal cord tumors can cause neurologic deficits; intraluminal tumors can limit or obstruct passage of materials; tumors surrounding the gut may gradually narrow the lumen, causing blockage and reflex inhibition above the blockage; large abdominal tumors (e.g., ovarian tumors) can decrease the efficiency of abdominal muscles; painful anorectal ulcerations or perirectal abscesses cause the individual to resist evacuating feces (Peterson, 1983).

Surgery
Surgery involving manipulation or alteration of the gut may cause temporary alterations in peristalsis. Anesthesia and analgesia in the perioperative period plus immobility and restrictions in diet during the pre- and postoperative days all combine to create risks of at least temporary constipation.

Chemotherapy
Vincristine sulfate has the side-effect of neurotoxicity, which can cause autonomic nervous system dysfunction (among other neuropathies). This, in turn, can result in constipation and paralytic ileus (Dorr and Fritz, 1980).

Daily Living Factors

Activities in Daily Living

The following activities in daily living are associated with the prevention or management of constipation:

Usual dietary patterns, particularly as they involve intake of fiber and fluids

Usual pattern of bowel elimination

Activities that cause the person to ignore signals of the need for bowel evacuation

Usual medication taking patterns (e.g., use of over-the-counter medications such as laxatives, heavy use of aspirin or constipating antacids)

Taking of prescription medications that may be constipating

Lack of exercise or physical immobility

Demands in Daily Living

Demands include self-expectations of what constitutes normal bowel patterns (e.g., a bowel movement every day regardless of food intake, or one every two or three days).

Environment for Daily Living

Environmental factors affecting constipation include:

Accessibility to and availability of toilet facilities when the person experiences the urge to defecate

Opportunity for privacy for toileting activities

Values and Beliefs

Many adults have developed special beliefs about what constitutes a normal pattern of bowel elimination, what happens if elimination does not follow this pattern, and what should be done to restore the desired pattern. The beliefs may or may not be congruent with present knowledge of bowel physiology and pathophysiology and may affect participation in a prescribed or recommended bowel regimen.

Functional Health Status

Strength

Physical strength is needed to get to the toilet or commode.

Strength of abdominal muscles is needed to evacuate the bowel if stool is harder or larger than normal.

Endurance

Physical endurance may be needed to complete the bowel evacuation if it is difficult or prolonged.

Cognition

Management of constipation may depend on the capacity to

Understand the relationship between diet, exercise, toileting patterns, and constipation

Attend to the urge to defecate and to understand that this sensation can be lost if it is regularly ignored

Adapt to treatment regimens that are not necessarily congruent with belief patterns

Emotions Depression, mental stress, short attention span, or cognitive impairment can limit attention to elimination signals and needs (Heitkemper and Bartol, 1986).

Nursing Diagnosis and Treatment

Constipation can be a troubling problem to individuals under any circumstances. It an be even more worrisome and energy-draining when it is added to the stresses of initial cancer treatment. There is usually a desire for immediate relief.

Diagnostic Targets Targets for diagnosis include the person experiencing the constipation, the person who prepares the food, and individuals who share the bathroom.

Risk Factors Persons who are at risk for not effectively managing constipation and its prevention and treatment in daily living include those who:

Have long-standing laxative or enema patterns as a means of controlling bowel movements

Are very distressed with any change in bowel patterns regardless of changes in diet or other circumstances

Do not eat or enjoy foods containing fiber, such as raw or cooked fruits and vegetables and whole grain products

Have problems with teeth or dentures or have friable ulcerated oropharyngeal and esophageal tissues that preclude mastication or swallowing of foods containing fiber

Restrict or are restricted in the amounts of fluids they can ingest

Have strongly held belief patterns that are incongruent with the treatment plan

Take large amounts of aspirin or other constipating drugs

Are very sedentary or immobilized

Have serious problems with fatigue or pain

Currently ignore or have developed a pattern of ignoring body signals indicating the need to have a bowel movement

Diagnostic Areas Inadequate ingestion of fiber or fluids R/T:

Lack of knowledge concerning their relationship to the presenting constipation

Previous, preferred dietary patterns that do not include fiber, leading to unwillingness to change

Fragile oropharyngeal or esophageal tissues or poor dentition that prevents chewing and swallowing of high fiber foods

Pain on masticating or swallowing

Ineffective antacid use R/T knowledge deficit of the constipating effect of calcium carbonate and aluminum-based antacids (e.g., Alkets, Camalox, Alka-2, Titralac, Tums, Dicarbosil, Amphojel, Basaljel)

Progressive weakening of sensation of urge to defecate R/T:

Procrastination in defecation when urge is felt associated with fatigue, pain, or preoccupation with other activities

Lack of prompt access to toilet facilities

Undesired changes in activities in daily living R/T increasing discomfort and preoccupation with lack of bowel movements

Manifestations   Reported:

Concerns about infrequency of defecation

Increase in hardness, dryness, or size of stool

Discomforts of and preoccupation with constipation interfering with usual patterns of daily living (specify which activities are involved)

Difficulty in defecation R/T fatigue, pain (specify nature and location and its relationship to defecation), loss of abdominal muscle tone, or lack of privacy

Delaying of defecation when urge is felt because of pain, fatigue, preoccupation with other activities, or lack of access to toilet

Lack of understanding of link between failing to defecate when the urge is felt and the gradual loss of the strength of the reflex

Use of constipating antacids or other medications (anticholinergics, aspirin, opiates, or tranquilizers)

Failure to include adequate fiber and fluids in diet because this is a deviation from usual or preferred eating patterns of self or food preparer, or because of difficulty in chewing or swallowing

Observed:

Decrease in frequency of bowel movements

Difficulty in bowel evacuation; increased size and dryness of stool

Decrease in appetite

Increase in frequency of trips to the bathroom

Complaints of nausea, headache, abdominal cramping, or abdominal distention, as these are different from previous physical status (Heitkemper and Bartol, 1986)

Changes in mental status that could create greater difficulty in maintaining attention to effective bowel patterns and an appropriate diet

Prescription of constipating medication regimens

Fecal impaction (on rectal examination)

Laboratory findings or medical treatments predictive of physiologic basis for serious fatigue

Depression or anxiety

Prognostic Variables

Poor prognosis for managing daily living to minimize constipation or to manage it is associated with:

The need for regular use of aspirin, opiates, or tranquilizers

The inability or unwillingness to ingest dietary fiber and adequate fluids daily

The ignoring of or lack of ability to attend to urge to defecate

Inadequate access to toilet facilities

Fatigue or pain that interfere with physical ability to defecate

Depression

Complications

Complications of unmanaged constipation include fecal impaction, discomfort, and interference with quality of daily living.

Treatment Guidelines

Knowledge deficit regarding dietary fiber and fluid requirements and their relation to constipation

Provide verbal and written guidelines on use of a high fiber diet and increased fluids to relieve constipation. (See High Residue Foods column in Table 6-3.)

Explore patient's and family's current diet and fluid intake. Determine what adjustments are needed that are acceptable to the patient, given the patient's current symptoms and preferences.

Ask patient to plan to give feedback (use a food diary if the patient or care giver is willing) on changes made, their acceptability, and outcomes.

Failure to ingest adequate fluid and fiber R/T dental problems, fragile oropharyngeal tissues, dysphagia, or esophagitis

See section on Difficulties in Eating, under Treatment Guidelines, for interventions related to pain control and dysphagia.

Table 6-3.   Low and High Fiber Foods

	Low Residue Foods*	High Residue Foods†
Beverages	Low fat milk products, tea, soft drinks	Fruit juices and nectars
Breads	Breads, crackers, and rolls using white flour	Bread products using whole grains
Cereals	Cream of wheat, corn or rice cereals, strained oatmeal	Whole grain cereals
Desserts	Jello, custard, tapioca, rice puddings	Fruit-based desserts
Fruits	Apples (peeled, raw or cooked), bananas	Any fruits and juices
Meats	Tender cuts of all meats and poultry (skinned), white fish (canned or fresh), clams. Avoid frying in meat preparation.	Any meats
Other protein sources	Eggs (not fried), low fat processed cheeses	Peanut butter
Other foods	Clear broths, strained cream soups	Bean or pea soups, soups with fibrous vegetables, barley, brown rice, all types of grains
Seasonings, condiments	Salt, sugar, jelly, honey	All other seasonings, jams, conserves, pickles, olives, nuts, dried seeds, catsup, mustard
Starches	Pasta, white potatoes (peeled), white rice	Sweet potatoes, brown rice, pasta with tomato sauce
Vegetable	Well-cooked green beans, carrots, squash	All raw vegetables, cruciferous vegetables

*For diarrhea, choose the foods and fluids in the low fiber column and avoid those in the high fiber column. Also avoid caffeinated beverages; cocoa or chocolate; tough, smoked or spicy meats; dairy products; sauces; and other foods high in fat.

†For constipation, unless contraindicated, use foods in the high fiber column in preference to those in the low fiber column.

Instruct patient to use a blender to include fresh fruits in milkshakes or fruit juice drinks, and vegetables in soups. Dip whole grain breads in liquids to soften them (e.g., coffee, cocoa, or tea). Use well-cooked whole grain cereals.

Use of constipating antacids R/T lack of knowledge of alternatives

Gather data on current patterns of antacid use. If needed, provide a list of calcium- and aluminum-based antacids to be avoided and a list of the preferable magnesium antacids, which are not constipating (see Table 6-4).

Table 6-4. Antacids: Effects on Constipation and Diarrhea

Antacids That Can Have an Effect of Constipating

Calcium Carbonate-Based
   Alkets, Camalox, Alka-2, Titralac, Tums, Dicarbosil

Aluminum-Based
   Amphojel, Basaljel

Antacids That Can Have an Effect of Diarrhea

Magnesium-Based
   Milk of Magnesia, Chooz Antacid Gum

Antacids That Can Have an Effect of Either Constipation or Diarrhea

Magnesium and Aluminum Hydroxide-Based
   Maalox Suspension or Tablets, Mylanta Liquid or
     Tablets, Gelusil, Aludrox, Di-Gel Liquid or Tablets,
     WinGel

Procrastination in defecating after feeling the urge, leading to (L/T) blunting of reflex

Gather data on:

Patient's awareness of urge to defecate and any past behavior that may have decreased it

Current circumstances that cause the patient to delay going to the toilet when the urge is felt (e.g., pain, fatigue, lack of access to toilet)

Explain how delaying defecation after feeling the urge to do so results in decrease in this important body signal and the normal bowel evacuation reflexes (Heitkemper and Bartol, 1986)

Where pain is a deterrent to defecation, negotiate with physician for analgesia that can be used to make defecation less painful. If the patient has a time when defecation regularly occurs, propose taking of analgesia in advance of that time to bring maximum relief.

When anorectal pain is present following defecation, recommend sitz baths or warm moist compresses for additional comfort.

When fatigue interferes with remaining on the toilet long enough to defecate in the presence of constipation, arrange for some form of physical support for arms and upper body (e.g., small table or pillow).

If access to the toilet is difficult because of its use by others, work with an appropriate person to gain priority for the patient's needs.

Disruptions in daily living associated with constipation

Gather data on the particular problem the patient is experiencing.

Plan a schedule for the taking of laxatives or use of suppositories or enemas that fit best with energy levels and other activities.

Explore alternatives in scheduling other activities.

Evaluation

Patient response to nursing intervention can be evaluated in terms of:

Return to more normal patterns of defecation

Reduced concern about the problem

Status of fiber and fluids in diet

Patterns of response to urge to defecate

Resolution of deterrents to defecation

Satisfaction with constipation treatment strategies (laxatives, suppositories, enemas)

Alteration of daily living schedules that better accommodates to bowel problems

---

Living With Diarrhea

Mild to severe diarrhea can be a symptom associated with a limited number of cancers and, more frequently, with certain forms of cancer therapy. Managing daily living in order to minimize its occurrence and deal with its discomforts and disruptions can be an important dimension of nursing care.

Medical Perspective

The medical perspective focuses on diarrhea as a possible manifestation of cancer and also as an expected side-effect of certain treatments. There is concern in medical treatment to maintain fluid and electrolyte balance as well as nutrition.

Nursing Perspective

Nursing focuses on diagnosing and treating any problems the patient may have

In modifying the diet to minimize the diarrhea

In managing the requirements of daily living around the discomforts and disruption of frequent or urgent defecation

In managing fecal incontinence so as to participate in the requirements of daily living and maintain self-esteem

Nature of Diarrhea

Diarrhea is a condition of increased frequency of bowel movements, greater in number than three times per day. The stools are semisolid or watery in consistency. It may be intermittent or ongoing. Abdominal cramping may or may not accompany diarrhea (Peterson, 1983).

Diarrhea can be caused by the tumor itself. It can also be related to medical treatment, emotional stresses associated with the cancer experience, diet, and medication taking. Diarrhea can be a preexisting condition that may be exacerbated by the cancer and its treatment.

Diarrhea can have a major impact on daily living associated with the discomfort, the need to have access to toilet facilities on short notice, and the risks of fecal incontinence.

Underlying Mechanisms

Pathophysiologic and Iatrogenic Factors

Tumor-Related Factors
Diarrhea may accompany carcinoma of the pancreas when the tumor blocks the ducts and creates lipase insufficiency. Villous adenomas cause excessive secretions in the intestines, resulting in a secretory type of diarrhea (Heitkemper and Bartol, 1986). Cancers causing partial intestinal obstructions can also have diarrhea as a symptom.

Surgery
Removal of portions of the intestine sufficient to cause short bowel syndrome can cause diarrhea. Vagotomy can result in an autonomic imbalance, with transient diarrhea. Gastrectomy can produce a dumping syndrome with associated diarrhea. Gastric and intestinal surgery tends to produce an osmotic type of diarrhea characterized by greater potassium losses and acidic stools (Heitkemper and Bartol, 1986).

Chemotherapy
The mucosal membranes of the intestinal tract are highly susceptible to antineoplastic drug-related mucosal toxicity due to their normal pattern of rapid cell proliferation. Antineoplastic drugs that particularly affect the intestinal tract and cause diarrhea are the antimetabolites.

Broad-spectrum antibiotics that change the intestinal flora (e.g., ampicillin, clindamycin, lincomycin, tetracycline, neomycin, and cephalexin) can also contribute to diarrhea.

Tube Feedings
Supplementary feedings via nasogastric tubes or gastrostomy tube feedings can cause diarrhea if the solutions are bacterially contaminated, high in osmolarity, administered too rapidly, or

too cold when administered or if the person has a lactose intolerance (Groenwald, 1987).

Radiation   Radiation of the abdomen in excess of 2000 rad will cause sufficient damage in intestinal mucosal cells to result in diarrhea of some degree of severity. For some it will be an increase in the number of normal stools; for others the diarrhea will be severe, with abdominal cramping and loose, watery stools. Abdominal radiation can be complicated by fistulas, ulceration, and proctitis. Chronic diarrhea related to radiation can occur as a delayed effect (Hilderly, 1987).

Psychologic Factors

Emotions, response to stress, anticipation of an event, or concern about problems can cause diarrhea (Heitkemper and Bartol, 1986).

Daily Living Factors

Activities in
Daily Living   Activities in daily living that are of concern in the presence of diarrhea include:

Usual dietary patterns and preferences, particularly as they affect participation in dietary changes to restrict fiber and to increase fluid intake and possibly high potassium foods

Antacid taking that has involved use of magnesium-based antacids that are laxative in their side-effects (see Table 6-4)

Home, social, and work responsibilities or travel that may limit the person's ability to reach a toilet quickly enough to prevent fecal incontinence

Usual patterns of dress that may impede rapid removal in case of an urgent need to defecate

Use of protective items to manage fecal incontinence

See also section on Sexuality in this chapter.

Events in
Daily Living   Events of concern are:

Oncologic treatments that increase the acuity of diarrhea

Social or work obligations that may be difficult to meet because of discomfort or acuity of diarrhea

Demands in
Daily Living   Self-expectations regarding control, particularly bowel control, may be violated by the severity of the diarrhea and risks of fecal incontinence.

Usual family and social role implementation may be impaired by severe diarrhea.

Work-related demands can increase stress, which may increase the diarrhea, or the diarrheal problems may generate concerns about meeting work requirements.

Environment for Daily Living

Distances, stairs, or other environmental barriers to easy, rapid access to toilet facilities at home and in public facilities, gas stations, airplanes, and so on may create worries, difficulties, or episodes of fecal incontinence.

Values and Beliefs

Values related to personal cleanliness and control of odors affect the person's ability to manage daily living with diarrhea.

Functional Health Status

Functional capacities affected or needed for managing daily living involve physical strength and mobility, cognition, sexuality, and emotions.

Strength

Physical strength and mobility are needed to move to the toilet area and to remove clothing quickly if necessary.

Flexibility is needed to cleanse and protect perianal skin areas (or areas surrounding an ileostomy or colostomy).

Cognition

Management of diarrhea requires the capacity to understand:

The underlying bases for the diarrhea and its effect on other body functions (e.g., fluid and electrolyte balance)

The relationship between high fiber in the diet and diarrhea (when this is a risk or problem)

Strategies for eating a low fiber diet that is adequate in nutrients

The need to increase fluids to replace those lost

How to increase potassium in the diet (if needed)

How to adapt daily living—work, transportation, and dress—to accommodate to the degree of diarrhea being experienced

The capacity to recognize and heed body signals warning of the incipient need to defecate is also required.

Sexuality

Decrease in libido or reduced willingness to engage in intercourse associated with risks of an episode of diarrhea may occur.

See also section on Sexuality in this chapter.

Emotions

Stressors in daily living may increase the incidence or severity of diarrhea.

Depression, shame, guilt, or a change in body image or self-confidence can occur with worry about risk or actual experiences of loss in bowel control.

Nursing Diagnosis and Treatment

Diagnostic Targets

Targets for diagnosis include the person experiencing the diarrhea or risk of diarrhea, persons who share bathroom facilities, and persons who prepare food and do the laundry.

Risk Factors

Persons who are at risk of not managing daily living well with diarrhea are those who:

Are having or have had treatment that causes particularly severe diarrhea and abdominal cramping

Have restricted strength, mobility, or body flexibility

Must continue to work during treatment

Must use public transportation

Do not have easy access to toilet facilities

Diagnostic Areas

Decreased control of diarrhea R/T knowledge deficit of low residue diets, effective use of antacids, or need for increased fluids

Failure to maintain potassium levels R/T knowledge deficit regarding potassium content in foods and beverages or risks of hypokalemia

Painful skin excoriation R/T failure to cleanse skin adequately and apply protective emollients

Inadequate control of fecal material from incontinence R/T failure to wear protective garments

Ineffective laundering of clothing or bedding R/T:

Lack of knowledge on disinfection in laundering and procedures for removing fecal stains

Personal inability to deal with fecally soiled clothing and bedding

Fecal incontinence R/T:

Lack of easy availability of toilet facilities (specify the difficulty)

Architectural barriers (specify) to reaching toilet

Clothing barriers

Reduced mobility and strength for getting to toilet

Feelings of shame, guilt, or depression R/T fecal incontinence

Disturbed relationships with sexual partner R/T reluctance to be sexually active because of discomfort or fear of episode of diarrhea. (See section on Sexuality in this chapter.)

Increased risk of infection R/T ineffective hand washing after bowel movements

Manifestations   Reported (by patient or care giver):

Presence of increased number of bowel movements per day, stools that are semisolid or watery, abdominal cramping, or urgency in defecation

Inability to delay defecation until a toilet is reached

Pain in perianal or ostomy area due to skin excoriation

Continued use of magnesium-based antacids

Continued inclusion of higher-than-desirable levels of fiber in the diet

Inadequate fluid intake

Lack of knowledge of how to increase potassium in the diet or lack of money for high potassium foods

Lack of knowledge on how to increase potassium without increasing fiber

Concern over fecal incontinence interfering with specified activities or events in daily living

Lack of knowledge of or money for protective garments or supplies

Revulsion at having to launder clothing or bedding that contains fecal materials or stains

Lack of knowledge of how to launder fecally contaminated and stained clothing or bedding safely and effectively

Environmental or clothing barriers that delay toileting

Lack of strength or flexibility to remove lower garments quickly

Lack of access to the toilet when it is urgently needed

Shame, loss of confidence, depression, or anger over loss of control related to defecation

Dissatisfaction (self or partner), with altered patterns of sexual activities associated with the occurrence of episodes of diarrhea or fear of such episodes

Observed:

Urgent need to use toilet facilities

Difficulty in removing clothing

Fecal stains on clothing

Ineffective hand washing after a bowel movement

Excoriation of skin surrounding anus or ostomy

Missed appointments for outpatient treatment

Documentation of higher fiber than appropriate in eating diaries

Patient or care giver's lack of knowledge about fiber in foods, potassium in the diet, or the importance of fluids

Change in patient mood indicative of a less positive self-concept (not explained by other events)

Lower serum potassium values

Signs of dehydration

Prognostic Variables

Poor prognosis is associated with:

Severe and protracted diarrhea

Decreased anal sphincter control

Lack of physical and mental energy for managing the changed activities in daily living

Restricted mobility and strength

Barriers to toilet access related to environmental or people-related factors

Lack of adequate laundry facilities or services

Lack of ability to understand the relationship of diet to diarrhea

Lack of physical or mental ability to care for perianal or ostomy skin areas

Problems in finding appropriate transportation to work or treatment sites

Complications

Complications of failure to manage diarrhea effectively in daily living can include:

Fluid and electrolyte imbalance

Skin excoriation and associated pain

Inability to carry out requirements of daily living (e.g., work, relationships, travelling to treatment site)

Shame and depression over loss of control

Treatment Guidelines

Knowledge deficit of low residue diet, fluid requirements, and side-effects of antacids

Gather data on fiber in usual and preferred diet and current pattern of fluid intake.

Provide information on the relationship between fiber and diarrhea and on fluid replacement in the patient's presenting situation

Provide written information on the low residue diet (see Table 6-3). Ask patient to compare it to usual and preferred diet and to indicate what adjustments could be made at breakfast, lunch, and dinner to decrease usual fiber intake.

Ask patient about comfortable, feasible strategies for increasing fluid intake (commensurate with degree of fluid loss being experienced).

Provide information about the side-effects of antacids (see Table 6-4).

Schedule feedback sessions (by phone or in a clinic visit) on successes, questions, or problems.

Knowledge deficit regarding strategies for increasing potassium-rich foods in the diet (for patients with osmotic diarrhea)

Provide written information on foods high in potassium that could be included in a low residue diet (e.g., milk and milk products, yogurt, meat, potatoes, bananas). Note that many other good sources of potassium have high fiber (e.g., whole grains, legumes, winter squash, leafy vegetables, dried prunes, apricots, dates, peaches, raisins, cantaloupe, citrus fruits). Foods very high in potassium include salt substitute—1360 mg/$\frac{1}{2}$ teaspoon; canned tomato puree—1060 mg/4 oz; sardines in oil—1060 mg/4 oz; frozen dinners (e.g., Swanson's chicken dinner—731 mg) (Epstein and Oster, 1984).

Explore with patient or food preparer the strategies they would find acceptable for increasing the amount of potassium in the diet.

Failure to maintain skin integrity and comfort in perianal or ostomy regions

Where diarrhea is a known iatrogenic risk, instruct patient to:

Cleanse the skin area at risk with mild soap (or plain water), rinse carefully, and pat dry

Apply a protective ointment (e.g., Vaseline, A and D ointment, zinc oxide ointment) following bowel movements—even before any skin irritation occurs

Apply protective ointment prior to an anticipated liquid stool to give added protection in case the earlier application has rubbed off on undergarments

Use local anesthetic creams or ointments (e.g., Nupercaine) where excoriation has occurred and the area is painful

Ineffective management of fecal incontinence

Where severe diarrhea is an expected iatrogenic risk or is appearing, talk with the patient about managing the problem, so that there is an awareness that diarrhea is not uncommon.

Gather data on any barriers to access to toilet facilities (e.g., travel distance to treatment site, stairs, and distance to the bathroom in the home).

Talk about clothing and ease of removal in case there is little warning of the urge to defecate.

Advise patient that where access to the bathroom in the home is inconvenient or unpredictable (others may be using it), it may give peace of mind to have a commode available in an accessible, private area.

Provide information about the types of protective garments that are available, including sources and costs. Inform patient of the availability of reusable plastic panties with disposable liners as well as the totally disposable protective garments. Discuss options for protecting bedding—Chux, pieces of old sheeting over a piece of rubberized fabric or plastic. (Absorbent supplies are expensive, so consider alternatives if money is a problem.)

Where travel to and from the treatment site is long, or when diarrhea becomes frequent, suggest that toilet facilities (e.g. gas stations) be "spotted" en route in case they are needed

Knowledge deficit regarding laundering of fecally soiled garments or bed linen

Instruct patient to:

Rinse and brush off removable fecal material in cool water (e.g., in toilet bowl)

Place in a covered receptacle in warm water in which $1/2$ cup of Borateem has been dissolved. Soak for at least 30 minutes. For small stains or only occasional leaks, treat with a prewash stain removal product.

Wash in hot water (120°F to 130°F) with adequate amount of detergent or soap

Feelings of shame or depression related to fecal incontinence

When patients are having severe diarrhea and incontinence is a risk, make opportunities for the patient to talk about what is happening (e.g., "Some of our patients who have had this treatment have had real problems in not being able to control their diarrhea—it has been physically and emotionally difficult").

Be genuine and sensitive in acknowledging the specific difficulties and the feelings that accompany the loss of bowel control after so many years of having been "toilet trained." Describe what other patients have said about the experience and what they did to maintain their self-esteem. (One man continued to work driving trucks on long-haul runs and dealt with the expected fecal "accidents" with humor. Many patients would not have the ego strength to take this approach.) If there are current support groups meeting in which one or more members have dealt with the problem of fecal incontinence, suggest that the patient may find it helpful to participate.

Assist in working through measures to offer greater control of the incontinence and more satisfactory management of incontinence episodes.

If the diarrhea will be of a known duration (e.g., it will stop within *x* amount of time after radiation or antimetabolite therapy is over), note that this is a temporary condition (but do not be specific about the length of time or underestimate it!).

Disturbance in sexual relations

See section on Sexuality in this chapter.

Faulty hand washing

Stress the importance of careful hand washing after each bowel movement and after handling of soiled linen because of vulnerability to infection at this time. (See section on Vulnerability to Infection in this chapter.)

If patient or care giver has never had instruction in safe hand washing techniques, give instructions or demonstrate. Identify soaps or detergents that would be most effective. If needed, ask for a return demonstration.

Evaluation   Patient response to nursing intervention can be evaluated according to:

Reports of status of the diarrhea and its management in the requirements of daily living, including funds for and availability of supplies

Reports of ability to stay on low residue diet, maintain fluid intake at the needed level and, if needed, increase the amount of high potassium foods without increasing residue

Reported strategies for handling any episodes of fecal incontinence and the patient's related emotional status

Reported comfort and safety in managing laundering of fecally stained garments and linen

Reported status of relationship with sexual partner and of any problems in sexual relationsips associated with the presence of diarrhea

Status of observed fluid and electrolyte balance (observed through laboratory data and physical signs)

Absence of fecally based infections

Living With Fatigue

Fatigue, like anorexia, is often an initial and ongoing symptom of cancer. It is exacerbated during periods of active treatment as well as in advancing neoplasia.

Medical Perspective

The medical perspective on fatigue tends to be related to its pathophysiologic significance. It may also be viewed in terms of the effect it has on the capacity of the patient to participate in further medical treatment or monitoring activities. Treatment may be directed toward identified underlying causes, such as anemia or altered electrolytes.

Nursing Perspective

The nursing perspective on fatigue relates to:

Specific areas of diminished personal energy levels for meeting the physical, emotional, social, and cognitive requirements in daily living

Specific problems in daily living arising from these diminished capacities

Daily living requirements or environmental barriers that place extra demands on limited energy resources

Access to support systems to assist with the requirements of daily living

Nursing's focus for diagnosis and management addresses problems in managing the individual's and family's requirements in daily living as effectively and comfortably as possible in the presence of current or predicted energy deficits.

Nature of Fatigue

Fatigue is a directly experienced state. It is a normal response to use of energy. Problems tend to arise when it extends over periods of time. Fatigue can range in severity from mild lassitude to utter exhaustion. Manifestations of fatigue include:

Subjective complaints of weakness, tiredness, lack of energy, weariness, lassitude, exhaustion, drowsiness, disrupted sleeping patterns, tiredness on awakening, dullness, becoming tired when thinking or talking, and difficulty in concentrating, planning, and making decisions and complaints that "eating is a chore"

Observable manifestations of pallor, increased sighing, decreased smiling, decreased attention, apathy, lack of enjoyment of previously enjoyed experiences, increased forgetfulness, decreased caring about or ignoring of things that were previously important, irritability, shallow respirations, making more mistakes than usual, decreased initiative, worrying, tearful episodes, slower speech responses, short answers, dull tone of voice, progressive anxiety, antisocial behavior, tendency toward depression, and anorexia (Aistars, 1987; Billings, 1986)

Daily living can increase fatigue. Patterns of daily living or requirements that increase fatigue include:

Distress over disruption in daily living associated with the patient's current and projected energy deficits

Environmental and architectural features that require use of more energy

Role requirements and demands of others that exceed energy resources of the patient

The unavailability of people to give needed assistance

Deficits in needed support services (e.g., transportation, shopping, equipment, supplies)

Fatigue can affect daily living. Daily living tasks requiring physical strength and stamina, cognitive tasks, and work and social obligations must be adjusted in order to accommodate changes in energy levels. Relationships can also be altered by low energy.

Underlying Mechanisms

Pathophysiologic and Iatrogenic Factors

The pathophysiologic factors that underlie fatigue in cancer are complex, interactive, and currently poorly understood. Fatigue frequently precedes and accompanies the diagnosed presence of malignant neoplasia (Theologides, 1982). It accompanies all of the cancer therapies.

Tumor-Related Factors

Malignant neoplasms can cause:

Metabolites (lactate, hydrogen ions, and end products of cell destruction) to accumulate (Piper et al, 1987; Taylor, 1987)

Marked increases in Cori cycle activity (anaerobic gluconeogenesis that uses more than normal amounts of energy and produces more lactate) (Young, 1977)

Muscle force to be impeded by the hydrogen ions produced as lactate accumulates (Karlsson et al, 1981; Nakamura and Schwartz, 1972)

Degradation of skeletal muscle related to protein imbalances, caused by altered protein metabolism, protein losses, and tumor need for increased glucose (Lopes et al, 1983)

Increased metabolic rate as growing tumors burn more calories (DeWys, 1982; Knox, 1983)

Altered neurotransmission and force of muscle contractions. This occurs with fluid and electrolyte abnormalities, which are associated with the disease processes and nutritional deficits (Akerstedt et al, 1982).

Changes in oxygenation and reduced oxygen carrying capacity of the blood when hemoglobin drops to low levels

Fluid and electrolyte imbalances, hypercalcemia, hyperuricemia, hyponatremia, and hypokalemia. These occur with particular tumors and alter neurotransmission and muscle contractions (see above).

Other manifestations associated with the cancer that may compound fatigue include nausea and vomiting, diarrhea, pain, dyspnea, muscle spasms, and itching (Piper et al, 1987). Sleep disruption may contribute to fatigue (Hauri et al, 1985).

Anxiety, hopelessness, and grief can affect energy levels, just as lower energy levels can, in turn, depress psychologic responses (Britton, 1983; Piper et al, 1987).

Sensory underload from home and treatment setting environments as well as changes in the person's mobility can create inadequate sensory stimulation of the reticular activating system. One manifestation of this reduced stimulation can be fatigue (Aistars, 1987).

Diagnostic Tests

Persons who undergo medical diagnostic testing during the active treatment stage encounter activities and stressors that engender fatigue through disruption of eating and elimination patterns in preparation for tests as well as through the discomforts of the actual procedures. News that the response to treatment is not encouraging can cause feelings of increased anxiety or depression, which further engender fatigue.

Surgery

Many aspects of surgery may be synergistic in producing fatigue. These include sedation, anesthesia, decreased ventilation, inadequate normal sleep cycles, analgesia, restricted nutrition and mobility, the physical trauma produced by the surgery itself, plus the continuing effects of underlying disease before and after the surgery (Rhoten, 1982)

Chemotherapy

Fatigue is a major iatrogenic effect associated with chemotherapy. Cell destruction end products, nausea, and vomiting are thought to be contributors. Drugs that cross the blood–brain barrier and those that have neurotoxic properties may affect neurotransmission and thus produce fatigue (Piper et al, 1987).

Radiation

Fatigue is also a major problem with radiation (Haylock and Hart, 1979). The specific mechanism is not known, but possible explanations are the accumulation of cell destruction end products together with the increased metabolic rate needed to dispose of them, toxic metabolites that inhibit cell functioning, anemia from the shortened life of erythrocytes, or the body's mechanism to slow down activity in order to conserve energy (Haylock and Hart, 1979). Another factor compounding fatigue may be the energy demands involved in making the daily trip to the health care setting for the treatments over a period of 4 to 5 weeks (Hilderly, 1987).

Biologic Response Modifiers

Biologic response modifiers have fatigue as a consistent side-effect. The fatigue is not dose dependent, but is cumulative and is sufficient to affect the capacity of the individual to carry out activities of daily living (Mayer and Smalley, 1983).

Daily Living Factors

Any degree of energy deficit affects the managing of requirements of daily living. Conversely, many aspects of the activities, events, and demands in daily living, as well as barriers in the institutional or home environment, can create demands on already compromised energy levels. When fatigue is extreme the external resources of people and services become crucial to effective management of daily living. The perspective on the patient's daily living thus also involves concern about the daily living and status of support figures—their interest, availability, and physical and emotional capacities, their staying power in the valley times as well as in the good times.

Activities in Daily Living	Physically demanding activities in daily living, mental activities requiring concentration (e.g., balancing the checkbook, filling out the income tax, and preparing shopping lists), and emotion-laden activities (e.g., interaction with family members or health care providers and social situations) that may be stressful all are areas for nursing assessment when energy is low.

Events in Daily Living

Events in daily living that consume energy and can contribute to fatigue include:

> Personal and social events requiring extra energy expenditure for personal grooming, travel, social interaction, food preparation, or eating

> Medical events that physiologically cause further energy depletion; create stress, anxiety, or depression; or require energy expenditure for preparation, waiting, travel, or interaction with multiple health care workers

> Past events whose memories create depression or anxiety (e.g., losses, past chemotherapy experiences)

> Anticipation of future events that create stress and anxiety (e.g., waiting for the next bone marrow test to determine the status of cells) or signs of separations or future losses

Demands in Daily Living

Self-expectations: These demands can involve the person's self-requirement to maintain, modify, or relinquish usual patterns of grooming, home maintenance, and family, work, and social role obligations.

Expectations of others: Others may expect the patient to either continue or be released from previous standards, role activities, role behaviors, and relationships. Institutions may demand that the patient be involved in activities that require energy expenditures (e.g., participation in preventive or rehabilitative activities following treatment, or self-care activities such as pulmonary hygiene or ostomy care).

Possessions: Possessions such as pets, car, home, or yard make demands for expenditure of energy.

Environment for Daily Living

The institutional, home, or work environment may generate sensory underload or overload, stressors, or immobilization, thus contributing to fatigue.

The person's environment may compound fatigue by requiring extra expenditure of energy to accomplish activities in daily living (e.g., stairs, distances, lack of facilities or conveniences, and difficult terrain).

Values and Beliefs

Personal values play an important role in managing daily living with fatigue. Some previously held standards for self-care and home maintenance can no longer be maintained because they require energy expenditures beyond one's currently available resources. Previously held and valued social roles, control over lifestyle, and goals that require energy expenditure may all be in jeopardy during cancer treatment.

Societal beliefs that can affect energy expenditure include those dealing with patient obligations to maintain, modify, or relinquish role obligations during illness or treatment. These can be particularly troublesome when no visible signs of illness are present or when energy levels wax and wane over prolonged periods of time during the course of chemotherapy.

Functional Health Status

Functional capacities for meeting the requirements of daily living when fatigue is a problem include physical strength and endurance, cognition, sexuality, and emotions.

Strength and Endurance

Fatigue associated with cancer and its treatment affects one's capacity to engage in physical, mental, and emotional work and one's endurance to meet the required activities in daily living. Difficulties can be identified by balancing the patient's present and predicted energy status, based on pathophysiology, iatrogenic factors, and emotional status, with the identified requirements in the person's daily living in the present and future.

Cognition

Managing daily living with fatigue requires the capacity to understand (at the application level):

The causes of and predicted pattern for fatigue in the presenting situation

Strategies for managing stressors, sensory environment, activities, demands, and environmental features in order to keep them within the current and predicted energy levels

The usefulness of noting patterns of high and low energy levels as a basis for planning activities and treatments

The value to one's morale of investing energy to have at least one valued experience each day

Strategies for conserving energy within one's particular environment and daily living requirements

Strategies for mobilizing and maintaining external resources to cover tasks one no longer has the energy to perform

| | Interpersonal skills needed to renegotiate roles to make them congruent with current and anticipated levels of energy |

Sexuality   Depressed energy in the absence of other symptoms can decrease interest in sexual activity. This can, in turn, create stresses between the partners.

Emotions   Functional capacity can be affected by the patient's usual moods of optimism or pessimism in stressful and nonstressful times and by the moods in the present situation.

External Resources for Managing Daily Living With Fatigue

Fatigue can interfere with meeting even the basic requirements of daily living. Therefore, the status of availability, acceptability, and usability of external resources in the forms of people and services is an important consideration.

People   The availability of others to assist the patient may be determined by asking:

What support persons are available?

What is the status of their physical and emotional strength and endurance?

Do they have a working knowledge of helping strategies in the presenting situation?

Services   Support services may be assessed with the following questions:

Are transportation and other energy-conserving services available, and does the person have sufficient financial resources to purchase these services?

What types of services will the patient and family accept?

Nursing Diagnosis and Treatment

Diagnostic Targets   Targets for diagnosis and treatment include not only the person who has the cancer, but also those care givers who may be called on to provide support services (e.g., nurses, family members, or other care givers).

Risk Factors   There are increased risks of difficulty in managing daily living because of fatigue for the person who:

Has neoplasia with an early and high incidence of fatigue (e.g., leukemia, mediastinal lymphomas)

Receives aggressive medical treatment

Has complications such as infection, anemia, vomiting, or diarrhea

Has many physical, mental, and emotional demands in daily living (e.g., the need to continue working in or out of the home during treatments)

Lives or works in environments containing barriers to energy conservation (e.g., stairs, long distances from the bedroom to the kitchen or bathroom or from the clinic entryway to the treatment room)

Lacks available support figures

Lacks financial resources to purchase services

Lacks private transportation services; must travel long distances to public transportation

Is depressed or hopeless; has given up

*Diagnostic
Areas** Inability to meet (specified) requirements of daily living R/T specific changes in physical, mental, or emotional strength and endurance

Ineffective planning for meeting daily living requirements with reduced energy R/T lack of understanding about the basis for the fatigue and its usual pattern during the treatment phase

Exacerbated fatigue R/T (specified) elements in daily living that create excessive energy demands

Ineffective energy conservation R/T (specified) environmental barriers (home, institutional, or work)

Ineffective management of (specified) requirements in daily living R/T deficits in the availability or usability of support persons and services

Ineffective management of the requirements of daily living R/T lack of knowledge regarding options and strategies for keeping requirements within energy resources

Disturbed interpersonal relationships R/T lack of understanding of the impact of fatigue on communication patterns and priorities

Neglect of specific, crucial aspects of daily living R/T inadequate energy (e.g., failure to eat or take in fluids, take care of monetary matters, maintain hygiene, prevent infections, monitor oneself, or keep health care appointments)

Exhaustion, frustration, fear, or anxiety R/T constraints that make it impossible for the patient to be relieved from work and home responsibilities during the course of treatment

Disrupted relationships with sexual partner R/T lack of energy for or interest in meeting partner's sexual needs (see section in this chapter on Sexuality)

---

* Many of these diagnoses can apply to the care giver as well as to the patient.

Manifestations	Failure to manage daily living in the face of fatigue may be manifested in a variety of ways, including:

Deterioration in appearance, grooming, hygiene

Weight loss

Apathy

Disinterest and reduced participation in decision making regarding activities in daily living and health care

Flattened affect

Reduced or less animated speech, more mumbling

Increased sighing and respiratory rate

Decreased smiling

Episodes of tearfulness

Irritability

Progressive anxiety

Failure to engage in prescribed treatment regimen

Failure to keep appointments

Increased need for sleep and rest

Increased preference for quiet environment

Increased preference for being alone

Concern about family and work obligations

Concern about relationships with important others

These manifestations may appear in the patient, but also may become apparent in care givers who begin to burn out.

Prognostic Variables	Poor prognosis for managing daily living effectively with fatigue is associated with:

Prolonged periods of severe low energy

Hopelessness

Sensory underload or overload

Environmental barriers to energy conservation

Lack of support persons to provide needed services

Lack of transportation

Lack of money to purchase services

The need to continue to work or maintain home responsibilities during treatment

Complications	When fatigue is sufficient to interfere with carrying out the basic requirements of daily living, such as eating, participating in treatment regimens, self-monitoring for side-effects of treat-

ments and changes in health status, and performing hygiene to prevent infections, the person's health is in greater jeopardy. A downward spiral in participation in maintaining one's well-being can ensue. Depression is a risk. Disruption of relationships with support persons can also be a complication.

Treatment
Guidelines

Where fatigue is a problem, nursing treatment deals with several major factors. These include reducing fatigue-exacerbating elements in daily living, modifying activities and demands in daily living to reduce energy expenditure, modifying demands and role obligations to conform to energy levels, scheduling activities in accordance with documented highs and lows of energy, modifying the environment to reduce energy demands, mobilizing external resources to take over some activities and support the patient's energy levels, legitimizing behavioral or emotional responses to low energy, and helping to structure self and others' expectations to be congruent with the pattern of energy and its manifestations.

Changes in functioning related to reduced strength and endurance that negatively affect areas in daily living

Gather data on:

Specific areas of changed functioning the patient is experiencing (physical, mental, and emotional)

Daily patterns of high and low energy

Critical areas of daily living being affected by the changed functioning (physical, cognitive, and interpersonal tasks) and the value they have for the patient and others who are closely involved

Explore options (at the hospital or at home) to:

Alter the timing of activities from low to higher energy times

Omit or reduce the frequency of lower priority activities

Utilize possible shortcuts

Obtain assistance in completing some tasks

Build in greater flexibility in scheduled activities

Plan for rest intervals within and between tasks (determine the amount of time needed for restoration of energy after particular activities)

Alternate tasks requiring high and low energy

Assist the patient (and care giver), as needed, to plan a schedule that makes acceptable alterations in patterns in daily living based on the data on requirements, patterns of energy, opportunities for rest, and sources of assistance. Negotiate for a trial period and an opportunity to give feedback on its effectiveness and satisfaction with outcomes. Modify the plan based on subsequent evaluation.

Lack of understanding of basis for fatigue and its duration

Gather data on the status of the patient's understanding of the reason for the fatigue being experienced and expectations regarding trajectory and duration.

Offer information on the possible physiologic and psychologic explanations for fatigue. Point out its legitimacy in the presenting situation and describe the usual trajectory of energy level associated with the particular form of therapy and pathology. (Note: Some patients require 12 to 16 months to recover energy, and 37% to 56% of patients may not recover their previous energy levels [Cella and Tross, 1986; Fobair et al, 1986]).

Offer contacts with other patients and family members who have experienced comparable energy deficits and energy requirements in the same treatment situation as a means of reducing the sense of aloneness and as a possible source of options for managing daily living.

Fatigue-exacerbating factors in daily living (hospital or home)

Gather data on frustrating or irritating experiences in patterns of daily living. Examine patient situation for sensory underload or immobilizing features (e.g., radiation implants, protective isolation, living alone) that may increase sense of fatigue and boredom. Examine for sensory overload (e.g., hospital noises, constant activity in the patient's hospital room, children playing in the home, radio or TV programs chosen by others that distress the patient).

Reduce sensory underload or overload situation or help patient to develop strategies for doing so.

Help patient and others, as needed, to develop and test strategies to reduce frustration, irritation, and stress in presenting situations.

Environmental barriers to energy conservation

Gather information on distances to bathroom, laundry, bedroom, and stairs, and availability of conveniences for cooking, laundry, and personal and home maintenance in patient environment; in the hospital, note placement of needed articles and food, and distance to bathroom versus commode.

Help the patient to develop temporary or long-term options for removing or circumventing barriers (e.g., moving the bed to another location, using a commode, relocating supplies or equipment). Encourage the patient to plan ahead so that one trip can accomplish several tasks.

Lack of available support persons

Explore preferences in accepting or recruiting assistance from others. Identify individuals who might be available and acceptable as sources of help. Propose other possible resources (e.g., chore services, church or club members, friends, and neighbors). Engage the health care system or other bureaucracies to provide help.

Difficulty managing tasks within energy resources

Encourage self-monitoring for signs of increasing fatigue during activities, and taking of rest periods when needed. In hospital, check with patient regarding energy levels and try to adjust schedule to accommodate changes in patterns and levels of energy.

Encourage patient to schedule heavier tasks during predicted times of higher energy.

Propose trying to get more done on the "good" days and then easing back on the "down" days.

Encourage patient to think of the least energy-demanding approach to each task (e.g., sitting instead of standing when tasks permit this, omitting the nice but unnecessary steps, and thinking ahead to combine tasks where possible).

Praise the patient for working "smart" instead of working "hard." Begin to set this pattern during hospitalization.

Disrupted interpersonal relationships related to fatigue

Indicate to patient that it is quite normal to be more easily irritated, angry, or tearful in the presence of fatigue.

Help patient to develop scripts (planned verbal approaches) for alerting others when fatigue is likely to create interpersonal stresses. Train care givers to observe for cues of rising fatigue.

Help patient and care givers to develop strategies for structuring presenting situations when fatigue threatens to become disabling or disruptive.

Legitimize the patient's behavior to key family members and explore ways in which they can make daily living encounters easier for the patient and themselves within the normal dynamics of their family. (For example, "Irritability, changed communication patterns, and crying are normal symptoms of fatigue and are the result of the treatment or the disease. Therefore, these manifestations should be viewed in the same way one would view sneezing with a cold. They are the product of the disease or treatment, not a personal attack.")

Neglect in self-care that threatens health status

Identify the areas of self-neglect that are most threatening to the person's health and well-being.

Explore the reasons why these activities are not being carried out in order to rule out factors other than fatigue (e.g., not valuing the activities, wanting to die, not having money for them, having other priorities, or not having support from the family to engage in the activities).

When the major factor in self-neglect is lack of energy:

Explore scheduling options that may enable the activities to be undertaken during times of higher energy. Ask or help the patient to develop a tentative schedule of self-care or monitoring activities for a designated trial period. Set a time for feedback and modify as needed or as circumstances change.

Explore the possibility of recruiting support persons to assist in self-care and monitoring, or relieving the person of other tasks so that self-care is possible.

Continuation of work and home care responsibilities during active treatment

Explore any possible energy-saving and rest possibilities that may be possible under the circumstances (e.g., a ride to and from work as opposed to public transportation, food preparation short cuts, a place to lie down during breaks and lunch periods, or resting at home before the evening meal).

Explore the possibility of cutting out as many noncrucial activities as possible to increase rest time for the duration of the treatment and immediate post-treatment period.

Evaluation
PATIENT

Response to nursing treatment can be evaluated in terms of the following factors:

Appearance, movement, and patterns of speaking

Reported satisfaction with meeting requirements of daily living (home and work), interpersonal relationships

Patterns of self-care and self-monitoring related to the treatment regimen

Existence of ongoing or new problems associated with low energy

FAMILY

Reports on:

Their own energy level in relationship to the requirements of daily living

Satisfaction with management of their interpersonal relationships with the patient as these have been affected by fatigue

Status of their management of patient self-care and home maintenance

---

Living With Vulnerability to Infection

One of the side-effects of certain neoplasms, advanced neoplastic disease, and treatment of malignancies is an increased vulnerability to infection. Infections can be the first indication of a cancer and are a major concern during active treatment.

Medical Perspective

The medical perspective focuses on both immunosuppression and infection. With chemotherapy, neutropenia is produced by the therapy and can be used as a measurement of body response to the therapy. At the same time, there is concern with minimizing the risk of infections during high risk periods, monitoring for the earliest signs of infection, and providing the most effective treatment to resolve the infectious process, reduce morbidity, and avoid mortality.

Nursing Perspective

Nursing's focus for diagnosis and treatment addresses the knowledge, functional capacity, and environmental resources the patient and family need in order to:

Manage activities in daily living and the environment to minimize the risk of infection

Recognize the earliest manifestations of infection

Communicate effectively about signs and symptoms with the health care system

Manage the medical treatment regimen and requirements of daily living in the presence of infections

Nature of Vulnerability to Infection

Daily living with increased vulnerability to infection involves:

Altered host resistance associated with some types of neoplasia, with advanced cancers, and with some forms of medical treatment

Altered manifestations of infection, in that the classical signs and symptoms of infection are muted or initially absent

Altered course of infection with rapid movement to full-blown, often life-threatening pathology

Host capacity to observe, recognize, and report earliest manifestations of infections

Activities and environments in daily living that bring added risk of infection or can reduce the risks

Host or family capacity to engage in activities to reduce infection risks in daily living

Alterations in lifestyle associated with reducing risks of infection that reduce the quality of life

Host or family capacities and resources for integrating the treatment of the infection into daily living

Underlying Mechanisms

Pathophysiologic and Iatrogenic Factors

Vulnerability to infection is increased by several host factors. It is also affected by some forms of oncologic treatment.

Tumor-Related Factors

Certain neoplasias (e.g., Hodgkin's disease) are associated with abnormalitites of cell-mediated immunity, which is related to increased risk of infections involving intracellular pathogens (e.g., herpes zoster, infection with *Cryptococcus neoformans*) (Robichaud and Hubbard, 1987).

Advanced neoplasms (e.g., lung cancer and brain tumors) seem to decrease sensitivity and ability to respond to the challenging antigen, causing the host to fail to mobilize body defenses (Armstrong et al, 1971; Pitot, 1986).

Leukemias and several lymphomas infiltrate bone marrow and alter production of mature granulocytes, leading to impaired phagocytosis.

A decrease or alteration in circulating globulin of host origin, seen in some lymphomas and leukemias, increases susceptibility to bacterial infections (Armstrong et al, 1971).

Tumor progression may create ulcerations of skin or mucous membranes, creating new portals for entry of organisms.

Nutrition

Anorexia is an early and often recurring feature of neoplastic disease, decreasing the intake of carbohydrates and protein needed to maintain the immune system (Nixon et al, 1980). Cancer-related nausea and vomiting may further reduce infection-fighting resources of the host.

Tumors take priority in using glucose for their own growth. With low carbohydrate and protein intake, glucose stores become depleted and body reserves of protein are drawn upon (Groenwald, 1987).

Losses of protein-rich exudate occur through cancer-caused ulcers; fistulas and cancers of the gastrointestinal tract can further reduce resources for production of immunosuppressive elements in the patient.

Age

Predictable and characteristic immunodeficiency is associated with aging (e.g., T lymphocytes are less mature and the ratio of

T helper cells to suppressor cells is increased; B lymphocytes are significantly decreased in both number and differentiation) (Goldman, 1986; Jeppeson, 1986; Weksler, 1981).

Infection-Related Factors

Earlier or current infections can result in immunosuppression through depression of lymphocytic and monocytic functioning, making the person more vulnerable to other infections (Robichaud and Hubbard, 1987).

Viruses such as those causing AIDS, influenza, and infectious mononucleosis; bacterial infections such as tuberculosis and bacterial pneumococcus; and fungal infections such as candidiasis and coccidiomycosis also can make the individual vulnerable to other infections (Gold and Armstrong, 1984).

Antibiotics used to combat infections create imbalances in the internal environment, permitting normally innocuous organisms to grow and create infections.

Surgery

Surgery and associated treatment activities create new, abnormal portals for pathogens to enter the body (e.g., surgical incisions, intubation, injections, catheters, and infusions). Unclean respiratory equipment and indwelling urinary catheters also increase infection risks.

Surgical removal of lymph glands and channels, as with mastectomy, or splenectomy can compromise resistance to infection in a local area, such as the arm on the side of the mastectomy or the entire body in the case of splenectomy.

Exposure to the hospital staff and the pathogen-loaded environment of the hospital during the surgical experience creates additional infection hazards. Almost half of infecting organisms are acquired during hospitalization (Pizzo, 1981).

Radiation and Chemotherapy

Infection is the leading cause of death associated with radiation and chemotherapy.

Tissue trauma—moist desquamation or ulceration in skin and destruction of layers of mucous membranes—predisposes to infection.

Granulocytopenia, which may be associated with the effect of radiation and chemotherapy on the most rapidly reproducing cells in the host hematopoietic system, decreases the number of granulocytic cells available to resist infections. The lower the absolute neutrophil count, the greater the risk of infection. Counts of less than 500 indicate extreme risks for infection, but counts of 500 to 1000 still indicate serious risks. The greatest risk of infection associated with chemotherapy occurs 7 to 14 days after each course of therapy, when the neutrophil count is the lowest.

Normal barriers, such as flow of body fluids in some normal portals, may be reduced by radiation and chemotherapy, allowing pathogens to enter or flourish (e.g., reduction and thickening of saliva and incidence of parotitis and dental disease).

Infection risks can be linked to length of time since last radiation treatment, dose, and site (e.g., lung radiation carries higher risk of infection than does breast radiation)

Altered Manifestations of Infection
The classical local manifestations of infection—heat, redness, swelling, and tenderness—observed in the nonimmunosuppressed can be muted or absent in the immunosuppressed because of the absence of or decreased number of granulocytes (Robichaud and Hubbard, 1987). The course of the infection may be devastatingly rapid and severe. Infections that are normally rather innocuous can quickly become full-blown and life-threatening in the immunosuppressed.

Altered Capacity to Observe
At times the tumor or the treatment decreases the physical or mental capacity of the individual to attend to or observe the prodromal manifestations of beginning infections.

Daily Living Factors

Many aspects of daily living are affected by the person's increased vulnerability to infection. Conversely, activities in daily living and the environment in which daily living occurs can affect the incidence of infections. Functional capacities involving strength and endurance, flexibility, sense organs (e.g., eyes, ears, touch) and body sense (attention to body signals), cognition, and motivation can be factors influencing infection-reducing and self-monitoring behavior. The behavior of family members, sexual partners, and those in social and work-related situations can be influential.

Activities in Daily Living
During active treatment, medical treatment activities increase the possibility of exposure to contaminated equipment and persons who may be a source of infection (e.g., health care providers and other institutional workers, and other patients).

Daily activities bring patients into contact with family members, close associates, and persons in public transportation, stores, and churches, who may be sources of infection.

Infection is a risk in activities concerned with food shopping and preparation, laundry, hand washing, oral hygiene, and any activities increasing risk of skin breaks or trauma (e.g., gardening, sewing, use of tools, playing with or caring for animals or birds).

Events in Daily Living
Infection risks are increased by encounters with people (e.g., social events such as meetings, dinners, church services, parties) and animals, who may transmit pathogens, and by travel in

which one encounters people in close proximity in enclosed spaces or goes to unfamiliar geographic areas and is exposed to endogenous organisms to which one has not developed resistance). In patients with low neutrophil counts, even spores on cut flowers or plants and organisms in soil can pose a danger.

Demands in Daily Living

Stress may be linked to alterations in immune response. It may be produced by demands on the patient that exceed the supply of physical and emotional energy (Riley et al, 1981). Demands in daily living may also increase exposure to pathogens.

Self-expectations that may affect occurrence of infections include the setting of standards for home making, social and job performance, or care giving to others that exceed energy levels or increase exposure to communicable diseases in others; sexual behavior; lack of self-expectations for maintaining necessary personal hygiene and cleanliness in the environment.

Expectations of others that increase infection risks include role obligations to give care to others who have infectious illnesses (e.g., children, aging parents, ailing spouse); expectations of sexual partner for activities that increase infection risks; the need to travel at frequent intervals for treatment; participation in seasonal social demands (e.g., traditional holiday activities); and work demands.

Demands of possessions include maintenance of pets or livestock, home, yard, or car when others are not available to assist. These activities may place demands for energy that is not available or may expose the patient to trauma or pathogens.

Environment for Daily Living

Environmental factors that are important when vulnerability to infection exists include:

Protective barriers (e.g., masks, gowns, gloves, laminar air flow) or the lack of them

Access to effective hand washing and bathing facilities (in institutional and home setting)

Access to laundry facilities (hot water, clean equipment, and appropriate laundry products)

Heating or cooling equipment in the home that is functional and does not foster spread of organisms

Adequate food preparation facilities for washing, cooking, and refrigeration of foods to remove and prevent growth of organisms

Presence of plants, soil, cut flowers, pets, or vermin in the home as sources of pathogens

General cleanliness of the living environment (institutional or home)

Values and Beliefs

Values and beliefs that can affect daily living with vulnerability to infection include:

Status of belief in germs as a cause of infections

Belief in the efficacy of medical advice and care in the prevention and treating of infections

Beliefs about the merits of home and ethnic remedies in the prevention and treating of infections

Belief in one's obligation to continue to engage in behaviors that may increase infection risks

Value and priority assigned to personal hygiene

Valuing of control over lifestyle, self-care, treatment, and personal independence as it affects willingness to make adaptations to reduce infection risks

Valuing of survival

Functional Health Status

Strength and Endurance

Compromises can occur in physical strength, mobility, and flexibility needed to engage in personal hygiene, home maintenance, and food preparation activities needed to reduce infection risks, maintain optimum health, and permit self-monitoring for infections on an ongoing basis.

Cognition

The capacity to learn and apply knowledge needed to resist infections and sense earliest manifestations of infection is a critical function. The patient and family need to:

Understand what has happened to the patient's immune system and the implications these changes have for daily living, including risk factors and preventive measures

Be aware that classical early signs and symptoms of infection will be absent, and know the subtle symptoms that may be indicative of an infection in the immunosuppressed patient (e.g., increased lassitude, further loss of appetite—"just not feeling good")

Have the command of the language needed to recognize and report changes in status in a credible style

Know when and how to reach the health care personnel who will be most responsive to their situation

Motivation

Usual patterns of either giving serious attention to or discounting body signals and subtle symptoms (which now may be critical early indicators of infection) and the corollary—usual patterns of either seeking prompt medical attention for body changes or letting nature take its course in hopes that the

problem will go away, are an important functional consideration.

Nursing Diagnosis and Treatment

Diagnostic
Targets

Targets for nursing diagnosis include the patient and others,
who either expose the patient to increased numbers of pathogens or can reduce risk of infection by their behavior (e.g.,
health care providers, care givers, family members, close associates, sexual partners, and institutional or work setting personnel).

Risk Factors

Patients at risk of having difficulty in managing daily living with
increased vulnerability to infection are those who:

Have a white blood cell count of less than 2000 or an absolute
neutrophil count of less than 500 (even a count of 500 to
1000 presents serious risks of infection)

Have breaks in their skin or mucous membranes or have
abnormal body openings

Have leukemia or lymphomas

Are elderly

Have critical areas of dysfunction that limit effective participation in self-care, self-monitoring, or communicating
changes in their body status to appropriate health care providers (e.g., limitations in vision, body flexibility, cognition,
body sense)

Live in an environment where there is poor access to facilities
for maintaining cleanliness of self, clothing, bedding, towels
(e.g., water, water heating facilities, and laundry facilities)

Live in substandard, unclean, or verminous housing

Lack a phone in the home to contact the health care system

Lack consistent, competent primary care givers (if they are
unable to care for themselves)

Have a cultural background that does not incorporate belief
in pathogens as a cause of illness

Have a pattern of underutilizing health care services (e.g., "I
don't like to bother the doctor with little complaints, he's so
busy"; "Things have a way of taking care of themselves"; "As
God wills")

Diagnostic
Areas

Ineffective reduction of infection risks in daily living R/T:

Lack of understanding of immune status patterns and reasons
for need to alter lifestyle and environment

Lack of data on the current neutrophil count

Lack of understanding of areas in daily living requiring alteration to reduce infection risks and the nature of those alterations

Lack of (specified) resources (e.g., money, bureaucracies, policies, services) to make the (specified) alterations in daily living environment or patterns of daily living possible

(Specified) self-demands or priorities in daily living that either decrease body resistance (e.g., fatigue, nutrition) or increase high risk encounters (e.g., care of children with colds, sexual activities)

Unchangeable elements (specify) in daily living that increase infection hazards (e.g., presence of young children, specific risk elements in work, home, or school environment)

(Specified) cognitive or physical disabilities that restrict (specified) areas of participation in infection prevention or self-monitoring

Ineffective communication of significant change in body status R/T:

Unwillingness to "bother the doctor"

Lack of skills, language, communication equipment to report to the health care system

Ineffective infection control R/T (* specified) values or beliefs that interfere with infection prevention, self-monitoring, or participation in an infection treatment regimen. (* Identify the specific values or beliefs and the particular aspect of infection prevention or treatment that is affected.)

Manifestations   Manifestations of ineffective management of daily living to minimize infections or provide for early recognition and appropriate reporting include:

The presence and recurrence of infections when white blood cell count is not so low that they are unavoidable and treatment does not make them inevitable (e.g., presence of indwelling urinary catheter)

Patterns of ineffective reporting of signs and symptoms at an early stage

Inability to describe the risks and implications of normally innocuous infections or needed alterations in patterns of daily living to reduce infection risks

Absence of needed equipment (e.g., thermometer, mirrors to visualize body areas not directly viewable, and watch or clock with a second hand)

Observed or reported lack of skill in using self-monitoring equipment

Evidence of inconsistent self-monitoring (e.g., records that are not maintained or appear to have been written all at one time)

Reported or observed continuance of practices in daily living associated with increasing risks of infection:

Eating of lettuce and other raw greens

Ineffective practices in preparation of high risk foods (e.g., ineffective washing of raw vegetables and fruits; inadequate cooking time or temperature; failure to scrub surfaces, utensils, or hands after cutting or preparing raw poultry, fish, or meat)

Participation in social situations with high risks of infection (e.g., crowded rooms, association with people with colds, eating at sushi bars)

Wearing of contaminated clothing (self or care givers, including professionals)

Ineffective oral hygiene

Failure to wash hands after toileting and before eating, after care of wounds, and during steps of food preparation

Lack of skill in caring for abnormal body portals or breaks in skin or mucous membranes

Failure to wear masks when outside of own room while on protective isolation

Failure to ask visitors and others to wash hands and wear masks in their presence

Continued close interaction with pets

Presence of young children in the home and no alternatives for child care

High risk of infection in the work environment and no alternative work options

Cognitive disabilities that impair capacity to engage in prevention, self-monitoring, or treatment (e.g., confusion, altered level of consciousness, depression, and physical dysfunction, such as severe diarrhea, poor eyesight, restricted body flexibility and mobility, or severe fatigue)

Reported or observed behavior reflecting beliefs that attribute infections to something other than pathogens and host ability to respond to them

Prognostic Variables

Poor prognosis for managing daily living to prevent and control infections is associated with continued immunosuppression associated with the disease or treatment. Even normally innocuous endogenous pathogens become a source of infection when white blood cell counts are sufficiently low.

Poor prognosis is also associated with the presence of increasing numbers or severity of risk factors listed above.

Complications

Failure to manage daily living to prevent or control infections can result in increased morbidity and in death.

Effective management of daily living to prevent infections, in itself, can create unsatisfying changes in activities, events, environment, and personal relationships, further reducing the quality of life.

Treatment Guidelines

Lack of knowledge or understanding about infection risks and the dangers associated with infection

Provide information in language and in forms that the person finds usable. Offer input at times when the patient or care giver is most likely to be able to learn.

Where modification of the home environment seems to be needed, and verbal descriptions by the patient or family are inadequate, consider visiting the home for assessment, planning, or teaching, if this is acceptable to the patient.

Conflict between long-standing self-expectations and priorities in daily living and changes needed to decrease the patient's risk of infection

Explore the patient's and family's priorities, perceived role obligations, and valued activities that are linked to infection risks.

Explore acceptable adjustments the patient or other person (e.g., sexual partner) would be willing to try for a designated period of time.

Arrange for feedback contacts (e.g., by phone, or before or after clinic visit) in which the individual has the opportunity to evaluate the implementation of the plan and its outcomes in terms of health, and personal satisfaction with the resultant quality of life.

Adjust or refine the plan for an additional period of time and reevaluate as needed.

Lack of equipment or supplies

Gather data on equipment or supplies that are needed and those that are presently available in the patient's situation.

Mobilize resources to obtain needed equipment or supplies (e.g., teach patient or family how to obtain them or refer to social worker, local chapter of the American Cancer Society, or other community agencies for assistance).

Determine whether patient and family know how to use the equipment and supplies properly to reduce infection risks. Teach, demonstrate, and receive return demonstrations as needed.

Unchangeable elements in daily living

Where the person's living situation cannot be altered, encourage the person to take the best possible precautions and make the best, most satisfying adaptations under the circumstances. (This is similar to palliation in medical treatment.) Vary the supportive nursing treatment according to the presenting situation and external resources that can be mobilized. Almost any situation can be arranged to permit:

Effective hand washing and oral hygiene

Adequate washing and cooking of foods

Limits on contacts with adults or children who have upper respiratory infections or other infectious diseases

Limits on contacts with pets

Use of masks

Clearance of plants or flowers from the house

Cleanliness of the patient area

Restriction on activities that could result in trauma

Specific cognitive, emotional, and physical deterrents to infection control, self-monitoring, or participation in treatment regimen for existing infections

Identify (1) the specific deficits that do not permit effective infection control, self-monitoring, or participation in treatment of existing infection and (2) those activities that the patient is able to manage without assistance.

Consider the predicted duration of the deficits when planning for assistance.

Negotiate with the patient regarding the need for assistance, to gain acceptance and participation.

Explore strategies the patient may use to most comfortably incorporate activities (and care giver assistance, if needed) into patient's preferred patterns of daily living.

Assist in mobilization of other persons as needed to:

Help to monitor the patient' status according to a planned schedule in ways that are effective, and, as much as possible, acceptable to the patient

Carry out in ways that are acceptable to the patient specified activities in daily living that will reduce infection risks

Administer medications or treatments for existing infections

Diagnose and treat care giver's needs for teaching, training, and moral support.

Lack of language to recognize or report one's status

Offer verbal or written lists of quantitative values and descriptive words to the person who is to report to the health care system. Follow with examples (using the patient's own situation) of how the words and numbers can be used. Add to or revise the list as needed to incorporate language with which the reporting person is comfortable. Use checklists or analogue scales that are easy to complete.

Values or beliefs that interfere with infection prevention or self-monitoring

Recognize that values and beliefs do not change easily and do affect health-related behavior. Logic and explanations rarely effect change in strongly held values.

Mutually identify and nonjudgmentally acknowledge the values and beliefs that will influence patient, family, or care giver choices and behavior regarding infection control and treatment.

Where possible, incorporate the ideas and language of the beliefs into the infection risk reduction program and infection treatment activities. As possible, adapt the plan to incorporate the prevailing belief system.

Where the incongruence between the patient's belief system and that of the health care providers cannot be resolved and the disagreement has the possibility of creating disruption in relationships, identify the incongruence and plan on an interdisciplinary basis for consistent, therapeutic health care provider responses.

Lack of skill in making effective contact with members of the health care system

Give specific instructions about the number and extension to call, when it is best to call, the person (or backup persons) to be contacted, how to communicate in order to reach that person, how to communicate urgency, how to contact health care personnel on evenings, weekends, or holidays, and how to make oneself heard and have credibility in the system. (Note that these instructions must be tailored to take into account the norms in different clinical areas within the same health care system. Be sure to indicate the prevailing informal norms as well as the formal norms of the specific clinical area and personnel.)

Lack of confidence in managing social situations to minimize infection risks

Determine the nature of social situations involved in the pa
tient's current daily living.

Help the patient to develop a repertoire of behaviors and script
for limiting exposure to infection risks without losing the rela
tionships.

Evaluation

One cannot evaluate effectiveness of management of daily
living solely by the absence of infections. Under certain neo
plastic and treatment conditions, infections are almost inevita
ble regardless of the precautions. However, when these condi
tions are not present, the absence of infection may be a good
indicator of effective practices in daily living. Additional eval
uative data may include:

Feedback on teaching that indicates an understanding of

The risks and underlying mechanisms of infections

The elements in daily living patterns that are crucial to
prevention, and actions that can be taken to modify daily
living and the environment to make these accommoda
tions

Accurate, precise language used for self-monitoring and
reporting

Contacts with the health care system involving timely, ap
propriate, and effective reporting of infection-related situa
tions

Appearance of cleanliness: clean fingernails, hands
clothing, oral cavity, artificial orifices, or wounds

Reports of priorities and values as they affect prevention, self
monitoring, and treatment of infections

Observed effectiveness in hand washing related to eating and
toileting, and appropriate use of masks by self and visitors

Requests for assistance that give evidence of understanding of
needs related to risks of infection (e.g., transportation to
avoid riding crowded public transportation, or assistance
with shopping in the supermarket)

Descriptions of use of scripts or planned behavior to handle
interaction with high risk individuals and activities

Feedback on exploration of links between values, beliefs, and
knowledge and current health situation

Observed or reported activities in daily living or management
of the environment that reduce the risks of infection

Living With Pain During Initial Treatment

Cancer pain falls into two categories: acute and chronic. In the cancer experience *acute cancer pain* is usually associated with the treatment experience and abates when the therapy is completed and post-treatment healing has occurred. *Chronic cancer pain* is defined as pain that has been present for 6 months or more. It is usually associated with advanced cancer or post-treatment side-effects (Foley, 1987a). (See Chapters 7 and 10.) Some patients have the chronic pain of advanced cancer at the time of diagnosis, and thus may experience a combination of the acute pain associated with treatment and ongoing chronic cancer pain.

People experiencing even severe acute pain associated with initial cancer diagnostic or treatment activities tend to tolerate the pain experience remarkably well because they are sustained by the hope that the treatment will bring a positive outcome (Foley, 1987a). On the other hand, the pain experienced in the active treatment phase remains in long-term memory as a part of the person's cancer experience. It can affect interpretation and responses should acute pain occur subsequently (Coyle and Foley, 1985).

Medical Perspective

The medical perspective on pain takes on two dimensions. Pain is an important indicator in medical judgments about the patient's pathologic and pathophysiologic status—both in diagnosis of the neoplasms and in evaluation of responses to treatment. Pain management is also important in medical treatment, not only for the comfort of the patient, but also to permit the patient to participate in the treatment protocol and health care regimen in ways that give the best opportunity for a positive outcome. Medical management of pain during initial treatment usually involves the prescribing of analgesia, sometimes in combination with antianxiety or antidepressant medications.

Nursing Perspective

The nursing perspective addresses issues related to managing daily living in the presence of pain or with the prospect of pain. It can include a variety of areas and issues associated with both functioning and daily living.

Nature of the Pain Experience

The pain experience is made up of three components:

Perception of noxious stimuli: Stimuli are received by nociceptors in body tissues and organs, and transmitted by afferent myelinated or unmyelinated fibers to two neural systems within the ascending spinothalamic tract. One transmits spatial localization and sensory quality from small, defined receptor areas; the second transmits from wide fields and seems to carry diffuse autonomic and emotional components of pain to the brain stem and higher centers (Andersson, 1987; Billings, 1985; Maciewicz, 1982). The person having the experience is the arbiter of what constitutes noxious stimuli.

Interpretation of the meaning of the pain experience: The assignment of meaning to the pain experience will depend on previous experience and the context in which the pain is occurring.

Response to the pain stimuli: Pain response is composed of physiologic (sympathoadrenal, muscular, and affective responses) and behavioral components. Behavioral response to pain is learned and tends to be culture-based.

As a subjective, personal experience, pain has important properties that are central considerations for nurses in its diagnosis and management.* These properties of the pain experience influence nurses' thinking and behavior in data gathering and diagnosing of pain-related daily living and functional problems. They also serve as a rationale for nursing treatment in assisting patients and their families to manage daily living and functioning in the presence of pain and suffering.

Personal   It is the person's own pain and suffering and, as such, it cannot be physically shared. Thus, it can leave the person with an extreme sense of aloneness.

Private   It is a private, rather than a public, experience (contrast the private sensation of pain to the public sensation of light or noise). Because the stimuli are not available to others, there is a real possibility of disbelief and some risk in asking others to validate the pain experience.

In trying to enable others to vicariously grasp the nature of the pain experience, persons will often use concrete descriptive terms in hopes that they that will suggest something that the listener has experienced—a vise, a 50-pound weight, a knife or a needle, pounding waves, a scalding burn, a red-hot poker, bolts of lightning, etc.

There are no norms in pain. When the listener, by verbal or nonverbal behavior, signals doubt as to the reality of the pain or the degree of discomfort, this disbelief increases patient suffering.

Pain is often a check on what is real—"I have to pinch myself to believe this is real." When validation of that check on reality is not available, it can lead to increased anxiety, heightened awareness of the stimuli, and increased suffering.

Unitary   With pain, the whole person is involved. Pain involves physiologic, cognitive, emotional, and social responses. Failure to take a holistic perspective (i.e., focusing on the location of the pain rather than on the person experiencing the pain) can produce nontherapeutic outcomes.

Threatening   Pain threatens structural integrity, functional capacity, body image, and social abilities. Pain can threaten one's existence.

---

* The authors are indebted to the late Dr. Dorothy Crowley, professor, School of Nursing, University of Washington, for her contribution to knowledge of the properties of the pain experience.

Pain threatens one's self-concept with loss of control, limitations on functioning and the roles one can fulfill, potential decrease in ability to respond in culturally accepted ways, loss of autonomy, and perhaps loss of one's way of life and previous identity.

Pain in one person is a threat to others, reminding them of their own vulnerability. It may cause distancing in subtle or overt ways.

Health care providers' inability to control patient pain may threaten their sense of professional competence, leading to frustration and risk of subtle or overt nontherapeutic interaction with the patient.

Underlying Mechanisms

Pathophysiologic and Iatrogenic Factors

Tumor-Related Factors

Pain is not a predominant feature in most early neoplasms; however, when it does occur it can be constant and usually grows progressively more severe (Foley, 1987).

Pain associated with direct tumor involvement is the result of (Foley, 1979):

Tumor invasion of bone

Infiltration or compression of nerve roots, trunks, plexus, or other nerve structures

Occlusion of blood vessels with resultant vasospasm, venous engorgement, or tissue ischemia

Distention of pain-sensitive structures

Obstruction of the gastrointestinal tract, urinary tract, or uterus

See Table 6-5 for examples of tumor sites and types of pain.

Surgery

Incisional pain and phantom breast or limb pain accompany surgical treatment. Postoperatively, gas pains and discomfort from various tubes, dressing changes, and treatments are common. Rehabilitation to help in regaining mobility of parts affected by surgery can also cause pain.

Chemotherapy

Some chemotherapeutic agents can cause pain, primarily through biochemical injury of tissues (e.g., mouth pain with stomatitis, abdominal discomfort from intestinal response to injury to the mucosa, and local pain from extravasation of certain drugs). Chemotherapeutic agents causing neurotoxicity can result in headaches, leg pains, jaw pain, crampy abdominal pain, muscle pains, and burning pain in hands and feet. Bacte-

Table 6-5. Pain Resulting from Direct Tumor Involvement

Pathophysiology	Organs	Site of Pain	Type of Pain
Enlarging tumor, distending pain-sensitive structures	Liver	Right upper quadrant (local or diffuse), later radiates to right scapula	Vague onset, dull aching, increasingly troublesome, prevents sleep, aggravated by lying on right side or jolting movement
	Spleen	Left upper quadrant	Vague, feeling of abdominal fullness
	Kidney	Flank on affected side	Dull, aching
	Pancreas		
	Head	Early: Epigastrium Late: Radiates to right upper quadrant or dorsolumbar quadrant	Dull, intermittent Continuous, colicky, decreased by lying supine or sitting up and bending over
	Body	Epigastrium	Intense or excruciating, accompanied by vomiting, short in duration, frequent, most severe at night, relieved by sitting up and bending forward or lying on right side with knees drawn up
	Tail	Upper abdomen, radiates to back or left hypochondrial area	"Gripping," less frequent than in head or body
Occlusion of hollow viscus	Gastrointestinal tract		
	Esophagus	Epigastrium, substernum	"Heartburn"
	Stomach	Epigastrium, back, retrosternum	Vague, usually ignored, "stomach upset," feeling of fullness
	Right colon	Nonspecific	Vague, persistent
	Ureters	Flank	
	Bladder	Suprapubic region, rectum, back	
	Uterus	Pelvic area	Diffuse, crampy, progressive
	Blood vessel	Site beyond obstruction	Ischemic
Infiltration of tumor	Nerve roots, nerve trunks, plexus, other nerve structures	Local or referred	Constant, burning

Table 6-5.   Pain Resulting from Direct Tumor Involvement (*continued*)

Pathophysiology	Organs	Site of Pain	Type of Pain
	Bone	Local or referred	Dull, aching, deep, "quality of boring into the bone," worse at night, increases with size of tumor, may or may not be related to motion
		Metastatic	Constant, increasing, progressively worse during the course of the day, peaking at night
	Blood vessels		Spasms, diffuse aching, burning

rial, fungal, and viral infections, often a complication of neutropenia, can cause additional discomforts. Viral infections that currently can be neither prevented nor cured (e.g., oral or, less commonly, genital herpes or herpes zoster) can cause additional severe pain (Chapman et al, 1985).

Radiation   Radiation also causes pain through tissue destruction, with the pain being dependent on the area being irradiated and the dosage. When the radiation results in destruction of mucous membranes in parts of the gastrointestinal tract, it can lead to one or more of the following: oropharyngeal pain, painful swelling of the parotid glands, esophageal pain, abdominal cramps, local pain in the rectal area (proctitis), and excoriation of the skin in the perianal area from diarrhea. In the urinary tract, the discomfort is related to the symptoms of cystitis and urethritis. Dental caries and associated treatment can cause additional pain. Localized skin reactions in the irradiated area can range from mild erythema to moist desquamation comparable to a second-degree burn, with the associated pain.

When radiation involves lymph nodes in the cervical region, a transient myelitis may develop 2 to 3 weeks after treatment. The pain from this side-effect is that of a shocklike paresthesia radiating down the back and over the extremities when the neck is flexed. This is known as Lhermitte and McAlpine syndrome. Changing the neck position is thought to temporarily decrease the blood supply to the spinal cord (Hilderly, 1987).

Diagnostic Tests   Frequently during treatment, painful diagnostic tests such as bone marrow aspirations, spinal taps, venipunctures, and catheter placements add to the baseline level of discomfort. Even having to lie immobile for computed tomographic scans, bone or liver scans, or magnetic resonance imaging visualizations can be painful and anxiety-provoking.

Steroids   Withdrawal from steroids in the course of the treatment proto
col can result in pseudorheumatism with diffuse pain and ten
derness in muscles and joints.

Biologic   Biologic response modifiers tend to result in flulike symptoms
Response   involving the pain of headache and muscle aches plus the
Modifiers   discomfort of high fevers.

Daily Living Factors

Activities in   The activities in daily living affected by pain in the treatment
Daily Living   period depend on the location and severity of the pain, the
nature of the ongoing medical treatment, the requirements of
daily living, and the setting in which daily living is occurring.
During initial treatment, at least some of the daily living will be
taking place in the operating room, intensive care unit, surgical
unit, oncology unit, radiation room, laminar airflow room in a
bone marrow transplant unit, inside computed tomography or
magnetic resonance imaging equipment, and in outpatient
clinics. In each of these settings the activities and requirements
in daily living will be dictated primarily by a variety of health
care personnel. The pain being experienced by the patient will
tend not to change the diagnostic or treatment activity, but may
alter the effectiveness of patient participation in the activities
and requirements.

When treatment is given on an outpatient basis, the activities
in daily living to be carried out in the presence of pain will
include not only the medical regimen requirements but also any
role responsibilities at home, school, or work, and the activity
of travelling to and from the treatment site. (Activities associ
ated with eating, elimination, role obligations, and sex in the
presence of pain are discussed elsewhere in the chapter under
the headings Eating Difficulties, Diarrhea, Role, and Sexu
ality.)

Activities associated primarily with managing pain in daily
living include:

Behavior to reduce pain (e.g., positioning, moving, distrac
tions, taking analgesics)

Adjustments in the activities, events, and demands in daily
living to accommodate the pain experience

Activities involved in communicating the nature of the pain
experience to health care providers and others in such a way
as to influence their understanding and assistance in contro
ling the pain appropriately or adjusting daily living

Negotiations to adjust the role requirements of daily living to
keep them within the pain-affected capacities of the patient

Mobilization of resources to assist in managing the essential requirements and valued elements in daily living

vents in
Daily Living

Events in daily living associated with pain in the active treatment stage involve:

Medical activities that cause repeated or new pain. Past memories of painful events can increase anxiety and lower the threshold for pain in prospective repetitions of the procedures (e.g., venipunctures, bone marrow aspirations). They may even cause phobias regarding the treatment.

Medical activities that bring relief from pain

Completion of a treatment regimen, or healing that causes pain to cease

)emands in
Daily Living

Self-demands tend to involve:

Self-expectations as to the amount of pain that is accepted as tolerable, and acceptable behavioral responses to pain

The degree of participation in patient role activities in spite of pain (e.g., meeting the expectations of all of the health care providers involved in the treatment)

The degree of obligation felt to continue to participate in previous nonpatient roles or to continue treatment in the face of pain

Expectations of others tend to address:

Levels of pain that the patient is expected to tolerate

The level of pain relief that will be offered willingly

The pain-related behavior that is viewed as acceptable

The requests for pain relief that are viewed as acceptable

The adjustments that will be made in patient participation in the medical and hospital regimen on the basis of health care providers' perceptions of patient pain

The adjustments that will be made in patient participation in nonpatient role fulfillment based on others' perceptions of patient pain

'invironment
for Daily
Living

The physical and sensory environment can contribute to the effectiveness of management of pain. Sensory underload can permit or encourage the patient to focus on internal (pain) stimuli; sensory overload can jam already pain-loaded central nervous system circuitry, causing increasing disorganization and panic. Sights and sounds that are unfamiliar, threatening, frightening, or repulsive can increase anxiety, which in turn affects the response to pain. Sights and sounds that are familiar, relaxing, enjoyable, or distracting can decrease attention to pain.

Values and Beliefs

Values related to control of self, maintenance of one's identity, lifestyle, and survival all play a role in behavior to manage daily living when these valued components are threatened by the pain.

Societal and personal beliefs as to the meaning and significance of the pain will affect not only the person experiencing the pain, but the responses of others who interact with the person in pain (including health care providers).

Pain may be believed to have attributes of both retribution (associated with guilt for past activities) and salvation (redemption from past activities where guilt is felt). Such beliefs may cause the patient to endure the pain rather than seek relief (Lisson, 1987).

Societal beliefs about appropriate pain-related behavior can affect the way in which the pain experience is communicated and can cause misunderstandings when the persons in pain and those who interact with them come from different cultural backgrounds (Meinhart and McCaffrey, 1983; Mount, 1984).

Functional Health Status

Strength and Endurance

Acute pain in the active treatment phase is often accompanied by a variety of other iatrogenic responses, so that it may be impossible to attribute changes in strength and endurance to pain alone. Oropharyngeal and esophageal pain associated with side-effects of chemotherapy and radiation can reduce the capacity to chew, swallow, and talk. Anorectal pain can delay elimination.

Pain can cause fatigue and loss of sleep, which, in turn, can reduce the patient's tolerance for the pain.

Pain can and does limit desire and ability to engage in activities that increase the pain (e.g., coughing, moving, engaging in range of motion exercises, walking, or beginning to assume responsibility for self-care).

Motivation

Presence of acute, unmanaged pain can appreciably decrease the motivation to engage in activities of daily living crucial to a positive outcome (e.g., eating, mobility, or the will to survive). It can result in low priorities or interest in previously valued activities in daily living. However, in the active treatment stage, hope is a strong factor that promotes motivation to participate in activities in daily living associated with the treatment regimen.

Courage

Carrying out activities in the treatment regimen in the face of acute pain can require large amounts of courage and risk taking

Capacities for courage to face up to the requirements of daily living in the treatment phase vary among individuals.

Cognition   Cognition in the area of pain involves:

Memory of past pain and pain management

Capacity to understand the basis for the present pain and its meaning

Capacity to plan and implement strategies for managing daily living in the presence of pain

The cognitive approaches used in anticipating future painful experiences

Emotions   Anxiety, depression, and anger are emotions commonly present in individiuals experiencing cancer and its treatment. These emotions tend to heighten the suffering associated with painful experiences in the treatment phase, not only during the treatment itself, but during the period of anticipation of painful experiences.

Anxiety may be related to fear of pain, loss of control, loss of independence, being a burden, being abandoned, changes in body image, inadequate financial resources, or what the future holds.

Depression may be related to feeling hopeless or helpless, feeling alone and isolated, sensing that one's friends are withdrawing physically or emotionally, or fearing loss of previously valued roles and status.

Anger may be precipitated by unmet expectations of others, feeling that health care providers lack an appropriate sense of urgency, feeling that others do not understand or care, or believing that the situation is unfair.

Sexuality   Concern for sexuality and interest in and capacities for sexual activity can be markedly reduced by acute pain. (See section on Sexuality.)

Nursing Diagnosis and Treatment

Diagnostic Targets   The primary target for diagnosis is the person experiencing the pain. It also may become necessary to diagnose discrepancies in values and expectations between those who prescribe or administer analgesia and the patient when these discrepancies create unwarranted difficulties in daily living. Family members and companions who are frightened of the pain, inexperienced in living with someone in pain, or unskilled in participating in managing daily living with someone in pain also may need to be considered for nursing diagnosis. Failure to diagnose and treat such individuals may result in greater pain and suffering for the patient.

Risk Factors

The following factors increase the risk of difficulties in managing daily living in the presence of pain:

Anxiety, depression, and anger about the situation

The presence of multiple iatrogenic responses, including nausea and vomiting, fatigue, insomnia, and major alterations in body image

Earlier experiences of poorly managed iatrogenic pain (Howard-Ruben et al, 1987)

Expectations of severe pain experiences (Howard-Ruben et al, 1987)

Incongruence between patient's pain-related behaviors and attitudes and the attitudes and expectations of those who provide analgesia or who interact with patient in daily living where pain is a factor or issue (Mount, 1984)

Inability to communicate the pain experience effectively

Presence of concurrent, painful chronic disease (Foley, 1987)

Presence of concurrent psychiatric problems

Presence of chemical dependencies (Foley, 1987)

Daily living environments characterized by sensory under load or overload

Inaccessibility to distractions or lack of genuine interest in them

Ongoing role obligations with few options for relief

Reluctance to seek assistance from health care providers or others for fear of rejection

Fear that the limited amount of attention the patient believes that nurses, physicians, and others have allocated him will be used up if pain relief is sought and that it then might not be available if it were really needed (Lisson, 1987)

Diagnostic Areas

Inordinate anxiety/fear of anticipated painful experience R/T lack of realistic knowledge of what to expect

Inordinate suffering R/T:

Lack of understanding of the basis for the pain and the pattern it will take

Beliefs and cultural values that preclude or do not legitimize the seeking of pain relief

Ineffective communication of pain experience R/T:

Lack of vocabulary to describe experience

Pain-related behavior and communication different from what is expected or valued by those who prescribe or dispense analgesia or other comfort measures

Fear of rejection or misunderstanding by others

Fear of using up a presumed allotment of nurses' and doctor's attention and services

Belief that the pain has redemptive qualities

Ineffective management of daily living with pain R/T:

Lack of genuine diversion or distraction (sensory underload). Specify if it occurs only at a particular time (e.g., night).

Environmental sensory overload (specify nature and time elements)

Lack of respite from ongoing role obligations

Ineffective management of painful experiences R/T lack of knowledge or skill in cognitive or physical pain management options and strategies

Prognostic Variables

Poor prognosis for managing daily living with pain can be associated with:

Repeated painful treatments or iatrogenic responses

Unallayed anxiety and depression; psychoses

Loss of belief in recovery or loss of will to survive

Loss of credibility of the patient in regard to the pain experience with care providers, family, or companions

Loss of trust in health care providers' or care givers' concern over the patient's pain experience

Pre-existing painful chronic conditions

Multiple concurrent iatrogenic conditions that do not lend themselves to adequate relief

Substance abuse or dependency

Ongoing sleep deprivation

Lack of a comfortable sensory environment

Lack of adequate respite from ongoing role obligations

Complications

Ineffective management of daily living with pain in the initial treatment phase can result in failure to participate sufficiently in the treatment regimen to assure the best therapeutic out-

come. Failure to manage pain and daily living can negativel‑
affect the capacity to manage subsequent cancer pain experi‑
ences and can result in a downward spiral in patient participa‑
tion in care and in morale.

Treatment Guidelines

Nursing treatment in management of daily living and function‑
ing in the presence of pain involves using patient data to adjus‑
administration or self-medication of the prescribed analgesia i‑
such a way as to promote effective functioning and managemen‑
of the requirements of daily living. Note that nurses tend t‑
undermedicate for pain relief (Donovan, 1987). Sometime‑
nursing treatment involves negotiating with physicians to ob‑
tain adjustments in the analgesic regimen to provide mor‑
effective symptom control. It also involves adjusting the impor‑
tant or valued activities and events of daily living so that the‑
fall within the comfort time zones provided by the analgesia o‑
the times of freedom from pain. Beyond adjustments in pre‑
scribed medications and adjustments of daily living, specifi‑
nursing treatment related to acute pain will be associated wit‑
nursing diagnoses made as precise as patient data permit. Th‑
following treatment options, linked to some general diagnosti‑
categories, can be individualized according to the patient‑
particular presenting situation.

Inordinate anxiety or fear of anticipated painful experiences R/T knowledge deficit of what to expect; cognitive–behavioral options and strategies for dealing with painful experiences; or the basis for the iatrogenic pain and th‑ course it will take

Provide accurate information. This decreases uncertainty an‑
can increase patients' sense of control, since it enables them t‑
put the anticipated experiences into words that link them t‑
familiar experiences. It also permits patients to develop thei‑
own statements about the experience or to ask specific question‑
of care providers, who will give the precise information neede‑
to manage the experience (Fishman and Localzo, 1987).

Describe behavioral options for managing painful experiences‑
This gives a sense of additional control.

Provide information that centers on the sensations that will b‑
experienced. Use words that have precise meanings that lin‑
the upcoming experience to familiar sensations they have had i‑
the past (e.g., they may feel pulled or tight like a rubber band‑
cold and wet, stinging, pressure). Do not use general terms suc‑
as pain, hurt, uncomfortable, etc. (Syrjala, 1988).

Break the information about discomfort into the smallest tim‑
frames possible (Syrjala, 1988). For example, "You will feel
wet cold for a few seconds. Then you will feel a stinging sensa‑
tion for about 20 seconds. There will be about 30 seconds whe‑
you will feel nothing, then you will feel pressure for about 3‑

seconds. In the last step of the procedure you will have a feeling of pulling for about 5 seconds. The whole procedure will take about _____ minutes. I have told you the feelings you will experience and about how long they will last. In between these there will be times when you have no unusual sensations."

Suggest strategies of focusing that other patients have reported to be helpful during times of pain (Copp, 1974):

> *Counting:* Counting forward or backwards; counting objects—holes in acoustical ceilings, bricks, letters in words, flowers on the drapes, etc.

> *Repeating words or phrases:* Using control phrases—"I can make it," "I'm holding on"; intercession words—"Let it be over," "Help me"; memorized words—nursery rhymes, Bible verses, poems; repetitive words—short, nonsensical words; derisive phrases—"This is absurd"; evaluative phrases—"It's easing off," "It's almost over."

> *Thinking and visualization:* Taking the mind to a different place (e.g., thinking of what the family is doing, visualizing a pleasant place, remembering the details of a past experience)

> *Separating the mind from the body:* Putting the hurt somewhere else, denying being a part of one's body, pushing the pain away, letting the pain catch up with one

> *Distraction:* Listening to conversations, talking, watching TV, listening to the radio or tapes (Copp, 1974)

Observe for patient expressions (words) or actions that increase distress (e.g., "I can't stand it"; "I can't make it"). Teach substitution of more functional words or images (e.g., "I'm making it"; "The worst is over.") When patients become tense, suggest deep breathing and counting as they breath in and out, repeating a syllable, word, or phrase they have found helpful, or deliberate relaxation.

Touch the person to minimize the feeling of aloneness in the experience.

Talk about how well they are doing and that the procedure is going well—moving right along.

When patients are experiencing iatrogenic pain, provide information as to the basis for the pain—that it is an expected side-effect of the treatment. Indicate the pattern it will take (e.g., worse before it gets better, will disappear in about three days, will gradually get better). Indicate the analgesic and non-analgesic strategies to be used to control the sensations and manage the activities of daily living.

Ineffective communication of pain experience R/T lack of vocabulary

Help the person to find the words to describe the type of pain: its location, movement of pain, factors that make it worse or better, type of relief following analgesia, activities impaired by the pain. Follow the patients' lead in the kinds of words they feel comfortable using.

Use pain descriptor tools (for people who can read), and numbered (analogue) scales.

Communicate genuine acceptance of the reported pain experience as the patient's reality.

Fear of rejection or misunderstanding or lack of availability of time from health care professionals

Prior to the treatment that is expected to cause iatrogenic pain (e.g., surgery or treatments), indicate that the doctors and nurses expect patients to report their discomforts and that help will be given.

When patients indicate discomfort, help them to describe what they are experiencing, the problems it is creating for them, what they are doing to manage it, what has worked in the past, and what they think would help.

If pain management is important to effective participation in the treatment regimen, indicate its importance so that reporting of pain is seen as a legitimate part of the healing process.

Incongruence between acceptable pain-related behavior and communication of patient and health care provider or care giver

Gather data on the norms of pain-related behavior in the patient's family and culture.

If appropriate, describe pain-related behavior and communication that will be most effective in obtaining pain relief and needs attainment in the present health care situation.

If it is likely that the patient's pain behavior will create inconsistent or nontherapeutic responses in health care providers, write nursing orders prescribing nurse response to patient pain behavior so that there is consistency in attitude and intervention in all nursing contacts. Discuss findings and nursing treatment plan with physicians and personnel in other departments who are involved.

Ineffective management of daily living with pain R/T sensory underload

Gather data on the preferred sensory environment and comfort zone for sensory stimulation. Identify times when there is inadequate sensory diversion or distraction.

Arrange for sensory input that is desired or accepted by the patient (e.g., audio tapes, TV, videotapes; someone to read, to talk with, or to listen to; touching, stroking, or massage).

Schedule sensory stimulation for times of identified need (e.g., "the nights are so long and the pain gets worse then").

Ineffective management of daily living with pain R/T sensory overload

Gather data on aspects in the sensory environment that are creating undesirable or excessive sensory stimulation (e.g., roommate, visitors, children at home).

Identify times when sensory overload is most trying.

Negotiate with sources of sensory overload to modify input, or modify environment to reduce the amount of undesired stimuli.

Ineffective management of daily living with pain R/T lack of respite from ongoing role obligations

Identify patient's perception of current role responsibilities.

Explore options for feasible and acceptable change (e.g., delay or reduction in tasks, getting assistance).

Identify resources that patient may not have considered.

Assist in development of specific plans (if needed). Arrange for feedback.

Mobilize assistance from others in ways that are acceptable to the patient (e.g., spouse, children, other family members, or community resources).

Plan for feedback on effectiveness of plan and any ongoing problems.

Note: Acute pain can create difficulties in specific areas of daily living such as eating, elimination, roles, and sexuality. For specific diagnoses and treatment strategies, see the particular sections in this chapter.

Evaluation
Evaluation of response to nursing interventions related to management of daily living and functioning in the presence of acute pain can be made in the following areas:

Status of patient comfort in managing the requirements of daily living (e.g., participation in postoperative treatments—coughing, ambulating, engaging in range of motion activities)

Status of effectiveness of analgesic regimen (health care provider- or self-administered) in relationship to activities and events in daily living

Capacity to communicate understanding of the basis for the pain experience, the anticipated pattern of occurrence, and the place the pain experience has in normal and expected (versus unusual) context

Status of use of words to describe pain experiences that are specific and functional, rather than vague and stressing

Status of health care providers' accommodation to patient pain-related communication and behavior and resultant attitudes and behavior toward the patient and family. Status of patient credibility regarding communication of pain experience

Status of the patient's willingness to communicate the pain experience without inappropriate concern for staff work loads

Capacity to describe and evaluate strategies used to focus or distract attention during pain experiences

Status of sensory environment as it affects pain response—availability of distractors when desired and usable; maintenance of sensory stimuli within the comfort zone of the patient; control of overload situations

Outcomes from plans to alter role obligations to make them congruent with the patient's capacity as it is affected by pain during the initial treatment phase

Note: For evaluation of patient response to nursing treatment associated with pain-affected difficulties in eating, elimination, roles, and sexuality, see evaluation sections under these headings in this chapter.

Living With the Impact of Cancer and its Treatment on Sexuality

Human sexuality can be viewed broadly as individuals' views of themselves as attractive people capable of attracting the attention and affection of others. It also involves actual sexual functioning.

Cancer and its treatment can alter a person's feelings of being attractive in feminine and masculine ways (Cochran et al, 1987; Andersen, 1987; Andersen and Hacker, 1983; Schain, 1988; Schover et al, 1984; Schwarz-Applebaum et al, 1984; Sex and the Cancer Patient, 1984). It can also reduce comfort and effectiveness in sexual functioning. The changes that occur involve not only the person who has the cancer, but sexual partners, persons with whom there is a potential for intimacy, and other social or work-related contacts. The well-being of the patient may be closely related to effective diagnosis and management of cancer-related problems associated with self-perception of sexuality, sexual functioning, and relationships in which sexuality is a factor. Addressing the related problems of those most closely involved with the patient's sexuality can be crucial to the patient's well-being—as well as that of the partner.

Medical Perspective

The medical perspective on sexuality has tended to focus more on the physical, not the psychosocial aspects (Atwell, 1983). An obstacle to medicine's attending to issues of sexuality has been a general taboo of the discussion of sexual subjects between patients and their doctors (Schnarch, 1988). Often the medical perspective focuses on plastic surgery, prosthetics, or treatment to reconstruct or repair changes created by initial treatment so as to promote improved sexual performance or attractiveness.

Nursing Perspective

The nursing perspective acknowledges that sexuality can have an important and pervasive impact on daily living (Hogan, 1980). It involves:

How individuals feel about themselves from a feminine or masculine perspective

The desire to be with others in intimate and nonintimate ways and to have confidence in these contacts

The ability to interact comfortably and effectively with others at home and in the work place when issues involve sexuality, and the ability to give and receive affection in accordance with desires and needs

Comfort, confidence, and effectiveness in sexual activity

Thus, nursing's goal is to help patients find acceptance of themselves in terms of their sexuality in the midst of the cancer experience, find ways to feel and appear as attractive as possible, manage intimate relationships in ways that are positive, give and receive affection, and maintain their usual confidence in social and work interactions in which sexuality is a factor.

Nature of Cancer's Impact on Sexuality

The phenomena involved in sexuality include:

Self-perception: Cancer can affect one's ability to see oneself as a sexual human being with the capacity to be attractive to others. Self-perception often involves measuring oneself against standards of what constitutes attractiveness in a particular society or subculture. It also includes self-perception of one's "treasured parts" (e.g., head and body hair, breasts, testicles, facial and body features) (Heard, 1988). Another aspect is the impression one seeks to communicate to others, not only in matters involving intimacy or prospective intimacy, but also in work and social situations in which sexuality is a factor. Acknowledgement that one has a cancer can create negative changes in one's perception of one's sexuality—even with no symptoms and without the eventual effects of cancer treatment.

Interest in sexual activity: Usual levels of interest in sexual activity are often diminished by the emotional states that accompany acknowledgement of the presence of cancer in one's body and the prospect or actuality of its medical treatment. Additionally, the medical treatment can cause discomforts and change hormonal levels, reducing the desire to be sexually active. Intercourse may be contraindicated during certain forms of treatment. Other concerns and preoccupations growing out of the cancer experience may take priority for attention and energy over sexual activity.

Sexual functioning: The usual patterns and capacities for intercourse (e.g., desire, foreplay, arousal, lubricity, erectile capacity, ejaculation, comfort, orgasm) and other aspects of sexual intimacy can be changed by the tumor and structural or functional effects of the oncologic treatment.

Altered genetic functioning: Certain forms of oncologic treatment can alter genetic functioning for prolonged periods with potential risks to children conceived at this time (Murinson, 1981).

Infertility: Tumor-related or iatrogenic infertility can affect the developmental task of generativity as it relates to having children. One or both partners may go through a grieving experience over the loss of ability to bear children or the risk of producing genetically altered children. Infertility may also affect relationships between current or prospective partners in which having children is a goal. If the patient or spouse are committed members of religious groups in which child bearing is a valued goal in sexuality, there may be guilt at not being able to fulfill this expectation.

Underlying Mechanisms

Pathophysiologic and Iatrogenic Factors

Tumor-Related Factors

Tumors located in visible parts of the body (e.g., head, neck, skin, and extremities) can affect persons' self-perception and the responses of others. Tumors in the breasts or genital area are likely to affect not only self-perception of sexuality, but sexual performance as well. Physical changes associated with tumors in the pelvic or genital area can change pleasure in sexual activity as well as one or more components of sexual performance. Pain or bleeding during intercourse for females changes participation and can be a frightening, important diagnostic clue. Becoming aware of a lump on a testicle can also affect sexual interest and performance. Visible signs of Kaposi's sarcoma may be a major deterrent to the sexual interests of a human immunodeficiency virus-negative prospective partner.

Symptoms from tumors in other body areas can alter sexual functioning or give it a lower priority (e.g., brain tumors, spinal cord tumors, pain of bone or pancreatic tumors, overwhelming fatigue of blood dyscrasias, and dyspnea or cough of advanced lung tumors).

Surgery

Surgical procedures that have been found to significantly affect sexuality include hysterectomy, oophorectomy, pelvic exenteration, vulvectomy, mastectomy, abdominoperineal resections, cystectomy, orchiectomy, and prostatectomy. In addition, mutilative surgery affecting the face, neck, and head alter appearance and thus sexuality (Metcalfe and Fischman, 1985). Surgery can create alterations in structure as well as functioning. It can result in:

Loss of treasured body parts (e.g., breast, testicle, penis, uterus, ovaries, clitoris, labia, bladder, portions of the pelvis, leg, nose, portions of lips, and facial bones and tissue)

Creation of artificial orifices that may be repulsive to the patient or others and reduce sexual desire

Structural changes that alter expressions of intimacy and sexual functioning. Cystectomy can result in damage to the clitoris because of its proximity to the urinary meatus, altering sexual sensations; the vagina may be shortened and narrowed. With subsequent fibrosis and introital stenosis, penetration may become impossible. Pelvic exenteration can create similar problems. Vulvectomy removes sexually sensitive tissues. In radical prostatectomy, damage to both nerves and muscles can create dysfunction, with loss of erectile capacity and absence of emission and ejaculation. Abdominoperineal resection results in damage to nerve structures, causing sexual dysfunction in 100% of males and possibly delayed physiologic responses in females. Removal of portions of lips or facial bones can alter kissing. Mastectomy may alter the nature of foreplay.

Disruption of nerve pathways that affect vascular responses involved in sexual functioning (e.g., loss of parasympathetic nerves in radical pelvic surgery can delay physiologic responses; prostatectomy or abdominoperineal resections causes erectile dysfunctions)

Loss of sensation (e.g., perineum, skin over the breast following mastectomy, or the inner aspect of the upper arm following dissection of the axilla)

Loss of fertility or child bearing capability (e.g., oophorectomies, hysterectomy, orchiectomy, or prostatectomy that results in retrograde ejaculation)

Chemotherapy   Side-effects of chemotherapy that can affect sexuality include:

Swollen lips and mouth associated with stomatitis

Fatigue

Vulnerability to infection from sexual activity

Hair loss (head, body, axillary, or pubic)

Nausea, vomiting, diarrhea, weight loss

Weight gain with steroid use (males and females) (Knobf, 1983)

Placement of catheters (urinary, right atrial, and venous access devices)

Gonadal changes: Alkylating agents commonly have a profound effect on spermatogenesis (azoospermia may last many years, and recovery may never be complete). Females may expect amenorrhea with long-term treatment with cyclophosphamide or with use of busulfan. Alkylating agents accelerate onset of menopause, particularly in older women (Johnston and Stair, 1985).

Teratogenic and mutagenic changes in exposed eggs or sperm. (Note that normal offspring have been conceived and delivered following chemotherapy.)

Radiation

Radiation's effects on sexuality can include:

Severe fatigue

Diarrhea

Nausea and vomiting

Weight loss

Hair loss

Pain from inflammatory response (e.g., cystitis, proctitis, tenesmus—strong sensation of needing to evacuate bowel or bladder even when there is nothing to evacuate)

Permanent indelible tattoo markings of the radiation field plus less permanent purple markings that last for the duration of the radiation

Vaginal changes, including dryness (complete loss of lubrication), loss of elasticity, shortening or obliteration of the vaginal vault, friability of vaginal and labial tissues

Introital stenosis that makes penetration painful (Jenkins, 1986)

Erectile dysfunction with prostatic irradiation (Heinrich-Rynning, 1987)

Partial sterility in males. (A single dose of 15 to 400 rad results in transient sterility; recovery tends to occur within 9 to 18 months for 200 to 300 rad and 5 or more years for 400 to 600 rad. A single dose of 500 to 950 rad results in permanent sterility.)

Chromosomal damage in mature sperm ejaculated as long as 60 to 80 days following radiation. This can be manifested as dominant first-generation abnormalities (Johnston and Stair, 1985).

Permanent sterility in females. In women older than 40 years of age 600 rad produces menopause; in young women 2000 rad over 5 to 6 weeks has a 95% chance of producing sterility. Libido may be reduced due to loss of ovarian tissue (Johnston and Stair, 1985).

Hormonal Therapy

Estrogen therapy in males for prostatic cancer tends to produce decreased orgasmic experience and erectile dysfunction (Resnick, 1984).

Many patients undergo multiple forms of therapy—in succession or concurrently. In thinking about assessment and diagnosis of daily living problems associated with altered sexuality for a given patient, the nurse needs to consider:

The underlying mechanisms and iatrogenic effects of each form of treatment being planned or used

The potential or observed effects of individual treatments or combinations

The timing and aggregate of particular iatrogenic effects on sexuality produced by each treatment regimen

The aspects of sexuality for the patient and others that are likely to be or are being affected and the impact the changes will have on specific areas of their daily living

Daily Living Factors

When sexuality is viewed from a broad perspective, many facets of daily living become a part of the dynamics that must be understood in order to diagnose and treat the problems of patients and of others whose daily living has an impact on the patient.

Activities in Daily Living

Activities in daily living related to sexuality that are affected by cancer and its treatment include:

Daily dressing and grooming to minimize or mask changes created by the tumor or treatment (e.g., makeup to cover scars or discolorations; scarfs or clothing to cover, accommodate, or disguise tracheostomies, other artificial orifices, or catheters; hair styles, wigs, or scarfs to manage hair loss)

Shopping for clothing, makeup, and accessories to cover defects, accommodate ostomy bags (whether empty or full), and promote a feeling of attractiveness

Activities to reduce and manage discharge, odors, and noises from artificial orifices in day-to-day activities and in preparation for sexual activities

Placement of prosthetics to replace lost parts (e.g., noses attached to glasses, breast prostheses, prosthetic limbs, intraoral devices)

Interaction with current or prospective intimate partner associated with possible sexual activities

Expression of intimacy and affection in different ways

Adjustment of foreplay and intercourse to accommodate to structural or functional changes

Management of the questions and issues in social or work-related situations in which one's sexuality is an explicit or implicit factor

Events in
Daily Living

Events in daily living associated with cancer and sexuality can include both clinical and social aspects:

Seeing hair begin to fall out in chunks, eyebrows disappear, etc.

Seeing, after surgery, the area where a breast used to be or where the new ileostomy or colostomy has been placed

Dating

Addressing issues related to infertility or questions regarding genetic risks

Marriage

Engaging in an intimate relationship or the first intercourse after a major form of medical treatment in which structure or function has been altered

Becoming pregnant, child bearing

Job interviews

Returning to the workplace with changed appearance or functioning that alters one's former image of sexuality

Social events with groups in which sexuality is a consideration in interaction, status, or role relationships

Demands in
Daily Living

Self-demands relate to one's ideal body image and what constitutes attractiveness; the image one wishes to communicate to others in sexual, social, and work-related encounters; self-expectations regarding sexual roles and activities.

Others' expectations tend to be based on gender-related societal or personal standards involving acceptable appearance, sexual desire, cues in sexually oriented interaction, sexual dimensions of a job, and the nature of activities involved in sexual performance.

Environment
for Daily
Living

The environmental factors having to do with sexuality primarily involve the availability of privacy—place and time for intimate contacts or for managing one's personal appearance. The setting may be institutional or home-based.

Values and
Beliefs

Daily living involving sexuality is strongly influenced by both societal and personal values and beliefs. While each of the elements of daily living needs to be given distinct attention in assessment, clinical judgments will require appropriate *integration of findings from the various elements* in order to rule out problems or to make valid, precise diagnoses.

Societal beliefs regarding sexuality include the nature of acceptable sexual roles, and behaviors and goals as they apply to females, males, spouses, partners, friends, social acquaintances, and people in work settings.

Societal values regarding sexuality include standards for what constitutes sexual attractiveness (e.g., having a certain weight and body form; women having hair and breasts; men having appropriate muscular development and normal body hair distribution; having all of one's visible body parts; having no artificial orifices, disfiguring scars, or blemishes; emanating no noxious odors).

Norms for sexuality can vary according to the work environment in which the patient or partner is a member (e.g., corporate headquarters, an industrial plant, a modelling agency, a farm). Social groups can also vary in their values regarding sexuality (e.g., young singles groups, cancer support groups, extended family groups, senior citizen groups).

Personal values attached to attractiveness, general sexuality, sexual roles, and sexual activity can vary with individuals.

Religious values regarding the nature of acceptable sexual roles and behaviors and the strength of obligations for child bearing can affect patient and family responses to the cancer experience.

Functional Health Status

Many dimensions of functioning, both sexual and nonsexual, contribute to the management of daily living with altered sexuality. Each area of functioning requires special consideration from a sexual perspective in addition to the more generic viewpoint.

Strength and Endurance

Cancer can affect the strength of one's sexual desire and one's physical and emotional capacity to project sexual attractiveness and to participate in sexual activity.

Motivation

Desire to maintain sexual attractiveness and activity can be decreased by anxiety, fear, and depression, as well as hormonal changes and physical and environmental factors.

Courage

Courage is required for risk taking in:

Approaching others in interactions involving sexual attractiveness or sexual activities, given the possibilities of interpersonal distancing or outright rejection

Responding to the approaches of others

Courage affects the capacity and willingness to request or try new expressions of intimacy and sexuality.

Cognition

Cognitive competence to deal with altered sexuality includes the capacity to:

Anticipate and understand structural, functional, and emotional changes associated with sexuality in the cancer experience and to plan adaptations and adjustments

Plan scripts and behavior to manage interpersonal encounters in which questions of altered sexuality are an explicit or implicit factor

Communication

Communication skills are involved in the capacity to:

Communicate sexual attractiveness to others

Manage verbal and nonverbal cues involved in sexually oriented situations in the presence of altered sexuality (or the perception others may have of altered sexuality). Such encounters may involve intimate, potentially intimate, social, or work situations.

Communicate and receive affection

The above functional capacities are assessed in the patient, but some may need to be assessed in partners (or others) as well when their sexual functioning, expectations, or problems and their affection-giving behavior will be a factor in patient well-being.

Each functional area needs to be considered as a separate entity. Then functional capacities that are logically linked can be combined in order to identify functional strengths and deficits in the patient situation.

Nursing Diagnosis and Treatment

Diagnostic Targets

Targets for diagnosis and treatment can include patient, spouse or partners, companions, employers, or co-workers.

Risk Factors

At risk for having increased difficulty in managing sexuality in daily living are those whose:

Site of disease or treatment involves genital organs, breasts, head and neck, limbs, artificial orifices, anus, or parts of the body that are visible in public settings

Sense of femininity or masculinity is strongly linked to the affected organs and functions

Understanding of the structure and functioning of the reproductive tract is limited

Treatment or disease has altered structural or functional resources for maintaining sexual attractiveness or activity (e.g., hair loss, fatigue, nausea and vomiting, diarrhea, cystitis, proctitis, shrinkage or obliteration of the vaginal vault, loss of lubricity, erectile dysfunction, reduced libido, infertility)

Self-esteem is based on having a perfect body or being sexually attractive (Sinsheimer and Holland, 1987)

Partners equate sexuality with a perfect body and full normal capacity for sexual activity

Previous sexual activity has been unsatisfactory

Sexual behavior is rigid and limited in options

Marital or partner bond is unstable

Job or social roles depend on being sexually attractive

Expressions of affection in nonintimate ways have not been well developed

Diagnostic
Areas
PATIENT

Loss of confidence in sexual attractiveness R/T:

Iatrogenic factors—fatigue, nausea, vomiting, diarrhea, pain, insomnia, disfigurement, or loss of capacity to function sexually (specify nature)

Knowledge or skill deficit in compensating for changes in body appearance or function

Interpersonal distancing behavior of others

Fear of abandonment

Difficulty in establishing or maintaining intimate relationships R/T fear of rejection

Reluctance to discuss, consider, or attempt alternatives to usual patterns in sexual activity (e.g., self-stimulation or different positions during intercourse) R/T values that restrict options

Limitations in options to seek desired reconstructive or rehabilitative surgery (e.g., breast implant, vaginal reconstruction, penile implant) R/T lack of information, resources (technical or financial), or personal support for taking action

PATIENT OR
PARTNER

Grief or frustration R/T inability to participate in usual or desired sexual activity

Disparity of desire for sexual activity between patient and partner R/T:

Patient's loss of desire (libido)

Partner's lack of understanding of the severity of patient's symptoms or of the effect of the treatment

Patient's desire to resume activity and partner's revulsion over changes in the patient

Ineffectiveness in intercourse when structure or function have been changed by cancer or its treatment R/T:

Lack of knowledge of other options for expressing intimacy and affection

Lack of knowledge of alternative positions and functioning for intercourse

Unwillingness to try other options

Lack of knowledge as to how to communicate needs, desires or options to one's partner

Patient's fear of experiencing pain or causing tissue damage

Grief R/T loss of child bearing options

MALE OR FEMALE PARTNER TO FEMALE PATIENT

Fear, reluctance, or ineffectiveness in engaging in sexual activity R/T:

Lack of understanding of physical changes in female genitalia or breasts

Fear of causing pain or tissue damage

Lack of skill in accommodating structural or functional changes (identify specifically)

Inability to communicate in an effective way with partner in sexual matters

FEMALE PARTNER TO MALE PATIENT

Ineffective sexual activity R/T lack of understanding of how to provide sexual satisfaction when no erection or ejaculation is possible (coital alternatives).

CARE GIVER– SEXUAL PARTNER

Lack of satisfaction in sexual relationships R/T inability to fully shift from care giver role to sexual partner. (There is a particularly high risk of this problem when daily care involves a bowel and bladder regimen.)

MALE PARTNER TO MALE PATIENT

Ineffective, unsatisfactory sexual relations following abdominoperineal resections or rectal radiation implants R/T knowledge deficit of coital alternatives to anal intercourse.

OTHERS

Ineffective role relationships (specify) R/T:

Inability or unwillingness to control manifestations of revulsion over changes in patient

Lack of knowledge or skills in interacting with the patient in the presence of changed appearance or functioning

Belief that the diagnosis of cancer or effects of its treatment makes the individual unsuitable for previous roles

Manifestations

It may be difficult to obtain data on problems associated with sexuality and cancer. Many persons are reluctant to discuss their sexual problems with physicians, but may talk to nurses (Jenkins, 1986; Von Eschenbach and Schover, 1984). The willingness, skill, and ease of the nurse in approaching the subject of sexuality will be factors in the comfort patients feel in providing data needed to rule out problems or to make diagnoses of potential or actual problems in sexuality in daily living (Heinrich-Rynning, 1987).

PATIENT

Reported:

Loss of confidence or self-esteem related to sexual attractiveness because of *_____ (* specify related factors)

Dissatisfaction or unhappiness with appearance

Fear of rejection in sexual interaction

Unsatisfying relationships with others (specify role—e.g., husband, girlfriend, employer, member of social group)

Perception of interpersonal distancing behavior in others

Fear of causing damage, complications, or pain by resuming former sexual activities

Inability to talk with sexual partner about feelings, needs, fears, and concerns, or about partner's behavior, feelings, and concerns

Unhappiness with failure of others to demonstrate affection verbally or physically

Perception of lack of understanding or negative responses from sexual partner

Loss of interest or priority for sexual activity because of emotional status or iatrogenic effects and perception of sexual partner's responses to this change

Erectile failure

Retrograde ejaculation

Fear of loss of job or former social roles because of diagnosis or because of treatment-related changes in appearance or functioning

Reluctance to date because of perceived changes in sexuality

Concern over lack of resumption of usual phone calls, appointments, or invitations from friends, employer, or co-workers

Observed:

Changes in appearance, structure, or functioning that *could* affect sense of personal attractiveness or sexual functioning

Laboratory values that indicate major risk of infections in a sexually active patient

Negative attitude toward viewing body changes caused by disease or its treatment

Ineffective choices and preparation for *predicted* body changes (e.g., procuring of wig for hair loss, gaining knowledge regarding resources for prostheses or rehabilitation, planning for alterations in intimate activities, planning a different style of dress to accommodate to structural changes)

Lack of adjustment evidenced by nonuse of resources or clothing to disguise or minimize body changes and to maintain personal attractiveness

Partner does not visit the patient when such visits are realistically possible

Nonuse of privacy arrangements for patient and partner

PARTNER   Reported:

Lack of knowledge regarding physical changes from the treatment and its implications for sexual activity

Fear of causing pain or damage

Lack of knowledge about alternatives to previous sexual practices

Inability to talk with patient about sexual matters

Feelings of revulsion at the changes in structure or functioning of the patient

Lack of patterns for expressing affection verbally or behaviorally

CARE GIVER   Reported inability to shed the care giver role and enter wholly into the sexual experience

OTHERS   The manifestations of responses of others to the patient are more likely to be reported through the patient's eyes than by others talking to the nurse. The nurse may observe frequency of phone calls, numbers of cards and letters, and visitors' behavior during inpatient stays.

Prognostic Variables   Poor prognosis is associated with:

Self-esteem based primarily on personal attractiveness and sexual functioning in combination with cancers or treatments that mar that attractiveness and decrease capability or comfort in sexual activity

Partners, companions, employers who base their acceptance and esteem for the patient on physical attractiveness and sexuality

Side-effects of tumor or treatment that result in low capacity and priority for activities to maintain attractiveness or (if previously sexually active) to engage in sexual activity

Iatrogenic or tumor effects that, for long periods of time or permanently, mar appearance and create difficulties in sexual functioning

Unwillingness of patient or partner to accept or find satisfaction in alternative strategies for showing affection and engaging in sexual activity on a temporary or permanent basis

Lack of availability of or lack of resources for obtaining plastic surgery, prosthetics, rehabilitative services, appropriate clothing, and so on to remove or disguise body changes and help to make the patient feel attractive and functional

Complications

Failure to manage problems of sexuality in the presence of cancer and its treatment can result in decreased self-esteem or disruption or loss of marital, work, and social relationships. These losses and the negative psychophysiologic concomitants may decrease the patient's will to live, to participate in a lifestyle conducive to recovery, and to make a genuine commitment to the treatment protocol. Thus, the complications may affect not only the patient's sense of well-being, but his or her survival.

Treatment Guidelines

Loss of confidence in one's sexuality

Gather data on factors that contribute to this person's sense of sexuality and the changes that contribute to feelings of loss.

Genuinely accept as reality the loss the person feels. Legitimize it. Where the changes are of limited duration, indicate this and look to ways to avoid threatening situations or to compensate on a temporary basis (e.g., clothing to cover catheters, subtle makeup to cover paleness).

For women, suggest reading the book *Beauty and Cancer* (Doan-Noyes and Mellody, 1988).

Explore strategies that are within the physical and emotional resources, value system, and financial resources of the person that can realistically compensate for the losses felt (see The Mirror Exercise).

Help the patient develop strategies and scripts for satisfyingly managing interpersonal encounters in which sexual inadequacies are a concern (e.g., with sexual partner: "I really miss our loving. If we talked about what is getting in the way of our touching and having sex as we used to, it might make us both more comfortable"; with a new partner: "It may be important for you to know that I had leukemia a few years ago. I'm wondering how that might affect our relationship") (Schover, 1988).

Gather data regarding support persons available to the patient and assess the realistic risks of abandonment, weighing the nature of the previous relationships and the course of the disease.

Address the needs of the support persons as a means of reducing risks of their interpersonally or physically distancing from or abandoning the patient.

The Mirror Exercise

Purpose: To help in adjusting to iatrogenic body changes

Equipment: A full-length mirror

Study yourself critically in the mirror for several minutes and notice specifically:

The parts of your body you look at most

The parts of your body you avoid looking at

The negative thoughts you have about your appearance

Your best features

Any changes the cancer or its treatment has created in the way you look

Practice this exercise two to three times until you can identify at least three positive things about your looks.

When you are comfortable seeing yourself as a stranger might see you, repeat the exercise, dressed and looking like you would like to be seen by your sexual partner. Study yourself as you did in the first exercise. Give yourself at least three compliments on your appearance.

Finally, do the exercise when you are nude. Don't disguise any of the changes that the cancer or treatment have made. Give yourself time to get accustomed to the changes. Breathe deeply if you become tense. Continue the exercise until you have found at least three positive features or can remember the three compliments you paid yourself in the previous exercise.

These exercises can help you to feel more relaxed when your lover or other persons look at you. You can also remember them when you are feeling insecure.

(Adapted from Schover LR. Sexuality and cancer for the woman who has cancer and her partner. New York: American Cancer Society, 1988)

Offer the possibility of joining a support group in which some o the other members either have similar concerns or are willing to share their experiences in managing sexual issues.

Fear of rejection in new or ongoing relationships

Gather data on the nature of the patient's situation that create fear of rejection.

Recognize and reinforce attempts to initiate relationships. Use the patient–nurse relationship as a practice ground. Reinforce what the patient does well and talk about how he or she can build on those strengths.

Help the patient to explore options to maintain or regain self esteem. Try this exercise with the patient: Liken self-esteem to four bank accounts, with net worth in a *physical account* (how you look and function), a *social account* (how well you get along with others and the network of people you can count on), an *achievement account* (what you have accomplished—school, work, family, and personal achievements), and a *spiritual account* (religious and moral beliefs, values, and the support these give). The cancer treatment draws from the physical account, and possibly from the social account and even the spiritual account. Analyze the costs of the cancer in each of the accounts and attempt to make "loans" from the other accounts. If treatment has affected appearance and functioning, turn attention to the caring received from family and others. If work or school are interrupted, focus on enhancing some elements of social or spiritual life or other areas of personal growth in the cancer experience. In this way it is possible to avoid bankrupting the whole of one's sense of self-worth (Schover, 1988).

Explore options for compensating for changes the person believes are contributing to risk of rejection.

Develop and rehearse strategies and scripts for addressing specific situations for which the patient identifies risks of rejection. For example, rehearse various rejection scenarios with a friend, altering responses until there is some comfort with the behavior. Remind the patient that rejection in a relationship frequently occurs outside of the cancer experience for a variety of reasons (Schover, 1988).

Choices to seek or use options to compensate for iatrogenic changes limited by knowledge or resources

Gather data on:

Knowledge of options that are available to modify or compensate for body changes created by the treatment

Desire to use any of the options available

Status of physical and emotional energy to locate and obtain services and equipment or supplies

Finances to purchase services or equipment

Support from others for participation in rehabilitation programs or treatment

Provide information on resources that are congruent with the patient's needs and financial status (e.g., free loans of wigs from the local American Cancer Society). *If the patient wishes to pursue the options further:*

Arrange for contacts with patients who have used the surgery, prosthesis, equipment, or rehabilitation program

Check with local department stores for special consultants who may be available to help patients overcome physical changes from the cancer or its treatment

Where others are creating barriers to rehabilitation, explore options for changing the opinions or behavior of those who are nonsupportive, or strengthen patient's position for moving ahead with the rehabilitative services or equipment without their support

Lack of knowledge of the nature of changes and their implications for sexual functioning as a basis for sexuality in daily living†

Offer broad openings for the person to raise questions, concerns, and issues. This may be initiated even before treatment is begun. (For example, the nurse may say to the patient, "When a person has had *_____ [* identify the treatment], questions and concerns arise about sexuality and sexual functioning." The nurse should pause, and, if there is no response, give some examples of the concerns other patients or their partners have had.)

Provide candid information about changes that may be experienced after particular forms of treatment.‡ For example:

Males

Retrograde ejaculation associated with transurethral prostatic resection

"After your operation you may find during intercourse that your semen and secretions flow into the bladder, not in the usual direction. The feeling of ejaculation will be there even though the semen does not pass out through the penis. The semen will pass out of the body in the next urination and the urine will look a bit cloudier than usual."

Erectile dysfunction associated with abdominoperineal resection, and possibly with perineal prostatic resection or radiation, or fear of erectile dysfunction following prostatectomy

"Some men experience changes in their capacity for erection after *_____ (* specify treatment). If this should be a problem there are some procedures that can be done to restore this capability. Your doctor will be able to tell you about the options that are available if you should need them. There are also some references available from the American Cancer Society that give excellent information, such as *Sexuality and Cancer For the Man Who Has Cancer and His Partner.*' (Schover, 1988)

---

† Treatment for patient or partner

‡ The *PLISSIT* model offers a guide to the levels of therapeutic intervention that may be involved. It begins with what anyone can do and moves in complexity to intensive therapy that should be limited to the skilled trained sexual therapist. *P* = *permission*—giving permission to discuss sexual matters; *LI* = *limited information*—examples of this are given in this section; *SS* = *specific suggestions*—examples of this are given in this section and in the Schover, 1988 references; *IT* = *intensive therapy.* The level of intervention engaged in by any nurse will be determined by comfort in the area, knowledge, skill, and time available.

"Some men worry that they will have problems with erection after prostatic surgery. The nerves and the blood supply will have been left intact, so there is little physical reason not to function as before."

Reduced desire for sexual activity associated with orchiectomy or estrogen therapy

"You may find that you are not as interested in sexual activity as you have been before. Sometimes this is the result of the emotional impact of receiving news about your diagnosis; sometimes it comes from the side-effects of the treatment— you'll be more tired for a while. At times getting well and managing other aspects in daily living will take priority for your attention and energy."

"The medicines (or treatments) you are receiving to treat your cancer can have the effect of reducing your desire to be sexually active for a time."

Weaker or shorter orgasmic experience associated with estrogen therapy

"Once you feel like becoming sexually active again, you may find that your sensations during orgasm are not as intense or of as long duration as they were before. This is an expected effect from the medications you are taking."

Females

Dryness of the vagina, fragility of vaginal and labial tissues, and introital stenosis associated with pelvic radiation; or shortening and narrowing of vaginal vault with radiation or cystectomy

"During and after your radiation you will find that the tissues in and around your vagina will have become dryer, more tender, and more fragile. You may also notice that the vaginal space and the opening have become smaller. This is an expected effect of the treatment. If you are sexually active, it can and should make a difference in the way you and your partner approach your sexual activity." (See subsequent treatment guidelines for specifics.)

Legitimize the occurrence of sexual issues that will require resolution: "When patients have treatment such as yours, it is not at all unusual for them and their partners to have to make some adjustments in their intimate relationships. This is one part of the healing process for each of you. If you find you need or want help, there are a variety of resources available."

During the time when sexual intercourse is prohibited by the treatment or inhibited by patient symptoms, introduce the idea of the importance of increasing other forms of expressing affection and intimacy, such as hand holding, touching–stroking, kissing, being physically close to one another, and verbally expressing affection, caring, and support.

When symptoms abate and healing permits consideration of resumption of sexual activity, introduce such questions as, "Has the treatment or illness had an effect on your role as a *_____ (* man, woman, husband, wife, partner)?"; "Have you been thinking about resuming your sexual relationship?"; "Do you have any questions or concerns?"; "Have you and your partner been able to discuss resuming sexual activity?"

Indicate that there are some practical strategies for managing the changes.

Ineffectiveness in sexual activity R/T lack of knowledge of practical strategies for managing the changes

Provide information from the following areas as appropriate to the diagnosed needs and desires of patient or partner:

Male desire for intercourse during a time when it is not possible or advisable for vaginal intercourse

Suggest options such as manual manipulation or intercourse between woman's thighs or breasts.

Vaginal and genital dryness and fragility

Suggest strategies such as application of large amounts of water-soluble lubrication, but not Vaseline or oil-based products, which may promote yeast infections. It can be applied by the patient in private or as a part of foreplay.

Pain from narrowed vaginal opening and tender tissues

Once the physician has indicated that it is safe to engage in intercourse, advise the patient that:

Sexual activity should not be delayed or reduced because of discomfort, as this only compounds the problem

Sexual intercourse three or four times per week can help to keep the vaginal opening more flexible and can minimize the pain of penetration

Early use of a vaginal dilator (before shrinkage occurs) for a 10-minute period three times per week can prevent shrinkage and maintain vaginal size. It may need to be continued indefinitely and can make intercourse more comfortable (Schover, 1988).

During intercourse time should be given for adequate foreplay and arousal, as this raises the pain threshold and allows pleasurable sensations to emerge

An attempt should be made to relax the perineal muscles in spite of discomfort

The female superior position may give greater control

Shortened vagina

Advise patient that the following options have been found to be helpful: a rear entry position with the female's thighs held close together; a male superior position with pillows under the female's hips and the hand holding the base of the penis to limit depth of stroke. Advise trying other positions until the one with greatest comfort is found. If semen produces a burning sensation, advise seeking to delay male orgasm or using a condom (Jenkins, 1986).

Female need for sexual pleasuring when male partner has erectile dysfunction

Suggest the options of self-stimulation, use by the partner of oral or manual stimulation and penetration, or use of sexual aids such as a vibrator or dildo.

Need for pleasuring when there is diminished or absent sensation

Indicate that often other areas become increasingly responsive in erogenous ways. Suggest that partners explore alternate potentially sensuous erogenous areas—lips, ear lobes, breasts, and other areas.

Suggest use of manual stimulation and penetration.

Hemipelvectomy, mastectomy, other body changes that create a need to alter positions during sexual activity

Discuss the problems created by positional or balance difficulties and explore options such as other positions or use of pillows or other supports.

Inability to participate in sexual activity R/T repulsion over urostomy, ileostomy, or colostomy

If possible, make contact with partner during patient's hospitalization to legitimize and identify problems in sexuality commonly arising when the patient has artificial orifices or neurogenic bowel and bladder. Explore and legitimize concerns (e.g., "In my experience I've found that it is not uncommon for partners to have difficulty in looking at the stoma or imagine being close to it. It usually gets easier with time"). Identify resources that may be helpful, should the problem occur (e.g., reading, contact with another person who has experienced the problem, support groups, or anticipatory professional counseling).

Teach patient how to care for orifices prior to sexual activity in order to minimize secretions, sounds, and odors and to present an attractive appearance. Instruct patient to cleanse the area and clean and deodorize the pouch, making certain that it is securely fastened. Show pictures and samples of attractive feminine and masculine covers for ileostomy, colostomy, and ureterostomy bags. Discuss appropriate coverings for tracheostomy, gastrostomy, or catheters. Suggest that the patient consider positions in which the partner does not face the pouch.

Suggest that the patient offer the partner an opportunity to look at the ostomy at a time when the skin is intact and the area is clean and free of odor.

Try to make a contact with the partner to discuss the problems interfering with return to usual sexual relationships with patient. If strategies offered by the nurse are not acceptable, suggest participation in support groups such as CanSurmount, the local chapter of the United Ostomy Association, or professional counseling.

Female partner's difficulty in pleasuring the male R/T lack of knowledge of coital alternatives when male has erectile dysfunction

Suggest that they explore areas where sensual and erotic sensations occur, then use touch (e.g., manual, oral) to offer sexual pleasure. Suggest the use of feathers or soft fur, such as rabbit, for patients whose skin is too sensitive to tolerate other forms of touch.

Inability or decreased capacity for sexual activity R/T inadequate symptom management

Make patient aware that:

Sexual activity during the active treatment phase and while iatrogenic symptoms remain probably requires a some degree of planning so that a time is selected when fatigue is low.

If a period of intimacy is planned, medications can be taken to achieve relief from pain and nausea at that time. If the activity is spontaneous, medications can be taken and the initial activities can be prolonged to permit the medications to take effect.

Inability to explore alternatives in sexual behavior R/T own or partner's value conflicts

If intimacy is seen to be limited to the purpose of procreation rather than the expression of affection, or if certain positions or activities are proscribed, consider an open discussion of options with the least conflict to strongly held values as a way to help to offer comfort and promote better sexual relations.

Lack of skill and comfort in discussing sexual needs, concerns, and issues with partner

Explore the patient's difficulties. Identify communication strategies used in other areas of the relationship. Work with patient to develop a usable, feasible repertoire of nonverbal cues and scripts linked to particular presenting situations. Arrange for feedback.

Propose participation of patient and partner in support groups such as I Can Cope or CanSurmount, or contact with another patient or partner who may have faced a similar situation.

For the independent, self-help person, identify or offer reading materials such as the American Cancer Society pamphlets, *Sexuality and Cancer For the Woman Who Has Cancer and Her Partner* and *Sexuality and Cancer For the Man Who Has Cancer and His Partner* (Schover, 1988 and 1988a).

Grief over loss of former expressions of sexuality

Help the patient to identify the changes before they occur and plan strategies for substituting satisfying expressions of affection and intimacy before, during, and after the changes occur. Suggest that this may prevent or minimize the loss and help the partner feel cared about and involved throughout the cancer experience.

Where the situation does not lend itself to prevention, or the losses exceed the person's capacity to cope, grief responses may occur. The nurse can:

Help the person(s) to become aware of the grieving and its manifestations in the situation, and suggest that grieving takes time for resolution—it can't be foreshortened merely because one is aware of its presence and legitimacy

Legitimize the grief in terms of the loss that has been experienced

Wait to institute rehabilitative measures until the denial and anger stages of grieving have subsided. Then, depending on the situation and the loss, help the person institute measures to make the expressions of affection and sexuality more satisfying. See previous treatment guidelines.

Grief R/T loss of child bearing capacity

In terms of preventing the loss, when the man has a risk of becoming sterile as a result of cancer treatment, propose the option of sperm banking. For women, where it is legal, available, and financially feasible, suggest the possibility of eggs being taken from her prior to treatment and fertilized with the husband's sperm for surrogate mothering.

Suggest to the patient and partner the importance of recognizing that grieving, when it occurs, may be an added complication to the physiologic and psychologic stress of the disease and treatment.

Observe for cues indicating the current grief responses being experienced. Link grief manifestations to the other observed manifestations in diagnosing and treating the problems in daily living.

When the patient or partner recognizes the loss and the grieving being experienced, legitimize it as being normal, but a source of additional distress to be managed among the other requirements of daily living. Do not seek to rush the person through to resolution.

When the person is ready, propose exploring alternatives to child bearing, such as adoption, foster parenting, child-free lifestyle, volunteering for Big Brother or Big Sister programs—looking at the pros and cons of each—as a step toward healing. Offer information about RESOLVE, Inc. the national organization for people with problems of infertility (Address: 5 Water Street, Arlington, ME 02174).

Difficulty in shifting from role of care taker to sexual partner

Explore the factors in the situation that make the release of the care taker role difficult (e.g., patient symptoms, anxiety over effects of sexual activity on patient status, or the actual nature of the care giving required [outside of the sexual realm]).

Discuss the importance of closeness to both partners and the physical and psychologic benefits each can have from physical manifestations of closeness in this time of stress.

Suggest strategies for closing out the care taker role from one's thinking and moving more fully into the role of sexual partner (e.g., recruiting a home health aide to do the patient's bowel program, or giving attention to the fatigue level of the care giver).

Concern of others regarding their discomfort in interaction with or their avoidance of the patient in social or work roles

Gather data on what changes in the patient are disconcerting or frightening to the persons or what problems they are having during interaction.

If the appearance of the patient creates a problem, suggest that they send notes or cards with a personal note appended. Phone conversations constitute a step up in risks in interaction, but still do not present the visual cues. If the person "doesn't know what to say," help to develop some scripts and options.

In preparation for a face-to-face contact, prepare the persons for what will be seen and instruct them to deliberately plan where their eyes will focus (e.g., planning to look at the person's face and not allowing the gaze to drop to the breast area after mastectomy, or focusing on the eyes and not on the neck of the person with head and neck surgery). Instruct the person to be aware of the messages that facial expressions send and to practice some control using a mirror. This advanced planning offers the person a sense of some control. Suggest that the script for options in the conversation be planned and rehearsed in order to manage the first minute or two of the contact.

Help the patient to develop behaviors, strategies, and scripts that make it easier for others to overcome their initial discomfort. Use of humor, a direct approach about one's status, diversion such as discussion of other topics, or focussing on what is going on with the other person are options.

Instruct companions that most persons who are experiencing cancer wish to be treated as the persons they were before the diagnosis and the treatment. They do not want oversolicitude, the hearty "My how well you are coping," or excessive sympathy. Suggest that instead of "How *are* you?" a better question may be a more general, "How are things going?" or "How does it feel to be back?" followed by a genuine interest in and acceptance of whatever approach to the question the patient takes (whether short and noncommittal or a serious report on how he or she really feels). Recommend following the patient's lead in the conversation.

Where employment and job performance are concerned, recommend that the employer or co-worker gather data on how the patient would prefer to manage during the course of treatment, the limitations that may occur, and the accommodations that would be helpful. *Then,* negotiations can be made to mesh the needs of the job and the company with those of the patient. Remind the employer or co-worker that it is no kindness to persons undergoing cancer therapy to automatically relieve them of parts of their job. Since physical, mental, and emotional resources of the patient may wax and wane during the course of the treatment, advanced planning of mutually acceptable strategies for updating information on the patient's current status and any changes in work arrangements can make the employer, co-workers, and the patient more comfortable with the interaction.

If the employer, personnel manager, supervisor, and co-workers do not have the insight or skill to set up negotiations, help the patient to structure this interaction.

Evaluation

Because sexuality is so broad and pervasive when it is viewed in terms of daily living and functional health status, evaluation of the patient, partner, and others will be needed. Depending on the diagnosis and treatment focus, one evaluates the status of:

Patient self-esteem and confidence in sexuality

Comfort, skill, and effectiveness in interpersonal relationships involving sexuality or sexual functioning

Behavior to manage structural or functional changes affecting appearance and sexuality

Management of grief over sexual or child bearing losses

Partner's comfort, effectiveness, and satisfaction in accommodating changes in patient's sexuality

Others' comfort, effectiveness, and satisfaction in interacting
with the patient who appears or functions differently than in
the past

Living With Social Isolation
During Active Treatment

Some sense of physical or emotional aloneness—a feeling of separation from
others—occurs for every patient during initial treatment. Most obvious is the *physical*
separation associated with going to a hospital sometimes many miles from home. Other
visible barriers that create a sense of isolation include thick walls, closed doors,
television monitors instead of people in the radiation treatment room, masks and gowns,
plastic walls, and signs that warn others to keep their distance or take precautions. Less
obvious is the *emotional* separation from others. Some of this is associated with the
patient's having a potentially life-threatening illness that others don't have, and
symptoms they can't experience. (See also sections on Role and Sexuality in this
chapter.)

Those who are closest to the patient also experience a new sense of social isolation,
caused in part by physical and emotional factors associated with the patient. In addition,
there are emotional disturbances in themselves as they see threats to their own mortality
emerging from the patient's cancer diagnosis. The geographic distances, environmental
barriers, and emotional factors that isolate the patient create a sense of isolation for close
family and friends as well.

Persons experiencing cancer have times when they need to become more egocentric as they wrestle with acceptance of their disease, with changing priorities and values
and with the demands of the treatment. During such times it is not unusual for them to
emotionally close out those who want to share. Those who are not ill, but care a great
deal for the person who has cancer, will also experience some egocentricity as they too
seek to process the reality of threat to life and all its implications.

Medical Perspective

The medical perspective in cancer tends to involuntarily create social isolation
through the confirmation of the neoplastic diagnosis and the prescription and implementation of treatment that must, necessarily, create isolating conditions. Some physicians' behavior may also unwittingly contribute to patients' and families' sense of
isolation through their objective, scientific demeanor as they diagnose and prescribe

They can also send distancing messages by verbal and body language (e.g., sitting behind desks, standing behind chart carts), touching only for diagnostic or treatment purposes, and focusing on the organ, the tumor, or the response to treatment rather than the person whose life is being affected. Medical care too can be conducted in ways that isolate the patient (e.g., if the physician–teacher discusses pathologic phenomena and exhibits interesting phenomena involving the tumor or host response to treatment for each student to inspect as if the patient were only incidental). This is not to say that all physicians adopt these behaviors in their professional role, but only to identify isolating features that the patients and families may experience in the course of medical treatment.

Nursing Perspective

Nursing's focus is to acknowledge the reality that, to some degree, each patient and each close relative or friend of the patient will experience some feelings of social isolation during the cancer experience. Sometimes that isolation serves a useful purpose and shouldn't be interrupted, even though it is uncomfortable. At other times social isolation can be a serious problem and a deterrent to recovery. Diagnosis will involve identification of:

The isolating features in the presenting situation

The amount of discomfort being experienced by the person(s)

The impact the isolation is having on patient or family functioning and daily living

From such clinical judgments and diagnoses, treatment decisions can be made on how to relieve discomfort and mobilize resources to minimize dysfunctional isolation.

Nature of Social Isolation

Social isolation is a presenting situation in which a person experiences discomfort, dysfunction, or suffering associated with physical separation or emotional detachment from others. It can be a self-imposed condition, as in the case of emotional withdrawal from others to process the meaning of the cancer experience and to engage in decision making. It can be imposed by others either through physical barriers and geographic distances or by the erecting of verbal and behavioral barriers. The degree of social isolation can vary from insecurity or threat of an undesired change in a relationship to actual physical and emotional abandonment by one or more people or by an entire system. Social isolation can occur in one or more areas of a patient's life—within selected relationships in the family, social circle, neighborhood, school, work, or the health care system.

Social isolation is accompanied by emotional responses ranging from comfort to intense loneliness and panic. Some persons have lived their adult lives in a pattern of social isolation. They are comfortable in their solitude and are made uncomfortable by having their personal space invaded by anyone, much less a group of health care providers, even impersonal ones. Some people link their social well-being to their relationship with an animal, not another human being. Separation from that animal can bring the sense of social isolation in the midst of caring health care providers. Most human beings thrive and manage stress better when they feel a predictable, strong, secure, mutual connectedness with one or more individuals, and positive links with less close members of their social and health care network. Threat to or actual decrease in the quantity or quality of those relationships can bring emotional distress.

Self-Imposed Isolation

Many people who learn that they have cancer engage in periods of introspection as they seek to assimilate the cancer experience into their lives. The illness, the threat, the prospects, and the reality of treatment, and the sudden dramatic alteration in their lifestyle all seem to generate a need for times for reflection and adjustment. Some of these processing tasks are described by survivors as (Taylor, 1988):

Accepting the reality of the cancer

Revising life priorities

Adjusting values

Adjusting to and accepting limitations

Seeking a reason for the occurrence of the cancer

Considering the impact of the cancer and treatment on relationships with family and friends

Considering the possibility of death

The processing of these issues can vary in intensity and duration. There is no question that there are periods of time when processing of these issues is shared, but even those who share experience some time of egocentric isolation.

Isolation Imposed by Others

Physical Factors

The treatment of cancer tends to create physical distances and barriers between the patients and those they wish to have close to them. It even creates the need for barriers between the patient and health care providers—sometimes for the protection of the patient and sometimes for the protection of the health care provider. Thus, there can be strong visual signals of physical isolation and, for some, an awareness that they create dangers (e.g., radiation) to others. Being isolated because one is a danger to others creates not only a feeling of being alone and isolated, but even worse, of being a pariah.

Philosophical Factors

Unresolved differences in values and priorities can affect the interactions between physicians, nurses, and patients and generate feelings of isolation for the patient. Some oncology departments are cure-oriented, tumor-oriented, and research-oriented. Patients who feel that they are being viewed as hosts of the tumors, host responses to the treatment, or sources of data for the department's research projects can feel depersonalized and socially isolated. There can be a sense of abandonment when patients are informed that they have "failed the protocol" rather than that the treatment protocol failed them.

Patients who feel threatened may envision health care providers as their "hope insurance," and value close personal support from them. Doctors and nurses may value making a contribution to the patient's hope through oncologic knowledge and technical expertise, giving much lower priority to personal support. When depersonalization occurs, patients and families can be left with serious feelings of isolation.

Conflict can also occur when the patient does not give the same value and priority to the approach and goals of cancer care as the health care providers do. Some patients may seek palliative care and medical support during the remaining lifespan, while the oncologist may value ongoing aggressive treatment and monitoring of the neoplasia. When goals are discrepant between care provider and receiver, a sense of isolation or even abandonment can occur.

Emotional Isolation

One patient spoke of cancer as being "the loneliest battle" (Morgan, 1988). Another wrote of the separations involved in making the transition to "the land of the ill persons," where healthy people can only visit but never stay (Trillin, 1981).

Some patients learn that it is more difficult for friends and relatives who have been emotionally close in the past to retain that closeness. These people have more to lose from the patient's illness (e.g., previous patterns of shared daily living, meaningful relationships, and the sense of invulnerability now threatened by a perceived possibility of loss of the person), and thus are more threatened. Less close relatives and friends may emerge as being more supportive in cancer crises (Taylor, 1988).

At times the patients' closest support networks may be only marginally functional, even when little stress is placed upon them. Such networks tend to disintegrate in the presence of a major crisis (such as cancer). The network then offers only more stress rather than support (Roberts, 1988).

Patients who have experienced major recent losses in their personal support system (e.g., through death, divorce, or having close family or friends move to another area) and have not found replacements can enter the cancer experience already feeling bereft. The particular personal stresses and isolating features of the cancer experience can increase that sense of aloneness.

Social isolation can be influenced by the behavior and responses of people in many components of daily living, including family, friends, neighbors, employers, co-workers, and health care providers. It would be rare to find that a patient or family were experiencing social isolation equally in all areas. Patient and family well-being may depend on mobilizing increased support and closeness in some areas to compensate for losses and isolation in others.

Underlying Mechanisms

Pathophysiologic and Iatrogenic Factors

Tumor-related factors and all forms of oncologic treatment bring isolating features with them. Age can also be a contributing factor.

Tumor-Related Factors   Knowledge of the confirmed presence of cancer can create a sense of isolation in and of itself.

Tumors that "show" (e.g., enlarging Burkitt's lymphoma on the neck, visible skin cancers, or Kaposi's sarcoma) can make the patient feel different from others and therefore more isolated.

Fatigue, shortness of breath, and discomfort can interfere with participation in usual activities and can contribute to the sense of isolation.

Surgery

Cancer surgery requires the patient to go to a hospital for variable periods of time. Contacts with support system are attenuated by geographic distances, institutional restrictions, and environmental constraints.

The after-effects of surgery (e.g., losses of treasured body parts, disfiguration, or creation of ostomies) can make the person feel wary of rejection. (See also sections on Role, Sexuality, and Vulnerability to Infection in this chapter.)

Chemotherapy

Chemotherapy can isolate because of fatigue, nausea and vomiting, diarrhea, pain, baldness, difficulties in eating and in communication, and vulnerability to infection. Trips to the health care facility for intermittent treatments can be disruptive.

Radiation

External beam radiation brings total isolation during treatment, the only connection with therapists being the television camera monitor and the audio equipment.

Radiation implants require staff and others to limit contacts severely in terms of distance and time in order to minimize exposure to the radiation emanating from the patient.

Iatrogenic effects (similar to those in chemotherapy, depending on site and dosage) change one's capacity to relate to others.

Daily trips to the treatment site for 4 to 6 weeks, combined with the fatigue and other iatrogenic effects, can limit the capacity to participate in even the most ongoing relationships that normally do not require much effort.

Bone Marrow Transplant

Bone marrow transplants, with the associated aggressive radiation and chemotherapy and accompanied by stringent protective isolation, cause so much debility, restricted capacity to communicate, and vulnerability to infection that the initiative for overcoming social isolation tends not to come from the patient. Ongoing need for avoidance of infection precludes many activities and contacts even when the patient feels much better.

Patients and families often travel long distances to specialized centers for treatment, so links to usual support systems are attenuated.

Biologic Response Modifiers	Usually these treatments require hospitalization. The flulike effects, fever, and other side-effects are sufficient to cause the person to become more egocentric during treatment.
Age	In addition to the effects of treatment, the age of both the patient and personal network can have an influence on mobility and thus on the ease with which personal contacts can be made. Also, as the patient grows older, there can be a reduction in the size and functional capacity of the support network (Copstead and Patterson, 1986).

Daily Living Factors

The following factors in daily living can influence social isolation. They serve as a basis for assessment and diagnosis.

Activities in Daily Living	Any activity that offers opportunities for experiencing the support or rejection of people or cherished animals in one's personal network, employment situation, or health care provider group will be of concern in diagnosing the strengths or deficits in physical or emotional closeness.
	Any activity that interferes with the offering and receiving of genuine, willing sharing of the cancer experience is also of concern.
Events in Daily Living	Events related to health care that alter the nature of supportive relationships include hospitalization, daily travel for treatments, being placed in some form of isolation, receiving treatments in isolating settings, and the scheduling of medical events or treatments that the patient or family find highly threatening.
Demands in Daily Living	*Self-expectations* involve:

The amount and nature of interpersonal closeness needed for comfort and well-being—usually and in the current situation

Expectations as to what constitutes "personal support" (e.g., attitudes, verbal and physical behavior) from specific others in the current situation (family, friends, nurses, or physicians)

Expectations of others include:

The kinds of closeness or support they feel they *should* offer the patient

How they expect the patient to behave in terms of sharing or concealing the cancer experience

The degree of independence or dependence they expect the patient to undertake

Environment for Daily Living

Important environmental factors include those in the institutional, home, work, or school environments that support or deter personal closeness (e.g., laminar air flow rooms, the number of beds in the patient's room, chemotherapy cubicles, external beam radiation rooms, signs warning of infections or types of isolation, use of gowns, masks, and gloves, the level of nurse staffing and constancy of nursing personnel, the number and rate of rotation of house medical staff, and current research that could involve the patient in its population).

The effectiveness of technology to make the patients feel secure that their needs and calls for assistance will be heard or seen by health care providers can also be a factor.

Home environments that provide opportunities for privacy for some interactions and openness for others can make a difference.

Neighborhood, church, club, or work-related norms for support of their group members will influence social interaction for the patient.

Distances between neighbors or family members and between home and treatment site, and transportation systems will affect social interaction and risks for isolation.

Values and Beliefs

The influence of values and beliefs on the degree of social support or isolation the patient feels can be determined by asking the following questions:

What discrepancies, if any, exist in values related to independence versus interdependence or dependence held by the patient, family, and health care providers?

What incongruences, if any, exist between the patient's, family's, and health care providers' values regarding being alone—physically? emotionally?

What beliefs are held about cancer (e.g., cancer means death; cancer is contagious)? What beliefs about role obligations and role behaviors of persons in patient, family, and health care provider roles are affecting behaviors and role relationships? Are there any incongruences?

What are the philosophies and objectives of the medical and nursing health care staff as they affect professional relationships with the patient and the family? What are the congruencies and incongruences between the beliefs of the patient and the family as to the nature of services to be provided and the treatment milieus?

Functional Health Status

The functional capacities particularly involved in maintaining a desired degree of closeness with others are strength and endurance, cognition, mood, communication, and courage. These capacities will change at various points in the treatment phase, as will the demands on them.

Strength and Endurance

These capacities involve the level of physical and emotional strength and staying power needed:

To deal with the stresses of the cancer experience and the strains it places on individuals and relationships

To continue the work of bonding with important persons in one's support network and to forge bonds with new, potentially supportive people

The amount of vulnerability felt should be considered in relationship to isolating factors in the cancer experience.

The person's tolerance for "alone" time in treatment and non-treatment settings is an area for assessment.

It is important to know what the patient's ego strength is when infections, radiation implants, or stereotypes about cancer cause one to be or seem to be a danger to others.

Cognition

Cognitive capacity associated with social isolation involves the ability to understand:

The thinking and values of others that are shaping their relationships

The rationale for physical isolation (to protect others from harm or to protect oneself from the pathogens carried by others)

Mood

Important dimensions of mood involve the status of usual and current optimism or pessimism; state and trait anxiety; and any history of depression (endogenous or exogenous).

Communication

Communication for building or maintaining social relationships can involve the capacity to:

Make oneself understood in the presence of oral lesions

Convey to family members, friends, co-workers, and health care providers the level and nature of interpersonal closeness that is needed or desired at any given time

Courage

Courage related to social isolation involves the capacity to take risks in maintaining or building bonds with others in the face of others' possible discomfort, preoccupation, or rejection.

Nursing Diagnosis and Treatment

Diagnostic Targets

Targets for nursing diagnosis and treatment of social isolation include the patient, family, friends, health care providers (inpatient, outpatient, home care), co-workers, and the patient's "most significant other" (Gates, 1988). Individuals or groups are chosen for diagnosis and treatment when there is evidence of patient discomfort with the quantity and quality of interpersonal closeness or where this can be predicted.

Risk Factors

Social isolation and associated discomfort or dysfunction in daily living is a higher risk among persons who:

Have disfiguring cancers

Have cancer therapy with high potential for disfiguring and severe iatrogenic effects

Have active treatment that extends over weeks and months

Are isolated for their own protection or that of others

Come to the cancer experience with a dysfunctional support system or one that is barely functional when no stress is present (Roberts, 1988)

Have experienced loss of an important person(s) in their support network within the last 12 months

Have a passive, dependent approach in their own lives

Have a history of depression or loneliness

Already carry heavy emotional burdens and responsibilities (Gates, 1988; Green, 1986)

Live in areas where there are great distances between neighbors or members of the family or poor transportation options

Receive their major personal support from pets from whom they must be separated

Have treatment teams that focus on the neoplasia and its treatment to the exclusion of the day-to-day human elements of the cancer experience

Diagnostic Areas

The diagnostic areas listed below suggest possible focuses for diagnoses related to social isolation. In order to become working diagnoses that could provide a basis for individualized treatment planning, they would need to be made much more precise. This is done by incorporating the specific data on isolating factors, the person's response, and the impact on daily living, as these are present in the current situation.

Feelings of aloneness R/T difficulties in interacting with family, friends, co-workers, or health care professionals who do not have cancer

Feelings of aloneness by the "most significant other," family member, or friend R/T difficulties in interacting with the person who has the diagnosed cancer

Feelings of neglect and isolation from support (Zimberg, 1986) R/T:

Being in protective isolation

Being a woman with continuing disproportionate household and care giving responsibilities (Green, 1986)

Having a personal or health care provider support system that appears to be available, but in reality only exacerbates the sense of isolation because of their distancing behaviors

Deficits in ability to communicate needs or desires to care givers and health care providers in ways that are effective

Receiving inadequate attention or care from health care providers and care givers

Feelings of alienation R/T:

Being labelled as a danger to others during time of radiation implantation

Distancing from other members of the gay community due to visible manifestations of AIDS-related Kaposi's sarcoma

Feelings of isolation R/T:

Unfamiliarity with the surroundings and personnel

Inability to speak or understand the language of the health care provider group (e.g., English, medical jargon)

Fear of being abandoned R/T:

Incongruence of health care values with physicians or nurses

Being informed that one has "failed the protocol" or that the tumor is not responding

Inability to meet role expectations of significant other(s) (specify)

Manifestations   Reported:

Feeling different from others who don't have cancer or the side-effects of the treatment

Sense of alienation or aloneness

Feeling neglected by staff or others

Missing contact with certain individuals

Fear of possible abandonment by important others

Lack of energy to maintain relationships

Lack of knowledge for linking with possible support groups

Observed:

Sad, depressed, apathetic, or angry mood (rule out physical causes)

Limited command of English (speaking or comprehension)

Decreased participation in decision making and activities in daily living

Decrease in number of visits, phone calls, cards, and letters the patient receives

Increased superficiality in conversation (patient or others); increased emotional distance from others

Physicians make visits short and businesslike, use only procedural touch, or use an impersonal or condescending approach

Nurses make only task-oriented contacts with the patient, maintain businesslike approach, or fail to assign consistent personnel

Prognostic Variables

Poor prognosis for managing daily living with social isolation is associated with:

Previous patterns of isolation, dependence, or loneliness

Treatment that is aggressive and of longer duration

A weak or dysfunctional support system

Loss of significant other(s) within the past year

A high degree of cultural isolation

Complications

Complications of social isolation include depression, loss of motivation to participate, giving up, or discontinuing treatment (Molbo, 1986).

Treatment Guidelines

Feelings of social isolation as a person who has cancer in the midst of people who do not

Help the patient or family to link up with cancer support groups (e.g., CanSurmount, I Can Cope), in which all are sharing the cancer experience (Lieberman, 1988).

Feelings of isolation from the cancer patient because one doesn't have cancer

Link the partner or friend of the patient with someone in another patient's support network, or with a support group in which experiences of the partners, family members, and friends are shared and new insights and strategies are learned.

Feelings of neglect R/T prescribed isolation

Explain the reason for isolation (the need to protect either the patient from exogenous pathogens or staff, family, and friends from the danger of radiation from the implants in the patient).

Negotiate with the patient regarding the frequency or times of contact, whether for treatment or discussion of feelings.

Introduce the possibility of feelings of "being neglected"; indicate that they are not uncommon and that they are legitimate. Explore options for managing contacts in such a way as to reduce the feelings.

Discomfort with environment of isolation

Discuss the time-limited nature of the need for isolation. Encourage interest in white blood cell counts and differentials to determine the absolute neutrophil count as a gauge of need for protective isolation.

Encourage the patient or family to decorate the room with pictures, drawings, and objects of emotional importance.

Encourage the patient to ask for clarification if he doesn't understand what is being said or can't hear what is being said by staff or visitors wearing masks (Hennessey, 1988).

Loss of previous patterns of or opportunities for physical and emotional closeness with important others

Identify factors contributing to social isolation (e.g., medically prescribed, self-imposed, or imposed by others).

Gather data on factors contributing to self-imposed or other-imposed separations.

Make an opportunity for the patient to discuss losses in relationships by commenting on the commonness of feelings of social isolation in persons experiencing cancer and cancer treatment. If the patient does share the losses and the feelings being generated by them:

Be nonjudgmental in responding

Legitimize the losses and the patient's responses: "What you are experiencing is not at all uncommon, but knowing that doesn't make it any easier to go through."

Avoid giving advice

Explore possible and acceptable alternatives for expressions of closeness and affection in the presenting situation:

Letter writing, journal writing

Telephone calls

Talking about areas of interest to the patient

Being with the person

Touching, stroking

Involve the partner or a representative of the patient's family and friends in a discussion of alternatives available in the presenting situation (National Cancer Institute, 1986):

Identify factors that contribute to separation behavior (e.g., belief that cancer is contagious, feelings of discomfort related to helplessness, or not knowing how to talk to the person).

Address the deficits in knowledge; correct misinformation. Offer ideas and strategies for becoming genuinely and concretely helpful in the present situation. Work on and rehearse scripts to get conversations started and to keep them moving.

Arrange (with patient's permission) for a visit from a CanSurmount volunteer; invite the person to a scheduled meeting of an appropriate support group (e.g., I Can Cope program), in which the shared cancer experience reduces opportunities for social isolation.

Explore patient's perception of the reactions to his diagnosis of persons most important to him (e.g., "How do you think your * _____ [* spouse, friend] is handling the knowledge that you have cancer?"; "How do the people who are important to you treat you when they are with you these days?"). If patient identifies specific persons who are having difficulty, explore ways in which the patient thinks he might behave to help them to become more comfortable in the encounters (e.g., "Can you think of any ways you could help _____ to regain his usual comfort in relating to you?"). If the patient has no suggestions, try an approach such as, "What do you think would happen if you . . . ?"

Lack of ability to make needs known

Introduce the expectation that in this health care setting the staff want the patients to make their needs and concerns known—emotional as well as physical.

Discuss the communication difficulties experienced by other patients as they have tried to make their needs known to staff and particularly to individuals who are closest to them (Wabrek, 1987).

Explore the patient's values about asking for help or asking others to respond and behave in ways that would be helpful.

Explore any strategies the patient might find acceptable that would enable him to communicate his needs and desires to specific individuals. Explore the option of the nurse communicating for the patient in specific instances.

Ineffective support system

Identify the patient's "most significant other" and assess (if possible) that person's willingness, ability, and skill in main taining a close, supportive relationship with the patient during the cancer experience. Determine the kind of support the significant other needs to maintain personal resources and build the skills needed to serve as an effective support to the patient.

If no person can be found to serve in the "key support role" from among the patient's personal network, negotiate with the patient to gain permission to mobilize links with surrogates in support groups for both emotional support and supportive services such as transportation, food, food supplements, and supplies.

Fear of abandonment

Prevention

Provide realistic information to patient and family about how this particular medical and nursing system works. Identify patient and family strategies that will be effective in gaining optimum support from the system.

Provide information concerning patient fears to physician and nursing staff.

Offer the nurse's service as an advocate, if desired. (See discussion of treatment of powerlessness in role relationships in the section on Role in this chapter for four levels of nurse participation.)

Explore strategies for maintaining supportive relationships within one's personal network. (See also section on Role, under Treatment Guidelines, in this chapter.)

Where possible, work with the patient's "most important persons" to help them to understand the adjustment the person experiencing cancer is undergoing, and his fears and reticence to share. Explore actions and behavior the support person may undertake to minimize fears of emotional or physical abandonment.

Actual abandonment

Gather data on the patient's perception of the abandonment (e.g., who has abandoned the patient, the area of abandonment [emotional or physical], and the degree of abandonment [partial or total]). Try to gather substantiating data on the presenting situation (e.g., tumor not responding to treatment, iatrogenic effects resistant to treatment, physician becoming more impersonal, nurses rotating the patient daily, no visitors, cards, or phone calls, patient having to give self-care at home).

Where health care staff are the focus, negotiate to improve their approaches to patient.

Where members of the personal network are concerned, gather data on past strength of the network. Mobilize support for members of the network, if there is potential for giving patient support. If there is little hope of mobilizing support from the personal network, place emphasis on linking patient with support groups and the building of new networks.

Alienation from partner, family, or friends R/T representing a danger to them

Prevention

Provide patient and important others with information about realistic risks versus myths about the risks of maintaining close contact with a person who has the patient's type of cancer or treatment. Answer questions honestly.

Suggest options and strategies for maintaining a genuinely supportive relationship with the patient without incurring any risks (e.g., in the face of radiation implants, AIDS-related Kaposi's sarcoma).

Actual alienation

See treatment guidelines above on "ineffective support system." See also section on Sexuality in this chapter.

Cultural isolation R/T English as a second language or medical–nursing jargon as an unknown language

Seek a representative of the ethnic or cultural group to provide information to the staff on critical issues in the care of the patient to minimize cultural isolation (e.g., diet, values, language, key words, or use of touch).

Arrange for ethnic or preferred food to be brought in, if it is not available through the institutional food service.

Incorporate cultural norms into planning for visits and family or friends remaining with the patient (as much as the patient's condition and the setting permit).

Where English is a first language, but medical language is "foreign," translate what has been said into the person's own language or vernacular.

Make arrangements for an interpreter to be present at times when informal as well as formal consent is needed and when instructions are being given (e.g., before treatment and for discharge planning).

Evaluation

Response to nursing treatment for social isolation can be evaluated in the following areas:

Reported feelings of continued isolation or feeling closer or more comfortable in critical relationships

Status of comfort and participation in the cancer experience of persons in the support network

Status of ability to report feelings, activities, and events associated with social isolation and to take action to prevent or manage them; status of outcomes of these actions

Supportive and nonsupportive behavior of health care providers

Status of adjustments in the implementation of health care to take into account the cultural factors; patient and family responses

---

Other Problems Having an Impact on Daily Living During Initial Treatment

Living With Fear and Anxiety

Initial cancer treatment usually occurs right on the heels of a confirmed diagnosis of cancer, when patients and families are still experiencing the stress of learning of a possibly life-threatening disease. Patients may be in early stages of grieving (denial, anger) over the sense of loss of confidence in their body and their health, even though they may be relatively symptom-free. Diagnostic tests have introduced them to the loss of privacy over their bodies and information about themselves that accompanies encounters with the health care system. Becoming a patient has also added the stresses of entering into new required roles and environments, and a sense of change in personal control over daily living.

Then the treatment protocols are proposed, with life and death decisions on the line. Consent forms and accompanying explanations spell out in explicit language the effects the treatment can have. Physicians may share information regarding prognosis without treatment and the statistics for recovery associated with the various forms of treatment. Even though the patient may be too stressed to be able to comprehend everything and even though the words can never equal the reality of the experience, the impressions created are enough to generate an increase in fear and anxiety during the period of anticipation of the treatment and the emergence of iatrogenic effects.

Fear and anxiety are both psychobiologic responses in which the emotional state is one of apprehension or foreboding. They may coexist. Either one can range in intensity from mild discomfort to disorganized panic.

Fear is the label given to the response when a specific focus for the response can be identified (e.g., fear of needles, of pain). *Anxiety* is the diagnosis when the response is to a diffuse threat to the integrity of the person (e.g., threats to survival, to cherished roles, to functioning, to values). It is a response to the unknown and unknowable.

Nursing Diagnosis and Treatment

Diagnostic Targets   Diagnostic targets may include the patient, family, or those who are sharing the anticipation and the waiting with the patient and watching the patient's response to the treatment experience.

Diagnostic Areas

Diagnoses related to fear and anxiety will include several elements.

FEAR

The presence and level of fear

The specific focus(es) of the person's fears, (e.g., pain, the introduction of the cytotoxic drug into the body, being alone in the radiation therapy room)

Areas in which the response to fear is interfering with effective management of requirements of daily living (including the medical regimen) and with life satisfaction

ANXIETY

The presence and level of anxiety

The person's perception of possible threats to personal integrity (life, functioning, roles, values)

Areas in which the response to anxiety is interfering with effective management of requirements of daily living (including the medical regimen) and with life satisfaction

Treatment Guidelines

Determine the presence and level of fear and anxiety.

Differentially diagnose between them by determining if there is a specific focus for the unease (fear) or a diffuse sense of threat (anxiety).

If the emotional status permits cognitive functioning, help the patient or family member to put the focus of the unease or concerns into words. Assist in identification of realistic goals that can reduce the concerns. Help, as needed, in the development of plans to mobilize resources or undertake strategies to achieve as much of the desired goals as possible. *

If fear or anxiety is based on knowledge deficit or misinformation, give reality-based information using short sentences and simple vocabulary, in amounts the person can take in without "shutting down." (Remember that *knowledge can increase fear and anxiety* as well as decrease them.)

Use touch as an adjunct to the verbal messages, if this appears to be acceptable to the person and the level of emotional response is not at the panic level.

Seek feedback gently to determine what the person has actually heard and understood, being careful not to give messages that the nurse thinks the person is incompetent or stupid.

When fear or anxiety are at high levels, modify the environment to reduce the number and level of stimuli, particularly stimuli seen as threatening. Reduce the numbers of health care

---

* Remember that fear and anxiety that are greater than modest levels reduce the person's usual capacity for cognitive functioning and fine muscular coordination, so more than normal assistance may be needed.

providers with whom the person must interact. Recruit a companion or care giver to be with the patient—one who is caring and empathetic but not easily infected by the patient's fear or anxiety. Do not try to teach or problem solve; instead, serve as an advocate on the person's behalf. Use previously enjoyed distractions (e.g., TV or preferred type of music) if this proves helpful.

Evaluation   If fear or anxiety is reduced, the person will appear less tense and the pulse and respiration rate will be slower. The person may indicate having greater peace of mind.

Living With Threats to Hope

Hope is a crucial life force for patients and their families in the cancer experience. The issue of hope emerges (in the context of cancer) when a desired and anticipated future appears to be threatened by the diagnosed disease. *Hope involves a concurrent awareness of both a precious expectation and a realistic threat.*

Hope has been characterized as being neither a passive waiting nor an unrealistic forcing of circumstances that can't occur (Fromm, 1968). Rather, it is a positive state of mind that brings an inner readiness for action and participation. Hope is an important internal resource as the patient and family undertake the rigors of oncologic treatment; it can help to maintain them through the difficulties of some of the more aggressive forms of treatment (Hickey, 1986).

Hope is not a steady state; it can be fragile and tenuous. Where cancer is the threat, hope is subject to the influences of:

Long-held beliefs about cancer outcomes

Remembrances of persons experiencing cancer and its treatment earlier in one's life and during the present experience

Pre-existing well-being or depression

Personal losses from which there has not been time to recover

Good or bad news from the physician

Faith in the health care providers or one's own ability to withstand suffering, and religious or existential beliefs (Miller, 1985)

Symptom emergence or abatement

Reports and observations of others experiencing cancer and similar treatment

Messages related to the degree of hope in the presenting situation as they are actually perceived and interpreted. These include unspoken messages (attitudes, body language, subliminal cues) sensed from health care providers, family, and others, as well as verbalized messages.

The genuine and sustained hopefulness or hopelessness of significant others

Hope can be responsive to the behavior of others, including their continuation of usual contacts, alteration in contacts, or unusual solicitude or distancing, whether it is evidenced in subtle attitudinal changes or actual physical distance.

Hope can be either realistic or false. Even false hope can serve a purpose for a time by offering respite or an interval in which to regroup inner resources for again facing the demands of reality.

Hope can focus on both long- and short-range targets. It can concern ultimate survival, but it can also be so mundane as to hope for a good night's sleep or a visit from a cherished friend.

Realistic fears and expectations combined with hope can mobilize body psychobiologic resources to respond to the treatment and achieve the best possible outcome.

Nursing Diagnosis and Treatment

Diagnostic Targets

The patient, family and companions who share the illness and treatment experience, and health care providers (nurses, physicians, others) are all possible diagnostic targets.

Diagnostic Areas

Diagnoses focusing on hope will contain several elements. These include:

The presence and degree of hope or hopelessness; its tenuousness or sturdiness

Factors that contribute to the current status of hope or hopelessness (e.g., signs and symptoms, information received from health care providers about prognosis and ongoing response to treatment, status of trust in health care providers, past experiences with persons who have had similar cancer and treatment, beliefs about the curability of cancer in general or this type of cancer, cues indicating hope or hopelessness in family and close companions, the strength and appropriateness of the personal support system)

Observed impact or potential impact on capacity to participate in treatment regimen

Manifestations

Hopelessness is manifested by some degree of:

Reported feelings of being "drained," vulnerability or helplessness, being overwhelmed, expecting the worst, being in despair

Observed decrease in activity, social or emotional withdrawal, increased irritability and tension (Miller, 1985)

Treatment Guidelines

PATIENT, CARE GIVER, OTHERS

Where hope is very tenuous or hopelessness is present:

Share patient data that can promote hope, or report on situations in which other patients have had similar experiences and are later doing well (where such information is realistically available). With patient permission, schedule a visit by CanSurmount volunteers who have had similar experiences and have managed.

Help the person to identify elements that create a new appreciation for life—elements that are realistically possible to enjoy. Consider, but do not limit options to aspects of daily living that have been enjoyed in the past. Where cure is questionable, look for pleasurable experiences rather than cure.

Support the finding of important reasons for living by helping the person to discover aspects in his or her present life that may have been taken for granted. Use ongoing daily contacts with the person to talk about past or present life activities, what is important to the person, what has given pleasure in the past, and what will now give pleasure. Coordinate this activity specifically in the nursing plan so that not every nurse develops these conversations in a random fashion.

Negotiate realistic goals with the person (patient, care giver, or other) that consistently include some pleasurable or satisfying event or experience, no matter how small. Consider *short-term* goals for this contact, later today, or this week; *intermediate* goals for the next 1 to 6 months; and *long-term* goals for beyond 6 months.

Help the person to find ways to experience laughter and to be aware of the importance of laughter. Suggest watching videos of funny movies (old or new) or television comedies, sharing funny experiences with friends, and hearing new jokes.

Encourage participation, even quiet participation, with friends, family, cancer support groups, or ostomy clubs.

NURSES One concern related to maintenance of hope among patients and families is the potential for erosion of hope among nurses. An overriding cynicism about prognosis can creep in for nurses who work in settings in which they see patients who receive initial treatment and then those who return when treatment is not successful, but not those who require no further treatment. It is important to anticipate, diagnose, and treat nurses' reduced capacity to genuinely promote hope in patients and families. Some of the strategies used by leaders on such units include:

Foster a sense of esprit de corps and a special group identity for the nursing team on the unit

Initiate support group meetings when needed

Arrange care conferences to plan sound, consistent nursing care for patients and families

Acknowledge and deal openly with guilt and grieving when patients regress or die after nurses have had prolonged contact over multiple admissions: ("We know that we nurses did everything we could.")

Celebrate life (birthdays, births, special occasions)

Create norms of genuine, dependable support from other nurses for individual nurses whose patient–family case load is emotionally and physically demanding

Hope is an important internal resource during the active treatment stage. Diagnosing deficits in this area for patients and families and helping to mobilize hope can be important, not only for their personal comfort, but also as a means of promoting the most effective host response and participation in the total treatment regimen.

Living With Noxious Odors†

During the initial treatment stage the most frequent noxious odors arise from iatrogenic oral lesions and ostomy stoma or pouches. These can affect the person's self-esteem and confidence in social and work relationships in daily living.

Frequent careful oral hygiene is the treatment for halitosis (see section on Difficulties in Eating in this chapter). Effective, regular changing, cleansing, and deodorizing of the ostomy pouch is the treatment for preventing ostomy odors (Brubacher and Schultz, 1988). After stripping out the contents of the ostomy pouch, warm water and possibly a mild cleansing solution should be poured into the open end and manipulated in the bag to remove any remaining material and cleanse the walls, repeating until the pouch is clean and odor-free. Then Osto-Zyme can be sprayed into it to control odors until the next emptying or changing of the pouch (Alterescu, 1982).

Living With Changes in Sleep Patterns

Unusual difficulties in sleeping tend to occur during the initial treatment stage as a result of (Brewer, 1985):

Emotional discomforts associated with knowledge of the diagnosis and anticipation of treatments

Physical discomforts associated with the disease or treatment

The hospital environment

At times, patients may be unable to sleep. Wakeful nights may be long, lonely, and filled with discomfort, fears, and concerns. At other times fatigue results in more than the usual amount of sleep. Sleep can become a way of escaping unpleasant symptoms such as nausea. Patterns of sleep may change and sleep may occur in shorter spans and at several times during a 24-hour period, when treatments, monitoring or other types of responsibilities permit. However, such unusual sleep schedules do not provide the same quality of sleep as that obtained during usual hours and can, in fact, lead to sleep deprivation (Brewer, 1985) and desynchronization (Richards and Bairnsfather, 1988).

The use of medications to promote sleep is not the ideal solution (beyond the most acute period), in that narcotics such as morphine sulfate or meperidine hydrochloride suppress REM sleep, while tranquilizers do not permit the person to reach the deepest levels of sleep (Kavey and Anderson, 1986). Thus medications are important during acute times of the treatment phase, but offer only abnormal sleep and are not long-term solutions.

Changes in sleep patterns of the patient can affect others as well. The person who shares the bed, bedroom, or patient unit, who may also be experiencing emotional tension, may find needed sleep disrupted by the patient's restlessness, getting up during the night, or seeking distraction in reading or television. At home, sleeping during the

---

† Noxious odors are also addressed in Chapter 10.

lay may impose restrictions on the daytime activities of those who share the home, such as children's play or vacuuming. In the hospital, ongoing activities may make daytime sleep difficult. The hospital environment, with its 24-hour approach to treatment and medical and legal obligations for monitoring, is not conducive to sleep (Richards and Bairsnfather, 1988; Wilson, 1985).

The physiologic and psychologic changes resulting from sleep deficits can affect management of daily living and functioning during active treatment. Responses to sleep deficits include:

Decreases in reasoning, judgment, association, impulse control, auditory and visual vigilance, motivation, and interpersonal effectiveness

Increases in anxiety, agitation, sensitivity, suspicion, irritability, mood disruption, emotional lability, fatigue, malaise, and sleepiness (Brewer, 1985)

There is some speculation that sleep influences healing via release of hormones that have anabolic functions (Brewer, 1985).

Thus promotion of as normal sleep as possible during the person's usual hours of sleep (both patient and care giver) can help the person to maintain basic resources to promote healing and manage the challenges of daily living during cancer treatment.

Nursing Diagnosis and Treatment

Diagnostic Targets

Diagnostic targets include:

Patient

Person sharing the bed, bedroom, or patient unit

Care givers, who also may become sleep deprived because of the wakefulness of the patient at night and care giving or other major responsibilities during the day

Persons who share the living space in the daytime

Diagnostic Areas

Note that the diagnoses may need to be revised several times during the treatment phase as patient status and other factors change.

PATIENT

Difficulties in sleeping R/T sounds of the hospital environment and monitoring and treatment activities for patient and others in shared space

Sleep deprivation R/T inadequate symptom management (e.g., pain, nausea, diarrhea, nocturia)

PATIENT OR PERSON IN SAME ROOM (*INSTITUTION* OR HOME)

Difficulties with occupying nighttime hours R/T sleeplessness

PATIENT OR CARE GIVER

Sleep deprivation R/T sleepless nights and child care or employment obligations during the day that prevent daytime naps

Difficulty in accepting the legitimacy of or adjusting schedules to sleeping in different time spans and at different hours than is usual R/T past patterns and beliefs

PATIENT,
OCCUPANTS
OF THE SAME
LIVING SPACE,
HEALTH CARE
PROVIDERS

Difficulties in adjusting the activities and schedules of others who share the living space R/T patient need to sleep in different patterns

TREATMENT
GUIDELINES

Institutional sleep deterrents

During night hours, keep non-nursing-oriented chatter to a minimum (Wilson, 1985), and essential verbal interaction at a low volume. Reduce other noises as much as possible. Provide patient with soft foam earplugs (Brewer, 1985).

Schedule treatment and monitoring activities so that they are grouped into one patient contact. Where in a double room, try to give scheduled care to both patients during one time span.

Inform patients at bedtime what the required schedule of monitoring and treatments will be. If possible, schedule around the hours when the patient says he usually sleeps the best (e.g., some sleep best the first part of the night, others later in the night).

Consider bringing wakeful, worried patients who are ambulatory or in wheel chairs to the nurses' station, where there is distraction, so that they won't lie in the dark and become increasingly distressed.

Other sleep-related problems

Determine available and desired alternatives to lying awake and doing nothing during the nights (in the institution or at home). Explore any deterrents to use of these diversions and seek alternatives (e.g., headphones for the TV or radio, a small reading light, lying on the recliner in another room).

Explore options for getting predictable periods of respite from child care or work responsibilities to permit a nap or rest in the daytime (for care giver or patient).

In hospital, try to schedule activities of patient care, housekeeping, tests etc. so that patient has opportunities for sleep at times that are desired or needed. Post a "Do not disturb" sign on door or cubicle curtain if needed and enforce it.

Legitimize the appropriateness of daytime naps or rest if this has not been a previous pattern.

Determine the ages and schedules of persons who occupy the living space during the day. Explore with patient and occupants the options available for managing the patient's need to sleep and the needs of others for activities. Help them to arrive at a tentative approach. Arrange for feedback and adjustments if needed.

Effective use of analgesics to relieve pain and sedatives to assist in sleep are two useful short-term medical interventions during acute phases of the active treatment period. Nurses, who usually have more accurate data on daily living, can negotiate with physicians regarding the need for medications for symptom control and can indicate the form of administration that will be best tolerated. Where treatment continues over prolonged periods, the ongoing problems of managing daily living with sleep difficulties or both the patient and others require nursing, not medical diagnosis and intervention. Such nursing management can become significant in maintaining well-being.

Summary

In this chapter, some common areas of dysfunction in initial cancer treatment, and the associated problems in daily living, have been addressed in terms of nursing diagnosis and treatment. Many of the areas will be approached again in later chapters, where they will be considered in terms of the differences that arise because the patient and family have moved on to a different stage of the cancer experience—post-treatment, survival, recurrence, or advanced cancer.

Accurate nursing diagnosis and effective nursing treatment initiated in the treatment phase may help patients to be more confident and competent as they subsequently encounter and manage variations on the same or similar problems. Strategies for problem recognition, consideration of options, and mobilization of resources and support systems learned at this point in the cancer experience by patients, families, and care givers should offer an ongoing repertoire of skills that will prove useful both to those who live with survival and those who face recurrence.

Bibliography

Role

Bartos O. Determinants and consequences of toughness. In: Swingle P, ed. The structure of conflict. New York: Academic Press, 1970.

Copstead LE, Patterson E. Families of the elderly. In: Carnevali D, Patrick M, eds. Nursing management for the elderly. 2nd ed. Philadelphia: JB Lippincott, 1986.

Casl SV, Cobb S. Health behavior, illness behavior and sick role behavior. Arch Environ Health 1966;12:246.

Murinson DS. Clinical pharmacology. In: Rosenthal SN, Bennett JM, eds. Practical cancer chemotherapy. Garden City, NY: Medical Examination Publishing, 1981.

Parsons T. Definitions of health and illness in the light of American values and social structure. In: Jaco EG, ed. Patients, physicians and illness. New York: Free Press, 1958.

Trillin AS. Of dragons and garden peas: a cancer patient talks to doctors. N Engl J Med 1981;304:699.

Loss of Desire to Eat

Behnke MC. Anorexia. In: Carieri VK, Lindsey AM, West CM, eds. Pathophysiological phenomena in nursing: human responses to illness. Philadelphia: WB Saunders, 1986.

Chance WT, Von Meyenfeldt MF, Fischer JG. Changes in brain amines associated with cancer anorexia. Neurosci Biobehav Rev 1983;7:471.

Coons H, Leventhal H, Nerenz D et al. Anticipatory nausea and emotional distress in patients receiving cisplastin based chemotherapy. Oncology Nursing Forum 1987;14:31.

De Wys WD. Pathophysiology of cancer cachexia: current understanding and areas for future research. Can Res 1982;42(suppl): 721.

Goo RH, Moore JG, Greenberg E, Alazraki NP. Circadian variations in gastric emptying of meals in humans. Gastroenterology 1987;93:515.

Hilderly, LJ. Radiotherapy. In: Groenwald SL, ed. Cancer nursing: principles and practice. Monterey, CA: Jones & Bartlett, 1987.

Holland JCB, Rowland J, Plumb M. Psychological aspects of anorexia in cancer patients. Can Res 1977;37:2425.

Lytle LD. Control of eating behavior. In: Wurtman RJ, Wurtman JJ, eds. Nutrition and the brain. Vol 2. New York: Raven Press, 1977.

Mayer D, Helrick K, Rigs C, Sherwin S. Weight loss in patients receiving recombinant leukocyte A interferon: a brief report. Cancer Nurs 1984;7:53.

McCorkle MR. Coping with physical symptoms in metastatic breast cancer. Am J Nurs 1973;73:1034.

Theologides A. Anorexia in cancer: another speculation on its pathogenesis. Nutr Cancer 1981;2:133.

US Department of Health and Human Services. Eating hints: recipes and tips for better nutrition during cancer treatment. Bethesda, MD: National Cancer Institute, NIH Publication 86-2079, 1986.

Williams K. Hunger. In: Carieri VK, Lindsey AM, West CM, eds. Pathophysiological phenomena in nursing human responses to illness. Philadelphia: WB Saunders, 1986.

Wurtman J. Effects of foods and nutrients on brain transmitters. Curr Concepts Nutr 1984;13:103.

Difficulties in Eating

Axelsson K, Norberg A, Asplund K et al. Training of eating after a stroke in a patient with dysphagia of pharyngeal type. Scandinavian Journal of Caring Sciences 1989;2:31.

Bersani G, Carl W. Oral care for cancer patients. Am J Nurs 1983;83:533.

Carl W. Oral complications in cancer patients. Am Fam Physician 1983;27:161.

Daeffler R. Oral hygiene for patients with cancer: parts I, II, III. Cancer Nurs 1980;3:347, 427; 1981;4:29.

Goodman MS. Head and neck malignancies. In: Groenwald SL, ed. Cancer nursing: principles and practice. Boston: Jones & Bartlett, 1987.

Goodman MS, Stoner C. Mucous membrane integrity, impairment of: somatitis. In: McNally JC, Stair JC, Somerville ET, eds. Guidelines for cancer nursing practice. New York: Grune & Stratton, 1985.

Grady RP, Farnen J, Ascheman P, et al. Nutrition, alterations in: less than body requirements related to dysphagia. In: McNally JC, Stair JC, Somerville ET, eds. Guidelines for cancer nursing practice. New York: Grune & Stratton, 1985.

Harwood A. The hot–cold theory of disease: implications for treatment of Puerto Rican patients. JAMA 1971;216:1153.

McNally JC. Dysphagia. Oncology Nursing Forum 1982;9:59.

Stroh R. Nutrition, alteration in: less than body requirements related to xerostomia. In: McNally JC, Stair JC Somerville ET, eds. Guidelines for cancer nursing practice. New York: Grune & Stratton, 1985.

Nausea and Vomiting

Ash D. The incidence, severity and frequency of nausea in cancer patients receiving cisplatinum. Second Conference on Cancer Nursing Research, A-28, England American Cancer Society (Abstract) 1981.

Bateman DN. Effects of meal temperature and volume on the emptying of liquid from the human stomach Journal of Physiology 1982;331:461.

Billings JA. Outpatient management of advanced cancer. Philadelphia: JB Lippincott, 1985.

Blacklow RS. MacBryde's signs and symptoms. 6th ed. Philadelphia: JB Lippincott, 1983.

Chase JL, Stagg RJ. Outpatient treatment of chemotherapy-induced nausea and vomiting. Outpatient Chemotherapy 1989;3:1.

Cotanch PH, Strum S. Progressive muscle relaxation as antiemetic therapy for cancer patients. Oncology Nursing Forum 1987;14:33.

Duigon A. Anticipatory nausea and vomiting associated with cancer chemotherapy. Oncology Nursing Forum 1986;13:35.

Dumas RG, Leonard RC. The effect of nursing on the incidence of postoperative vomiting. Nurs Res 1963;12:12.

Grant M. Nausea, vomiting and anorexia. Seminars in Oncology Nursing 1987;3:277.

Harris AL. Cytotoxic-therapy-induced vomiting is mediated via enkephalin pathways. Lancet 1982;8274:714.

Hilderly LJ. Radiotherapy. In: Groenwald SL, ed. Cancer nursing: principles and practice. Boston: Jones & Bartlett, 1987.

Hogan CM. Nausea and vomiting. In: Yasko JM, ed. Nursing management of symptoms associated with chemotherapy. Rev ed. Columbus, OH: Adria Laboratories, 1986.

Ignoffo RJ. Neoplastic disorders. In: Young LY, Koda-Kimble MA, eds: Applied therapeutics. 4th ed. Vancouver, WA: Applied Therapeutics, 1988.

Kennedy M, Packard R, Grant M, Padilla G. Chemotherapy related nausea and vomiting: a survey to identify problems and interventions. Oncology Nursing Forum 1981;8:19, 1981.

Koretz RL, Meyer JH. Elemental diets: facts and fantasies. Gastroenterology 1980;78:393.

Norris CM. Nausea and vomiting. In: Norris CM, ed. Concept clarification in nursing. Rockville, MD: Aspen Systems, 1982.

Rhodes VA, Watson PM, Johnson MH. Association of chemotherapy related nausea and vomiting with pretreatment and post treatment anxiety. Oncology Nursing Forum 1986;13:41.

Rhodes VA, Watson PM, Johnson MH. Patterns of nausea and vomiting in chemotherapy patients: a preliminary study. Oncology Nursing Forum 1985;12:42.

Rhodes VA, Watson PM, Johnson MH et al. Patterns of nausea, vomiting and distress in patients receiving antineoplastic drug protocols. Oncology Nursing Forum 1987;14:35.

Scogna DM. Nausea and vomiting: a significant problem for the cancer patient receiving treatment. In: Nursing care of the cancer patient with nutritional problems: report of the Ross roundtable on oncology nursing. Columbus, OH: Ross Laboratories, 1981.

Scott DW, Donahue DC, Mastrovito RC, Hakes TB. The antiemetic effect of clinical relaxation: report of an exploratory pilot study. Journal of Psychosocial Oncology 1983;1:71.

Tiedemann DE. Nausea and vomiting: a significant problem for the cancer patient receiving treatment. In: Nursing care of the cancer patient with nutritional problems: report of the Ross Roundtable on Oncology Nursing. Columbus, OH, Ross Laboratories, 1981.

Constipation

Dorr RT, Fritz W. Cancer therapy handbook. New York: Elsevier, 1980.

Heitkemper M, Bartol M. Gastrointestinal problems. In: Carnevali D, Patrick M, eds. Nursing management for the elderly. 2nd ed. Philadelphia: JB Lippincott, 1986.

Peterson M. Constipation and diarrhea. In: Blacklow RS, ed: MacBryde's signs and symptoms. 6th ed. Philadelphia: JB Lippincott, 1983.

Diarrhea

Epstein M, Oster J. Hypertension: practical approaches, p 179. Philadelphia: WB Saunders, 1984.

Groenwald S. Nutritional disorders. In: Groenwald S, ed. Cancer nursing: principles and practice. Monterey, CA: Jones & Bartlett, 1987.

Heitkemper M, Bartol M. Gastrointestinal problems. In: Carnevali D, Patrick M, eds. Nursing management for the elderly. 2nd ed. Philadelphia: JB Lippincott, 1986.

Hilderly L. Radiotherapy. In: Groenwald S, ed. Cancer nursing: principles and practice. Boston: Jones & Bartlett, 1987.

Peterson M. Constipation and diarrhea. In: Blacklow RS, ed. MacBryde's signs and symptoms. 6th ed. Philadelphia: JB Lippincott, 1983.

Fatigue

Aistars J. Fatigue in the cancer patient: a conceptual approach to a clinical problem. Oncology Nursing Forum 1987;14:25.

Akerstedt T, Gillberg M, Witterberg L. The circadian covariation of fatigue and urinary melatonin. Biol Psychiatry 1982;17:547.

Billings JA. Outpatient management of advanced cancer, p 125. Philadelphia: JB Lippincott, 1986.

Britton D. Fatigue. In: Yasko JM, ed. Guidelines for cancer care: symptom management. Reston, VA: Reston Publishing Co, 1983.

Cella D, Tross S. Psychological adjustment to survival from Hodgkin's disease. J Consult Clin Psychol 1986;54:616.

De Wys WD. Pathophysiology of cancer cachexia: current understanding and areas for future research. Cancer Res 1982;42(suppl):721.

Fobair P, Hoppe RT, Bloom J et al. Psychosocial problems among survivors of Hodgkin's disease. J Clin Oncol 1986;4:805.

Hauri P, Silberfarb P, Oxman T, et al. Sleep in cancer patients. Sleep Research 1985;14:237. Abstract.

Haylock P, Hart L. Fatigue in patients receiving localized radiation. Cancer Nurs 1979;2:461.

Hilderly LJ. Radiotherapy. In: Groenwald SL, ed. Cancer nursing: principles and practice. Boston: Jones & Bartlett, 1987.

Karlsson J, Sjodin B, Jacobs I. Relevance of muscle fiber type to fatigue in short intense and prolonged exercise in man. CIBA Foundation Symposium 82. Human muscle fatigue: physiologic mechanisms. London: Pittman Medical, 1981:59.

King K, Nail W, Kreamer K, et al. Patients' descriptions of the experience of receiving radiation therapy. Oncology Nursing Forum 1985;12:55.

Knox LS. Energy expenditure in malnourished cancer patients. Ann Surg 1983;197:152.

Lopes J, Russell D, Whitwell J, et al. Skeletal muscle function in malnutrition. Am J Clin Nutr 1983;36:602.

Mayer DK, Smalley RV. Interferon: current status. Oncology Nursing Forum 1983;10:14.

Nakamura Y, Schwartz S. The influence of hydrogen ion concentration on the calcium binding and release by skeletal muscle sarcoplasmic reticulum. J Gen Physiol 1972;59:22.

Piper BF, Lindsey AM, Dodd MJ. Fatigue mechanisms in cancer patients: developing nursing theory. Oncology Nursing Forum 1987;14:17.

Rhoten D. Fatigue and the postsurgical patient. In Norris CM, ed. Concept clarification in nursing. Rockville, MD: Aspen Publishers, 1982.

Taylor CR. Fatigue. In: Groenwald SL, ed. Cancer nursing: principles and practice. Monterey, CA: Jones & Bartlett, 1987.

Theologides A. Asthenia in cancer. Am J Med 1982;73:1.

Young VR. Energy metabolism and requirements in the cancer patient. Cancer Res 1977;37:2336.

Vulnerability to Infections

Armstrong D, Young LS, Meyer RD, et al. Infectious complications of neoplastic disease. Med Clin North Am 1971;55:729.

Gold J, Armstrong D. Opportunistic infections in patients with acquired immune deficiency syndrome. In: Ma P, Armstrong D, eds. The acquired immune deficiency syndrome and infections of homosexual men. New York: Yorke Medical Books, 1984.

Goldman R. Aging changes in structure and function. In: Carnevali D, Patrick M, eds. Nursing management for the elderly. 2nd ed. Philadelphia: JB Lippincott, 1986.

Groenwald S. Nutritional disorders. In: Groenwald S, ed. Cancer nursing: principles and practice. Monterey, CA: Jones & Bartlett, 1987.

Jeppeson, ME. Laboratory values for the elderly. In: Carnevali D, Patrick M, eds. Nursing management for the elderly. 2nd ed. Philadelphia: JB Lippincott, 1986.

Nixon D, Heymsfield SB, Cohen AE, et al. Protein and calorie undernutrition in hospitalized cancer patients. JAMA 1980;68:683.

Pitot HC. Fundementals of oncology. 3rd ed. New York: Marcel Dekker, 1986.

Pizzo PA. Infectious complications in the child with cancer: III. Complications of treatment and methods for prevention. J Pediatr 1981;98:524.

Riley F, Fitzmaurice MA, Spackman DH. Immunocompetence and neoplasia: role of nanxiety, stress. In: Levy S, ed. Biological mediators of behavor and disease: neoplasia. New York: Elsevier Biomedical, 1981.

Robichaud KJ, Hubbard SM. Infection. In: Groenwald SL, ed. Cancer nursing: principles and practice. Monterey, CA: Jones & Bartlett, 1987

Weksler M. The senescence of the immune system. Hosp Pract 1981;16:53.

Pain

Andersson S. Neurophysiology and biology of pain. In: Swerdolow M, Ventafridda V, eds: Cancer pain. London: Hastings Hilton, 1987.

Billings JA. Outpatient management of advanced cancer. Philadelphia: JB Lippincott, 1985.

Chapman CR, Syrjala K, Sargur M. Pain as a manifestation of cancer treatment. Seminars in Oncology Nursing 1985;1:100

Copp LA. The spectrum of suffering. Am J Nurs 1974;74:491.

Coyle N, Foley K. Pain in patients with cancer: profile of patients and common pain syndromes. Seminars in Oncology Nursing 1985;1:93.

Donovan M. Preface: pain control. Nurs Clin North Am 1987;22:645.

Fishman B, Loscalzo M. Cognitive–behavioral interventions in management of cancer pain: principles and applications. Cancer pain. Med Clin North Am 1987;71:271.

Foley KM. Cancer pain syndromes. Journal of Pain and Symptom Management 1987;2:513.

Foley KM. Pain syndromes in patients with cancer. In: Bonica JJ, Ventafridda V, eds. Advances in pain research and therapy. Vol 2. New York: Raven Press, 1979.

Foley KM. Pain syndromes in patients with cancer. In: Swerdolow M, Ventafridda V, eds. Cancer pain. London: Hastings Hilderly, 1987a.

Hilderly LJ. Radiotherapy. In: Groenwald SL, ed. Cancer nursing: principles and practice. Monterey, CA: Jones & Bartlett, 1987.

Howard-Ruben J, McGuire L, Groenwald SL: Pain. In Groenwald SL, ed. Cancer nursing: principles and practice. Monterey, CA: Jones & Bartlett, 1987.

Lisson EL. Ethical issues related to pain control. Nurs Clin North Am 1987;22:649.

Maciewicz R. Central pain pathways. Mediguide to Pain 1982;3:1.

Meinhart NT, McCaffrey M. Pain: a nursing approach to assessment and analgesia. New York: Appleton-Century-Crofts, 1983.

Mount B. Psychological and social aspects of cancer pain. In: Wall PO, Melzak R, eds. Textbook of pain. New York: Churchill Livingston, 1984.

Syrjala K. Stress and anxiety reduction: cognitive–behavioral therapies. In: Syllabus, general oncology update for physicians and nurses. Seattle, Washington Division of the American Cancer Society, University of Washington Schools of Medicine and Nursing, April 28–29, 1988.

Sexuality

American Cancer Society. Proceedings of the Workshop on Psychosexual and Reproductive Issues Affecting Patients With Cancer—1987. New York: American Cancer Society, 1987.

Andersen B. Sexual functioning complications in women with gynecologic cancer. Cancer 1987;60:2123.

Andersen B, Hacker N. Psychosocial adjustment after vulvar surgery. Obstet Gynecol 1983;62:457.

Annon JS. The behavioral treatment of sexual problems. Honolulu: Mercantile Printing, 1974.

Atwell B. Sex and the cancer patient: an unspoken concern. Patient Education and Counseling 1983;5:123.

Cochran S, Hacker N, Wellisch D, et al. Sexual functioning after treatment for endometrial cancer. Journal of Psychosocial Oncology 1987;5:47.

Doan-Noyes D, Mellody P. Beauty and cancer. Los Angeles, AC Press, 1988.

Fischer SG. The psychosexual effects of cancer and cancer treatment. Oncology Nursing Forum 1983;10:63.

Heard L. Care of the patient with modified radical mastectomy. In: Reiner A, ed. Manual of patient care standards. Rockville MD: Aspen Publishers, 1988.

Heinrich-Rynning T. Prostatic cancer treatments and their effects on sexual functioning. Oncology Nursing Forum 1987;14:37.

Hogan R. Human sexuality: a nursing perspective. New York: Appleton–Century–Crofts, 1980.

Jenkins B. Sexual healing after pelvic irradiation. Am J Nurs 1986;86:920.

Johnston LH, Stair JC. Sexual dysfunction: infertility. In: McNally JC, Stair JC, Somerville ET, eds. Guidelines for cancer nursing practice. New York: Grune & Stratton, 1985.

Knobf MK, Mullen JC, Xistris D, et al. Weight gain in women with breast cancer receiving adjuvant chemotherapy. Oncology Nursing Forum 1983;10:28.

Lamb MA, Woods NF. Sexuality and the cancer patient. Cancer Nurs 1981;4:137.

Metcalfe M, Fischman S. Factors affecting the sexuality of patients with head and neck cancer. Oncology Nursing Forum 1985;12:21.

Murinson DS. Clinical pharmacology. In: Rosenthal SN, Bennett JM, eds. Practical cancer chemotherapy. Garden City, NY: Medical Examination, 1981.

Resnick M. Hormone therapy in prostatic cancer. Urology 1984;5(suppl):18.

Schain WS. The sexual and intimate consequences of breast cancer treatment. CA 1988;38:154.

Schnarch DM. Talking to patients about sex: part I. Medical Aspects of Human Sexuality 1988;22:66.

Schover LR. Sexuality and cancer for the man who has cancer and his partner. Atlanta: American Cancer Society, 1988.

Schover LR. Sexuality and cancer for the woman who has cancer and her partner. Atlanta: American Cancer Society, 1988a.

Schover LR, von Eschenbach A, Smith D et al. Sexual rehabilitation of urologic cancer patients: a practical approach. CA 1984;34:66.

Schwarz-Applebaum J, Dedrick J, Jusenius K, et al. Nursing care plans: sexuality and treatment of breast cancer. Oncology Nursing Forum 1984;11:16.

Sex and the cancer patient. Editorial. Lancet 1984;1(8374):432.

Sinsheimer L, Holland J. Psychological issues in breast cancer. Seminars in Oncology 1987;14:75.

Von Eschenbach AC, Schover LR. The role of sexual rehabilitation in the treatment of patients with cancer. Cancer 1984;54:2662.

Social Isolation

Copstead LA, Patterson S. Families of the elderly. In: Carnevali D, Patrick M. Nursing management for the elderly. 2nd ed. Philadelphia: JB Lippincott, 1986.

Gates CC. The "most-significant-other" in the care of the breast cancer patient. CA 1988;38:146.

Green CP. Changes in responsibility in women's families after the diagnosis of cancer. Health Care for Women International 1986;7:221.

Hennessey S. Care of the patient with neutropenia. In: Reiner A. Manual of patient care standards. Rockville, MD: Aspen Publishers, 1988.

Lieberman MA. The role of self-help groups in helping patients and families cope with cancer. CA 1988;38:162.

Molbo D. Cancer. In: Carnevali D, Patrick M, eds. Nursing management for the elderly. 2nd ed. Philadelphia: JB Lippincott, 1986.

Morgan C. The loneliest battle. Surviving: A Cancer Patient Newsletter. Department of Therapeutic Radiology, Stanford University Medical Center, 1988;Jan–Feb:8.

National Cancer Institute: Taking Time. Bethesda, MD: US Department of Health and Human Services, NIH Publication 87-2059, 1986.

Roberts SJ. Social support and help seeking: review of the literature. Advances in Nursing Science 1988;10:1.

Taylor S. Ten issues that cancer patients have to teach. Surviving: A Cancer Patient Newsletter. Department of Therapeutic Radiology, Stanford University Medical Center, 1988;Jan–Feb:2.

Trillin AS. Of dragons and garden peas: a cancer patient talks to doctors. N Engl J Med 1981;304:699.

Wabrek AJ. Rehabilitative intervention: intervention with couples. In: American Cancer Society. Proceedings of the Workshop on Psychosexual and Reproductive Issues Affecting Patients with Cancer—1987. New York, American Cancer Society, 1987.

Zimberg M: Psychosocial isolation. In: Brown M, Kiss M, Mitchell-Outlaw E, et al. Standards of oncology nursing practice. New York: John Wiley & Sons, 1986.

Other Problems

Hope

Fromm E. The revolution of hope. New York: Harper & Row, 1968.

Hickey SS. Enabling hope. Cancer Nurs 1986;9:133.

Miller JF. Inspiring hope. Am J Nurs 1985;85:22.

Noxious Odors

Alterescu V. Osto-zyme. Journal of American Enterostomal Therapists 9:79, 1982.
Brubacher L, Schultz P. Care of the patient with colostomy. In: Reiner A, ed. Manual of patient care standards. Rockville, MD: Aspen Publishers, 1988.

Sleep

Brewer MJ. To sleep or not to sleep: the consequences of sleep deprivation. Critical Care Nurse 1985;5:35.
Lavey NB, Anderson D. Why every patient needs a good night's sleep. RN 1986;49:16.
Richards KC, Bairnsfather L. A description of night sleep patterns in the critical care unit. Heart Lung 1988;17:35.
Wilson TS. Sleep disorders in hospital (letter). Can Med Assoc J 1985;133:731.

7

Managing Daily Living During the Post-Treatment Phase

The post-treatment phase is quite variable in duration. It begins as soon as initial oncologic treatment is completed or discontinued. The ending, however, is less predictable in both time and direction. The post-treatment phase can end abruptly if the person experiences a recurrence of the cancer. Or, it can gradually, almost imperceptibly, slide into the phase of long-term survival when the vividness of memories of the diagnostic and treatment phases begins to fade, when preoccupation with and hypervigilance over body signals abate, and when the person picks up the strands of daily living in a more comfortable way and begins to once again address future-oriented plans and goals.

Expectations about the nature of the post-treatment phase and its reality can be quite incongruent. The patient and family, who have managed daily living with the tumult and assaults of surgical and/or medical oncologic treatment, often expect that life will return to normal when treatment ceases. In many cases this is not true. Some patients having low grade skin or cervical cancers with relatively mild treatment and high expectations of cure may be able to "walk away" from the diagnostic and initial treatment phases with little residual physical or emotional sequelae. But for most patients the cancer experience leaves an indelible effect (Mullan, 1985). The physical and emotional aftershocks make post-treatment adjustment a demanding, stressful task. Treatment sequelae, fatigue, physical dysfunction, attenuated will to continue to fight, depression, nightmares, fear that the cancer will return, and money worries make the patient realize that the fight against the disease is not over (Battrick, 1988; Mullan, 1985). The trek from the land of the ill back to the land of the well is still a long one, and the initial portions of the trek can be rocky.

Medical Perspective

The post-treatment phase is not a predominantly medical one. For the most part patients and families are left to fend for themselves as they seek to begin the return to the healthy world (Mullan, 1985). During the post-treatment phase physicians tend to be most concerned about repairing structural changes with plastic surgery or prosthetics, restoring functional deficits with rehabilitation, managing iatrogenic problems (e.g., dry mouth, short bowel syndrome, infections), and watching for recurrence. Patient contacts become attenuated as follow-up appointments occur at longer intervals.

Patients seem to sense that their problems of everyday living with post-treatment worries and dysfunctions do not have the same importance to physicians as their malignancies had (Battrick, 1988; Bergholz, 1988). Medical treatment plans rarely concern the psychosocial or physical problems of reentrance to the land of the well (Mullan, 1985).

Nursing Perspective

Unless the patient is scheduled for home care or some form of rehabilitation care, or joins a nurse-led support group, contact with nurses is also limited. Some patients continue to stay in touch with nurses who have provided care—by letter, phone, or with visits, but these are the minority. Present health care policies and financing limit the role that nurses can play in the convalescent period, even though their expertise and services might be needed. There are, however, opportunities for nurses delivering home care or working with the patient's oncologist or family physician to assess the patient situation in the home or when phone calls or physician appointments occur. Also, nurses from oncology clinics and inpatient units have been known to maintain phone contacts with patients about whom they have particular concern.

The content of this chapter is intended to alert nurses to high-risk problem areas in managing daily living during the post-treatment phase. This knowledge and perspective can be used:

During the latter stages of the active treatment phase to anticipate problems the patients and families will face and to help them to legitimize the problems and develop contingency plans

To sense and diagnose problems during short telephone or face-to-face contacts with patients and families during the post-treatment phase

To alert nurses who are delivering home or ambulatory care to high-risk problems, nursing diagnoses, prognostic variables, and treatment options

To create an environment in which high-risk challenges can be addressed in nurse-led support groups

The nursing perspective in the post-treatment phase addresses the physical and psychosocial problems in daily living that the patient and family have as a result of the cancer, the diagnostic and treatment experiences, and the persisting effects of the oncologic treatment. Some common problems include:

Feeling of a loss of protection when treatment is discontinued

Uncertainty about how to alter their lifestyle in order to prevent future cancer growth

Managing daily living requirements with residual low energy, low grade nausea, and/or depression

Anxiety associated with appearance of any signs or symptoms that might signal a recurrence of the cancer

Concern about symptoms that may suggest a life-threatening complication (e.g., pneumonia in the immunosuppressed)

Managing post-treatment changes in body structure and function as well as the technology that is involved

Difficulties in resuming role responsibilities, social activities, and relationships with family members, sexual partners, friends, employers, and co-workers

Residual financial problems associated with the cost of the cancer treatment

Finding a satisfying quality of life

Because the opportunities for contact with patients (and even more so with families) are limited in number and short in duration, it becomes crucial for nurses who care for patients and families in the post-treatment phase to be expert in predicting and sensing problems in daily living and functioning during this transition phase as a basis for helping patients and their families to prevent or more effectively manage the problems. While it may not be feasible for nurses themselves to be directly involved in providing the care, it is possible to help clients to recognize and more effectively utilize their own internal resources, their networks, and support sources in the community.

Nature of the Post-Treatment Phase

Several common challenges exist in daily living during the post-treatment phase as patients and family members make another transition in the cancer experience.

Inaccurate Expectations

Once the crises of the diagnosis and treatment have been managed, there may be an expectation that the post-treatment period will be one of respite from stress and relatively rapid, smooth recovery from the assaults of the therapy. Ideally, all patients were informed prior to treatment of the possibility of continuing side-effects related to the treatment. However, many were unable to take in this information and, for those who did, the reality of the sequelae often is more distressing than the impressions gained from hearing about them. Treatment-related pain (Table 7-1) can emerge and continue. Fatigue (Cella, 1983; Fobair et al, 1986) and nausea do not dissipate as quickly as anticipated once the treatment is ended. And for some, structure, appearance, and function are permanently altered. The reality and permanence of these changes and their impact on self-concept as well as on management of the requirements of daily living emerge unremittingly, situation by situation, day by day.

Separation Anxiety

Most patients look forward to the end of treatment with relief. There will be no more travelling to the clinic for therapy and tests. There will be time to heal instead of experiencing the additive debilitating effects of the treatment. It may come as a surprise, then, to feel frightened and anxious that the cancer treatment has been stopped and that the supportive attention of physicians and nurses has been simultaneously cut down. Both the patient and the family members may be wondering, "If the chemotherapy and radiation were holding the cancer cells at bay or killing them, will these cells begin to grow again now that treatment has been ended?"

Table 7-1. Post-Treatment Pain

Treatment	Pathology	Sites	Types of Pain
Chemotherapy			
Vinca alkaloids	Peripheral poly-neuropathy	Hands and feet (symmetrical)	Dysesthesia (numbness, tingling), increased by superficial stimulation
Steroids	Pseudorheumatism with steroid withdrawal	Muscles and joints	Diffuse muscle and joint aching
	Aseptic necrosis	Heads of femur or humerus	Shoulder or hip pain
Chemotherapy or Radiation	Postherpetic neuralgia	Path of herpetic lesion (e.g., dermatome pattern, nerve distribution—facial, eye)	Three distinct components; one to three may be present: continuous burning, intermittent shocklike pain, painful dysesthesias
Radiation			
Radiation of brachial plexus	Radiation fibrosis 6 months to 20 years after treatment	Hand and arm on radiated side	Dysesthesia and paresthesia of hand (pain, numbness, pins and needles)
Radiation of spinal area	Radiation myelopathy, radiculopathy	Localized area of spinal cord damage or referred to distant side	Dysesthesias below level of cord lesion, nerve pain of nerve root origin (sharp, stabbing pain increased by movement, coughing, or sneezing)
Radiation of tumor area	Radiation-induced secondary tumors 4 to 10 years after treatment	Site of earlier tumor and radiation	Painful enlarging mass (see Table 6-5 for tumor-related pain)
Surgery			
Mastectomy	Interruption of inter-costobrachial nerves (T-1–T-2) 1 to 2 months after surgery	Posterior aspect of axilla, inner surface of upper arm, radiating to anterior chest wall on operative site	Paresthesias (numbness, tightness, tingling, prickling, pins and needles, "crawling," itching sensation, feeling of wetness or dribbling), dysesthesias (burning, aching, stabbing, shooting pain), phantom nipple sensation, sense of tight band

Table 7-1.   Post-Treatment Pain (continued)

Treatment	Pathology	Sites	Types of Pain
Radical neck dissection	Injury to or interruption of cervical nerves	Distribution path of damaged nerves	Constant burning in area of sensory loss, intermittent shocklike pain, tingling, stinging
Amputation of limbs	Severing of nerves— phantom limb sensation (shortly after surgery); phantom limb pain (1 to 4 weeks after amputation in ±35% of amputees. Can become worse over the years in 5% to 10% of patients)*	Limb that has been amputated	Phantom sensation of continued presence of limb, pain comparable to that experienced before amputation (e.g., cramping, itching, hot pain). Severity relates to duration of symptoms before surgery.
	Traumatic neuromas	End of stump, phantom limb pain	Exquisite tenderness with pressure

Melzack R. The puzzle of pain. New York: Basic Books, 1973.

Coyle N, Foley K. Pain in patients with cancer: profile of patients and common pain syndromes. Seminars in Oncology Nursing 1985; 1:93. Personal communication. Laura Heard, RN, CCRN, MSN. Clinical specialist in rehabilitation nursing. 1989.)

Throughout the treatment experience, the patient and family were encountering doctors, nurses, and other health care providers who were concerned about their welfare and helped them to manage. Suddenly these people are no longer physically available on a daily basis (Mishel, 1987). The day-to-day physical and emotional problems, the procedures and equipment all have to be managed in the home setting—on one's own. Little questions and problems that could have been addressed with professionals as they occurred take on greater significance when it is more difficult to contact the nurse or doctor. The external resource of professional services has been abruptly reduced even though the physical and emotional problems have not necessarily diminished and may actually have increased because of the transition to the home environment.

Uncertainty About Strategies for Cancer Control

With the discontinuation of medical treatment comes a concern about assuming personal responsibility for keeping cancer at bay. Many of the genetic, environmental, physiologic, and lifestyle factors that permitted the initiation and promotion of the malignant processes in the first place are still present. How then can one act to prevent recurrence?

Studies show conflicting findings on the influence that psychosocial factors can have on modifying cancer recurrence or affecting survival time (Cassileth et al, 1988).

As a result, the American Cancer Society has issued a revised statement of policy indicating that currently available evidence does not support the theory that stress reduction techniques can change the risk of developing cancer or the duration of survival in humans. Therefore, the society does not recommend use of psychosocial interventions that claim to alter tumor growth or spread (American Cancer Society, 1989).

Professionals, professional and lay literature, and word of mouth offer an array of remedies, including diets, meditation, and visual imagery, as well as some less orthodox forms of treatment, including outright quackery (Cassileth et al, 1984). Patients and their families face decisions about what, if any, lifestyle changes or supplemental treatments they wish to undertake in an effort to maintain their health.

Hypervigilance in Self-Monitoring

One of the stressful aspects of the post-treatment phase is the concern about recurrence of the cancer. Signs or symptoms that the patient would have ignored before cancer now create fears that the cancer has recurred or spread (e.g., a cough, a little pain). One patient said she knew that she was on the road to recovery when she had reduced the number of times she palpated her other breast to only one time per day (Bergholz, 1988); another, a physician, found himself palpating lymph nodes during wakeful nights (Mullan, 1985). Patients say that it takes many months to begin to regain confidence that their bodies will not again betray them.

Stress of Scheduled Follow-up Appointments

Patients find that medical checkups create a high level of fear and anxiety; each checkup or scan is a new milestone to be crossed. Perhaps the blood tests will reveal new dangers, or the physician will find something that the patient hadn't noticed. One patient was so stressed by these appointments that she and her husband arranged that the husband would schedule them and not tell the wife about it until the night before. Another patient, more than usually anxious about an appointment, came early and sought out the clinical nurse specialist who had cared for her in order to gain the courage she needed to face the medical examination. Preoccupation with the threat of recurrence may abate as time passes, but can reemerge powerfully when the time for follow-up appointments approaches.

Adaptation to Changed Structure and Functioning

Most individuals who have had treatment for a malignancy experience change in structure and functioning. During the active treatment phase, these seem to be one part of the short-term challenge of surviving the cancer treatment. However, symptom distress does not abate just because the patient is discharged from institutional care. Rather, it may seem to increase when the care of the professionals has been sharply cut off. Discomfort from symptoms can persist for weeks after the treatment (Oberst and James, 1985).

In the post-treatment phase, when life is supposed to "return to normal" in the home setting, the stark reality of the long-term effects emerges. Body parts have been removed; muscles and nerves have been cut; tissues have been irradiated and subsequently continue to change in both structure and function (e.g., gonads cease to produce sperm or ova, brain structures are changed, the radiated breast becomes smaller and harder, salivary glands cease to produce saliva, intestines absorb less, the vagina shrinks and becomes dry, the penis fails to achieve erection); normal body orifices are closed or have become useless and new body orifices have been created; the immune system has been made less functional. In the post-treatment period the patient learns what it is like to live inside of this changed body 24 hours each day. It is a time of forming a new body image and reintegrating it into the self-concept and the ongoing requirements of daily living.

The post-treatment period is also a time when new skills in self-care associated with changed functioning and compensatory technology must be developed. If chewing and swallowing are long-term problems, then acceptable strategies for eating in various settings need to be developed. Effective, comfortable use of prostheses takes time, experimentation, and effort. Controlling excretions and odor with ostomies, learning how to dress in such a way as to accommodate drainage bags, gaining confidence in control, learning how to prevent accidents; all of these are learning challenges in day-to-day living of the post-treatment phase, even though patients may feel that they were well taught in the hospital (Oberst and James, 1985). Learning to communicate without a larynx or with a mechanical one is a slow and frustrating process. Learning new patterns of intimacy when appearance, structure, or function of organs associated with sexuality have been altered is a sensitive situation in which each partner learns over time. Each change in function or structure brings with it a need for alterations in daily living, and use of internal and external resources.

Incongruence of Perspective Between Patient and Others

Another challenge that many patients experience is the incongruence between their perception of the situation and that of family members and other support persons. Most individuals and systems seek to restore comfort and equilibrium as soon as possible. Thus, once treatment is completed, family members, friends, employers, co-workers, and even physicians and other health care workers may feel that the current cancer battle is over and it is time to get on with normal living. The patient, on the other hand, finds that only the battle of active treatment is over. The war to regain a sense of well-being is far from won. It is not possible to immediately return to preillness normalcy, much as the patient and everyone else might wish. Memories of the past stresses are too fresh, the current challenges are too overwhelming, the resources for managing are still not in place, and the future still contains a real threat. Even activities one formerly took for granted, such as the capacity to respond to others' worries and problems, has been changed by the patient's own cancer experience (Bergholz, 1988).

Incongruences concerning expectations about the pace and style of recovery can create additional challenges for the patient, plus a perception of alienation from the predictable support of others. This may even cause the person to be reluctant to share the realities of daily living and the feelings the experiences generate, and in turn cause feelings of increased isolation.

Incongruences in Expectations for Family

The spouse and family members are not immune from incongruent expectations. Most have managed the shock and stresses of sharing the patient's diagnosis and treatment experiences. Family members are supposedly the healthy ones, yet in the post-treatment period they begin to experience steadily increasing emotional distress that may peak at 2 months and continue for several months more. The anxiety of the treatment phase changes to reactive depression in the post-treatment phase (Oberst and James, 1985). Spouses have been found to experience an increase in somatic complaints, with fatigue, vague aches and pains, indigestion, and minor ailments such as upper respiratory infections (Oberst and James, 1985). Whereas everyone has concern for the symptoms and distress being experienced by the patient, much less notice is paid to the discomforts and illnesses of the spouse, care giver, or close family members. Those other than the patient (primary care giver, spouse, partner, family members) are expected to be healthy mentally and physically, even when this is not a reality for them.

Control of Roles, Participation, and Activities

PATIENT.   Renegotiating role responsibilities and relationships as the patient re-enters or partially resumes former roles or enters new ones is a requirement in daily living that may be carried out at either an overt or covert level. Initially, others, in the name of caring or kindness, may tend to take control of the life of the cancer survivor. They may make decisions on what the person can or cannot do, without bothering to check as to what the person wants or feels capable of doing. Should the survivor resist this type of "help" and seek to function independently, and then later come to a situation in which help is needed, it may be difficult to ask for assistance. For example, a waitress recovering from a mastectomy found her co-workers taking her trays out of her hands and carrying them for her; she physically resisted their efforts. They gave in, but obviously felt resentful that their well-meaning assistance had been rebuffed. When situations did arise in which the patient needed physical help, she became reluctant to ask for it.

By contrast, some survivors may seek to relinquish responsibilities they formerly held or initially resumed after treatment (e.g., selected household tasks). When this occurs, family members may become concerned that the change in behavior is a response to recurrence of the cancer or a new health problem. The patient is not the only one who is hypervigilant about cues that might signal recurrence or problems during the post-treatment phase; care givers and family members may be unusually attentive to them as well.

FAMILY.   The family as well as the cancer survivor is faced with the challenges of assimilating changes. Lifestyle disruptions continue, provoking a response of anger in some (Oberst and James, 1985). Mutually supportive and reciprocative relationships of the past may be changed to ones in which the spouse or family member continually gives to the survivor and receives little in return. The necessary grief occurs when he or she realizes that a previously accepted and perhaps cherished relationship is lost. In seeking restitution, there can be unevenness or difficulties in finding life rewards under the new circumstances. Like the patient, spouses and families have their up and down days too, as they grieve and seek to make adjustments.

Issues of sexuality and intimacy that initially arose during the treatment phase continue in the post-treatment phase. Body changes that occurred or began to occur during treatment often continue after treatment has been completed. For patients and partners who wish to be sexually active, the adjustment in role relationships and sexual practices continues to be an important and sensitive area for attention.

Problems arise in reestablishing roles and role relationships, in negotiating for the control that is needed, and in seeking assistance when it is needed. Strategies that take into account the concerns and sensitivities of both the patient and the significant others involved are important if these transitions are to be managed smoothly.

Underlying Mechanisms

The post-treatment phase is one of adjustment and transition (Northouse, 1984). The high drama of the diagnosis and the surgery or shorter forms of treatment is past; the grind of ongoing radiation and/or chemotherapy is over. Where treatment has been aggressive, emotional, physical, and financial resources may be depleted for both patient and family. There is a desire to return to normal daily living as soon as possible. Yet, as can be seen from the possible problems identified in the previous section, many challenges face both the patient and the family.

The underlying mechanisms of the post-treatment phase involve three major tasks:

Processing and assimilating the experiences of the diagnostic and treatment phases and their personal meaning

Dealing with the present in terms of:

Integrating the altered body structure and function into one's self concept—developing a new sense of "normal"

Meeting the current requirements of daily living with these constraints

Addressing feelings of isolation from those who have not had a comparable cancer experience

Moving toward a return to the land of the well by making any needed adjustments in resuming former roles, responsibilities, and relationships in home, work, and social spheres

Processing the Experiences of the Diagnostic and Treatment Phases

Patients and families often hope to be able to close the door on the diagnostic and treatment phases of the cancer experience once they are over. Most people are unable to do this, unless the cancer was a localized, unaggressive one and the treatment was limited. The emotional and physical assaults of the diagnosis and treatment can result in a response not unlike a post-trauma response, characterized by anxiety, nightmares, hypervigilance, flashbacks (occurring with stimuli of sights, smells, or sounds that may be experienced in a return to the doctor's office or clinic, the site of bone marrow aspirations or chemotherapy, and so forth), fear of recurrence, narrowed attention, avoidance of situations or activities that arouse recollection, and feelings of isolation from others who have not had the cancer experiences (Germino, 1989; Germino and Funk, 1989; Tanaka, 1988).

The return to daily living in the home situation and cessation of treatment tend to refocus thinking from the treatment of the tumor to the implications of the gestalt of the cancer experience: I am a person who has been diagnosed and treated for cancer. How have I been changed by the experiences? What does that mean to me? How does it affect my thoughts about the future? Have my values, goals, and priorities in life been changed? How will the post-treatment me relate differently to those who share my life? How will this affect them? (Simonton, 1984)

Many patients use cancer support groups to verbalize and work through the new realities in their lives (Taylor, 1988). Others think it through for themselves or find individuals who will listen and serve as safe, nonjudgmental sounding boards as they seek to assimilate the experiences and reemerge in their modified self-concept and life view. Some productively use a daily journal to help them think through their experiences and reactions.

Another factor to be processed is the realization that one is on one's own in trying to avoid the recurrence of the cancer. Physicians and medical science have done what they can. Questions regarding lifestyle factors that may have initiated or promoted the disease may resurface as the patient considers day-to-day living to minimize risks of recurrence. Beliefs about the causes of cancer or protective strategies, rational or not, may affect decisions about patterns in daily living and post-treatment lifestyle. The patient may feel obliged to try strategies and remedies that are proposed in lay literature or offered by friends, or guilty about deciding not to try them—"What if the macrobiotic diet really would prevent recurrence and I didn't try it?" Because there is no solid foundation of knowledge on how to prevent recurrence, the patient can feel an uncomfortable uncertainty (Mishel, 1987).

Feelings of isolation and alienation may occur as the patient perceives the personal nature of processing the cancer experience. Most oncologists and other physicians (other than psychiatrists or psychologists) concern themselves less with this personal assimilation of the ongoing results of the cancer and its treatment (Fisher, 1981). The patient's family, friends, and acquaintances who have not had the experience can empathize, but not fully share. Patients realize anew that the task of processing and integrating the cancer experience and its implications for their future is a personal one—others may help, but the patient is the only one who can actually accomplish the task.

Dealing With the Present

Dealing with the present during the days and weeks of the post-treatment phase involves several elements. These include:

Meeting daily living requirements with a body that has been structurally and functionally altered by the treatment

Learning by experience to interpret body cues with diminishing irrational fear

Taking initial steps in moving away from the sick role

Living With Altered Structural and Functional Status

The patient's physical status in the post-treatment phase is usually structurally and functionally altered. During treatment, the acute side-effects of the treatment were the focus. After it is over the more prolonged or permanent body changes become the reality. Fatigue can be severe and may continue for many months, particularly when hemotherapy has been used (Cella, 1983; Fobair et al, 1986). Low grade nausea can ontinue for weeks following radiation or chemotherapy. Altered sensations (par-sthesias and dysesthesias—see Table 7-1) emerge; the patient may be disconcerted to ealize that these may be constant companions in daily life.

Small and routine tasks in daily living that were once done without much hought—were taken for granted—now represent a conscious effort and a challenge; for nstance:

Masticating and swallowing without enough saliva

Planning meal schedules to accommodate a smaller stomach capacity following gastrectomy

Communicating without a larynx

Dressing to disguise a tracheostomy or colostomy

Working with reduced ventilatory capacity

Managing the bag care, odor control, diet, and accident prevention associated with a colostomy, ileostomy, or ureterostomy

Managing intimate relations with structurally altered genitalia or impaired genital nerve and blood supplies, or with a colostomy, mastectomy, facial surgery, or irradiated breast

Avoiding infection-producing encounters or activities when one is immunosuppressed

Managing new social contacts with facial disfigurement, with a history of cancer, etc.

In addition to managing daily living with the remnants of fatigue, possibly nausea, nd any other iatrogenic dysfunctions, there are often new skills to be acquired. The kills may be needed to compensate for body changes and to integrate any prostheses or echnology into the pattern of roles, role obligations, and relationships that constitute aily living during the post-treatment phase.

The extent of body changes, the successes and failures experienced in making djustments, and the degree of acceptance of the changes will affect the patient's motional status. Reactive depression is not an uncommon complication (Cella, 1983; Cross et al, 1984). The survivor's will to live and to keep on trying is vulnerable at this tage (Bergholz, 1988).

Concern About Recurrence—Hypervigilance in Self-Monitoring

Hypervigilance in self-monitoring is a common patient response to fear of recurrence in the post-treatment phase. It is not easy to regain confidence in one's body after he recent betrayal. Patients feel threatened by symptoms that would have caused no concern prior to the cancer diagnosis; for example: Is that swollen gland another ymphoma? Does the sore throat represent a recurrence of the leukemia? Is that lump in he remaining fibrocystic breast a metastasis of the breast cancer? Learning to assign ppropriate significance to body signs and symptoms is one of the tasks that is accomplished by experience during the post-treatment phase. The patient may gradually experience less emotional upheaval as time goes by and the body signals are found not to epresent recurrence. Immunosuppression tends to improve, and immunosuppressed patients gain experience and confidence in knowing which cues require treatment for atrogenic complications. By the time the person moves into the long-term survival phase, the fear and hypervigilance of the post-treatment phase tend to abate.

Movement From the Sick Role

The post-treatment phase is also a transition in terms of assignment of the sick role to the patient. Medicine's tasks of diagnosis and treatment have been completed; convalescence or recovery is now the perspective. Where the treatment has seemed to offer even a temporarily good prognosis, physicians (and nurses too) sometimes reflect an attitude that the patient should feel glad to have survived and been given the opportunity for a longer life; that the difficulties remaining should be of minor concern since the primary goal of current control of the cancer has been achieved.

Others' expectations regarding the pace at which the patient moves out of the sick role may be incongruent with the patient's capabilities or wishes. Fatigue, mental strains, and problems in adaptation to body changes and technology may cause the patient to need to remain in the sick role for a longer period than others might wish. Or the reverse may be true. Others may want the patient to remain in the sick role while the patient wishes to move out of it. These incongruent expectations can create alienation and stresses for both parties.

Patients may feel ambivalent about the degree of dependency being experienced. They may resist or rebuff solicitude or unrequested assistance. Yet on other occasions they may feel hurt that people are not perceptive enough to offer needed assistance or understanding (Bergholz, 1988). Patient response may seem perverse and unpredictable to those who are trying to be sensitive, supportive, and helpful.

Convalescence is not a smooth, steady trajectory for most patients; rather, there are peak days and valley days. For those who are seriously impaired, improvement may be so gradual that they may need to scan days or weeks to recognize it. Keeping a journal may offer evidence of progress.

Returning to the Land of the Well

The journey back from the land of the ill to the land of the well is a much slower one for most cancer patients than the sudden trip that took the patient to the land of the ill originally. Most patients do not expect it to take so long. This is particularly true if the treatment has been aggressive or prolonged. Some patients who experience near-death episodes and actually become prepared to die during the treatment phase find the journey to wellness bewildering. As one patient who survived aggressive, successful treatment for testicular cancer said, "I was supposed to die. I was ready to die. I was near death on several occasions. Now I'm going to live. I don't know what to do." Survival of the assaults of treatment can result in life taking on a new meaning. The land of the well may be viewed quite differently than it was before the patient entered the cancer experience.

From the patient's perspective, the nature of the return journey is affected by many factors. These include energy level, degree of depression, assimilation of the cancer diagnosis and its implications, a changed perspective on life's meaning, status of appearance and functional capacities, the nature of home and work environment, role responsibilities in daily living, and external resources.

Family members cannot escape the effects of the trauma they experienced during the treatment phase, if they were on a roller coaster of grief and hope as the patient's status shifted. They may well have begun anticipatory grieving when the outlook was grim. In the post-treatment phase they may feel guilty at having engaged in anticipatory grieving and having initiated separation behavior. It is possible to help families gain understanding and comfort from the knowledge that anticipatory grieving and beginning separation as a response to the possible death of the patient during the treatment phase is normal, and reestablishing of the relationship after anticipatory grieving usually takes time.

Persons who have experienced cancer and have integrated it into their self-concept often alter their priorities and values (Bergholz, 1988; Taylor, 1988). Having made it through the stresses and demands of the diagnostic and treatment phases, some patients feel that they have been given another chance at life. They see incentives for personal growth, opportunities to regroup and get new perspectives, and an occasion to re-examine their own and others' expectations (Mathews-Simonton et al, 1978). The priorities, expectations, and values of other people may assume less importance than they had before the cancer experience (Taylor, 1988). The resultant alterations in values and priorities, plus changed functional capacities, can make a return to former norms of roles and relationships impossible. This, in turn, can create new tensions in relationships with those who are affected because the patient is not the same as before.

Systems theory proposes that systems are intolerant of disequilibrium and act to return to a former or new state of equilibrium. Patients and those who share their daily living at home and at work are members of several established systems. These systems thus face the challenges of reestablishing equilibrium with a member (the patient) who is functioning, thinking, and feeling differently. Equilibrium can be reestablished, but it may be quite a different state from the precancer form. Members of the system may also sense that future disequilibrium is a serious threat, given the possibility of recurrence of the cancer or late iatrogenic complications. Just as the patient no longer has "seamless trust" in the future (Bergholz, 1988), so the family system too may share some level of uneasiness and wariness.

The patient and those who share daily living will overtly or covertly modify their roles and relationships to find adjustments that are acceptable or at least tolerable, given the system's requirements and members' personal values and capacities. A new basis for establishment of equilibrium occurs in the various systems that form the fabric of the patient's daily living. It may or may not be truly satisfying to one or more members of the system.

Health or wellness can be defined as a balance between the requirements of daily living and the patient's and family's internal and external resources for meeting those requirements in a way that promotes physical and emotional well-being and a satisfying quality of life. Even though patients and families may not achieve precancer levels of functioning and cannot escape the memory of the cancer experience, patients complete their journey back to the land of the well as they and their systems regain a new-found balance and comfort in their roles and relationships. The systems have defined a new sense of what is "normal" for them.

Nursing Diagnosis and Treatment

Most patients and their families manage the challenges of the post-treatment phase with minimal assistance from nurses. However, it is possible for nurses to offer support if they:

Diagnose high-risk challenges and post-treatment problems the patient and family may face, given the patient's and family's particular situation

Legitimize problem areas and develop contingency plans while patients and families are still in the latter stages of the treatment phase

Identify and document high-risk potential problems to increase nurses' perceptiveness to any subtle or overt cues indicating lack of effectiveness in managing those problems during the post-treatment phase, even though the contacts (phone or clinic visits) may be short and infrequent

Initial documentation of known problem areas or high-risk potential problems can heighten problem-sensing alertness by nurses who have contact with the patient or family. It is important, then, that these documented nursing diagnoses and concerns regarding future problems be transmitted across systems to nurses who will encounter the patients in other parts of the institution or health care system during the post-treatment and subsequent phases of the cancer experience.

Diagnostic Targets	The primary diagnostic targets are the patient and the family. Through them it may be possible to diagnose problem areas of relationships and functioning in work or social situations that the patient or family must manage but in which the source of the problem may be other people.
Risk Factors	Patients who are likely to have difficulty in managing the tasks of the post-treatment phase are those who:

Have had the most aggressive, prolonged treatment

Have major changes in structure and/or function

Were unable to realistically comprehend the nature and effects of sequelae of the treatment when they gave "informed" consent

Occupy roles in which a specific, now altered function was a crucial element to their performance

Continue to experience serious fatigue or depression

Tend to be pessimists or have a weak will to persist against difficulties

Lack a predictable, caring support person

Have family, health care providers, or co-workers who fail to negotiate effectively with the patient about desired assistance, support, and specific areas for dependence and independence

Have family, spouse, or significant others who are unwilling or unable to accommodate the patient's changed priorities and values or need to alter role relationships

Families or significant others at higher risk for ineffective management of tasks of the post-treatment phase are those who

Are dependent on the patient's continuing to occupy former roles (e.g., as provider of income, parent, primary care giver, sexual partner)

Have ongoing role responsibilities that leave little time or energy for meeting the patient's needs

Are repulsed by the structural or functional changes in the patient

Are themselves emotionally or physically dysfunctional, or are experiencing concurrent situational or developmental crises

Diagnostic
Areas

PATIENT

Ineffectiveness in managing daily living related to (R/T) severity of post-traumatic response, leading to (L/T) •_____ (•identify specific difficulties)

Uncertainty or emotional distress about undertaking strategies to reduce chance of cancer recurrence R/T:

Sense of loss of protection from discontinuation of treatment

Perceived lack of assistance or interest from health care providers

Lack of knowledge about what might be helpful—not harmful—or whether there is anything that can be done

Pressure from family, friends or acquaintances to undertake "prevention strategies" they favor

Decreased effectiveness in approaching the challenges in the post-treatment phase (specify) R/T:

Fatigue

Post-trauma response

Reactive depression

Lack of knowledge or skills (specify)

Lack of clarity of priorities, goals, and values

Inability to process and assimilate the diagnostic and treatment phases of the cancer experience R/T lack of:

One or more persons to listen and share

Desire or verbal ability to share what has been or is being experienced

Difficulty in modifying roles and role responsibilities (see Diagnostic Areas in the Role section of Chapter 6)

Difficulty in managing activities of daily living associated with intimacy and sexuality (see Diagnostic Areas in the Sexuality section of Chapter 6)

Hypervigilance in self-monitoring R/T fear of cancer recurrence or serious complications, L/T preoccupation with body signals and moderate to high levels of anxiety and fear. (Note that the spouse or other family members may also experience fears when they experience symptoms similar to those of the patient, wondering, "Do I have cancer too?" (Germino and Funk, 1989) and when they observe changes in the patient's functioning or behavior, wondering "Has there been a relapse or recurrence?")

Difficulty in interpreting signs and symptoms R/T lack of knowledge or experience with changed body functioning in the post-treatment phase, L/T inappropriate overreaction or under-reaction

Sense of isolation or alienation from others R/T:

Feeling that others who have not had the cancer experience cannot share or understand one's difficulties and feelings

Feeling abandoned by health care providers through lack of contact or because of cues indicating lack of interest in patient's "nonmedical" concerns

Incongruent expectations regarding patient's resumption of former role responsibilities

Difficulties in relating to others R/T one's own ambivalence and lack of clarity about areas of dependence and independence

Difficulty in moving from sick role to well role R/T:

Ongoing fatigue, symptoms, dysfunctions

Depression

Secondary gains from retaining sick role

Unwillingness of others to permit the transition

FAMILY

Hypervigilance in observing patient or questioning patient regarding health status R/T fear of cancer's recurrence

Difficulty in accepting patient's revision of behavior or role relationships R/T:

Pace of patient recovery being slower than family expectations

Feelings that patient doesn't sufficiently appreciate "being alive"

Patient's lack of sharing the basis for the changes

Inability to accept the new values and priorities the patient has evolved

Needs and goals that are incongruent with patient wishes or capacities

Lack of desire, capacity, or ability to assume role responsibilities that the patient is abdicating or is unable to perform

Ongoing distancing from patient R/T:

Grieving over the changes in the patient and the loss of the former relationship

Revulsion over structural and functional changes

Unwillingness to meet patient needs that would be required to be met in a closer relationship

Manifestations

Indications that the patient is not managing daily living well during the post-treatment phase include reports of:

Feeling ineffective in managing self-care and self-monitoring without the previous level of professional contact and supervision

Anxious hypervigilance of signs and symptoms that does not dissipate with time

Constant worry about whether the cancer is being controlled now that treatment has been completed

Uncertainty about making changes in lifestyle to try to prevent recurrence or spread of cancer, or undertaking new regimens that threaten health, finances, and well-being

Difficulties in resuming former roles because of the expectations or behavior of others

Discomfort or anger that the rate of recovery is incongruent with self-expectations or those of others

Depression, discouragement, or wanting to give up

Observed manifestations may include signs of depression, angry behavior, unusual apathy, prolonged serious fatigue, frequent calls or appointments with the clinic to discuss worrisome symptoms, failure to schedule check-ups at the designated intervals, deterioration of appearance and grooming from previous patterns.

Indications that family members are not effectively managing daily living with the patient in the post-treatment stage include reported or observed:

Frequent, anxious calling about the patient's signs and symptoms as possible signs of recurrence

Reports that the patient is not trying hard enough to recover, or is doing too much

Concern about cancer control remedies the patient is undertaking, or is failing to try

Frustration in trying to adjust to the patient's changed goals, priorities, communication, or behavior

Prognostic Variables

All patients and families eventually move from the post-treatment phase to the next phases of the cancer experience (long-term survival or recurrence). Some will have made a better adjustment than others. Patients that will have the greatest difficulty are those who:

Are unable to process the experiences of the diagnostic and treatment phases and place them in the past

Were diagnosed at a very advanced stage of malignancy in which cancer persists despite treatment or recurs after only a short remission

Have a need to retain the sick role

Have ongoing major dysfunction or lasting, visible, unrepaired disfigurement

Have dysfunctional families or support systems

Have strong self-identification with roles that cannot be regained or occupied with former effectiveness because of iatrogenic body changes

Families that will experience the greatest difficulty are those who:

Are dependent on the patient for crucial roles and functioning within their system and unable to find substitutes when the patient cannot fully resume the role

Are dysfunctional or experiencing serious concurrent situational or developmental crises

Lack usable external resources and supports

Have financial difficulties escalated by the costs of cancer treatment

Complications

When the tasks of the post-treatment phase are not well managed, each participant can pay an emotional and physical price. Relationships can be damaged, and family and other systems in which the patient is a member can become more dysfunctional. This can cause subsequent functioning in later phases of the cancer experience to be less effectively managed.

Treatment Guidelines

Difficulty (of patient or family) in processing the experiences of the diagnostic and treatment phases

Before the treatment phase ends, prepare the patient and family to anticipate a need to talk through the experiences of the diagnostic and treatment phases with someone who would be a good listener and with whom they would feel free to openly share their perceptions, feelings, fears, and current reactions or an ongoing basis. Indicate that sometimes unanticipated emotions (e.g., fears, anger, wanting to give up) emerge after treatment, and that it is easier and healthier to de-energize them by acknowledging them and then talking about them (Foa and Kozak, 1986; Hanser-McConnell, 1990) than it is to live with them. If appropriate, ask the patient and family to think of one or more individuals who might serve well in this role. Indicate that it can be done either in face-to-face or telephone conversations.

Encourage the processing of experiences by keeping a journal in which worries and concerns as well as activities are identified. This not only externalizes the worries rather than keeping them ruminating in one's head, but can also be used to identify the "baby steps" of progress so that, in review, the patient can track progress that may not be obvious from only a day-to-day perspective.

Help the patient and family to accurately identify the nature of professional care they can expect from the physicians and nurses who have been involved in the treatment phase as a basis for using them appropriately now that the treatment is completed.

Suggest the need to mobilize resources to help the patient and family to manage areas in which the more medically oriented experts would not be useful. (If possible, the nurse can determine whether this patient's oncologist, usual physician, or nurses in the ambulatory care setting tend to tune in to patient concerns other than those involved with pathology as a basis for suggesting how these professional resources can realistically be used.)

Identify local cancer support groups that could also serve in helping the patient or family to process the cancer experience. Give place, dates, and times of meetings and offer to have someone contact them if desired.

Hypervigilance in self-monitoring

Alert the patient to the fact that this is a common post-treatment experience, particularly in the earliest period, and that it probably will abate as time passes and he or she becomes more comfortable with the post-treatment status.

Tell the patient that it is OK to call in and talk to the nurse or doctor when fears or worries about symptoms occur, and that this is much better than worrying unnecessarily.

Where there are genuine risks of health problems associated with certain symptoms (e.g., a cough or other signs of infection in an immunosuppressed patient), teach the patient about the earliest signs and the importance of reporting them. Suggest that it is safer to overreport than to delay. Teach the patient how to report in a manner that will convey credibility and receive appropriate attention from the health care system.

Uncertainty about self-care to minimize recurrence risks

Indicate that:

It is positive and healthy for the patient to be involved in health promotion

It is understandable that there is uncertainty about adjusting lifestyle in such a way as to promote health after having experienced cancer

It is common to feel uneasy about not having the protection of continuation of treatment and the more constant presence of health professionals.

Suggest reading or audiovisual materials that may provide safe and useful ideas on positive and safe approaches the patient may undertake.

Alert the patient and family to the reality that:

Many well-meaning acquaintances and friends may recommend treatment, diets, activities, etc. that may or may not be helpful. Help the patient and family to develop scripts to respond to such offers that will not alienate the person but do not offer acceptance either; for example, "Thank you for bringing this to my attention. Several people have been making suggestions and I'm going to give them careful consideration."

There are entrepreneurs offering alternative, untested forms of treatment who are seeking to make money from patients who have had cancer. Suggest checking with the Better Business Bureau, with their doctor or nurse, or with professionally-led support groups to gain perspective on the usefulness of alternative forms of therapy. The American Cancer Society also provides information to individuals on alternative forms of therapy.

Difficulty in negotiating changes associated with new priorities and values

Indicate to the patient that one of the activities that patients often engage in during the post-treatment phase is the reexamining of priorities, life goals, and values. It is not unusual for life to take on new meaning (Taylor, 1988). The results of this reexamining can range from little or no change in values to a rather major reordering of priorities and goals. When values and priorities do change, the patient's behavior and role relationships are also altered. Unless others are made aware of the changes, they may not understand and can become disturbed by them.

Suggest that the patient think through what, if anything, he or she wishes to change in priorities and goals (a counselor may be very useful in values clarification). If the person does not have access to a counselor, making a written list of ideas may be useful. This should result in greater clarity when changed values and priorities are discussed with others who will be affected. An ounce of prevention in role changes is worth a pound of treatment for role disruptions and conflicts.

Feelings of isolation

In the latter portion of the treatment phase, alert the patient to the common experience of others of feeling isolated and alone in their post-treatment adjustments.

Determine whether the person has previously been comfortable with sharing experiences and whether there is a current relationship in which it is possible to comfortably share the cancer experience. Indicate the importance of maintaining the type of interaction in which the patient can say aloud (face to face, by telephone, or in writing) exactly what is being experienced, without regard for whether it seems rational or odd, positive or negative. Suggest that the patient can structure the other person's behavior (e.g., "I know you haven't had an experience with cancer and that perhaps some of my reactions may seem odd, but it would be so helpful if I could just talk about what is happening in me to someone who would be comfortable listening to me and asking questions to help me clarify my responses, but not giving too much advice").

Suggest that some patients (and families) find comfort in support groups, in which they can meet with others who have struggled or are struggling with similar issues and experiences. Give examples of these groups: American Cancer Society (ACS) I Can Cope and CanSurmount volunteer visitors and Make Today Count (mutual support group for people with life-threatening illness), National Coalition of Cancer Survivors, and groups developed by cancer treatment facilities. In addition, there are often local support groups for people with specialized problems, such as International Association of Laryngectomees (ACS), United Association of Ostomates, Reach to Recovery (ACS) for mastectomy rehabilitation, Leukemia Society of America, and, in some places, locally developed groups for women who have had breast cancer.

Difficulty with role negotiations

See Chapter 6, section on Role, under Treatment Guidelines

Problems with sexuality and intimacy

See Chapter 6, section on Sexuality, under Treatment Guidelines

For ostomates, recommend writing to the United Ostomy Association for helpful publications. (*Sex, Courtship and the Single Ostomate* and *Sex and the Female Ostomate* are available for $1.00 each through UOA, 2001 West Beverly Boulevard, Los Angeles, CA 90057-2491.)

Evaluation   Evaluation of patient management of the post-treatment challenges will involve self-reports on the status of:

Frequency of self-monitoring and degree of anxiety over innocuous body signals

Feelings of competence and success in reporting health concerns to physicians

Satisfaction in relationships with physicians in ongoing management of medical problems, and success in locating and using other support systems for addressing nonmedical concerns

Processing of the diagnostic and treatment phases and their sequelae, and development of post-treatment values, goals, and priorities

Capacity to manage the requirements of daily living and the physical and emotional deterrents that still exist

Expertise and comfort in accommodating, managing, or disguising structural or functional changes on a day-to-day basis

Any ongoing manifestations of post-traumatic response syndrome and success or failure of attempts to manage them

Ongoing feelings of isolation from significant others; trigger situations and strategies for managing

Success of strategies for negotiating alterations in role responsibilities and relationships in keeping with post-treatment priorities, goals, and capacities

Feeling that they are returning to the land of the well

Evaluation of family management will involve self-reports on the status of:

Level of anxiety over patient's health status

Satisfaction with meeting perceived patient needs and goals

Adjustment to changes in patient's role and role relationships and the development of a new definition for "normal" in the family system emerging from the patient's post-treatment status and the participation and functioning of the family as a system

Satisfaction with own quality of life in the family system and in relation to the patient in the post-treatment phase

Ongoing concerns and issues

Bibliography

American Cancer Society. American Cancer Society statement of policy: effects of emotion on cancer. CA 1989;39:A-9.

Battrick C. Before and after. Surviving: A Cancer Patient Newsletter. Department of Therapeutic Radiology, Stanford Medical Center, 1988; Jan-Feb:7.

Bergholz E. Under the shadow of cancer. New York Times Magazine, p 73. December 11, 1988.

Cassileth BR, Lusk EJ, Strouse TB, Bodenheimer BA. Contemporary unorthodox treatments in cancer medicine: a study of patients, treatments and practitioners. Ann Intern Med 1984;101:105.

Cassileth BR, Walsh WP, Lusk EJ. Psychosocial correlates of cancer survival: a subsequent report 3 to 8 years after cancer diagnosis. J Clin Oncol 1988;6:1753.

Cella D. Psychosocial adjustment over time to the successful treatment of early versus late stage Hodgkin's disease in young adult men. Ph.D. thesis, Loyola University, 1983.

Fisher RA. A patient's perspective on the human side of cancer. Proceedings of the American Cancer Society Third National Conference on Human Values and Cancer. Washington, DC, April 23–26, 1981.

Foa EB, Kozak MJ. Emotional processing of fear: exposure to corrective information. Psychol Bull 1986; 99:20.

Fobair P, Hoppe RT, Bloom J et al. Psychosocial problems among survivors of Hodgkin's disease. J Clin Oncol 1986;4:805.

Germino B. Concerns and communication issues in families with newly diagnosed cancer. Presented at the 11th Annual Oncology Nursing Symposium, Puget Sound Chapter Oncology Nursing Society, Seattle, Washington, February 11, 1989.

Germino B, Funk SG. Development of the family concerns inventory. Unpublished report. Grant funded by National Center for Nursing Research, National Institutes for Health 1RO1BRO1331-01A1, 1989.

Hanser-McConnell J. Fear. In: McFarland G, Thomas M, eds. Psychiatric mental health nursing: application of the nursing process. Philadelphia: JB Lippincott, 1990.

Mathews-Simonton S, Simonton OC, Creighton JL. Getting well again. New York: Bantam Books, 1978.

Mishel MH. The experience of uncertainty after treatment ends. Presented at the International Nursing Research Conference, ANA Council of Nurse Researchers, Washington, DC, October 13–16, 1987.

Mullan F. Seasons of survival: reflections of a physician with cancer. N Engl J Med 1985;315:270.

Northouse L. The impact of cancer on the family: an overview. Int J Psychiatry Med 1984;14:215.

Oberst M, James R. Going home: patient and spouse adjustment following cancer surgery. Topics in Clinical Nursing 1985;7(1):46.

Simonton SM. The healing family: the Simonton approach for families facing illness. New York: Bantam Books, 1984.

Tanaka K. Development of a tool for assessing posttrauma response. Archives of Psychiatric Nursing 1988;2:350.

Taylor S. Ten issues that cancer patients have to teach. Surviving: A Cancer Patient Newsletter. Department of Therapeutic Radiology, Stanford University Medical Center, 1988; Jan-Feb:2.

Tross S, Holland JC, Bosl G, Geller N. A controlled study of psychosocial sequelae in cured survivors of testicular neoplasms. Abstract C-87. Proceedings of the American Society of Clinical Oncologists 1984;25:74.

8

Living With Long-Term Survival

The survival phase of the cancer experience, unlike earlier phases, does not begin abruptly.* Rather, it occurs gradually, almost imperceptibly, as weeks, months, and finally years pass with no manifestations of relapse or recurrence. The worry about recurrence becomes cordoned off, but remains an ever-present sword of Damocles (Bergholz, 1988; Koocher and O'Malley, 1981). It rises in focus and power on special occasions, such as anniversaries of the diagnosis and visits to physicians, or when threatening symptoms appear, but retreats to the background when these events pass without incident. Self-monitoring becomes less compulsive, less hypervigilant. At some level, survivors accommodate the residual iatrogenic structural changes and dysfunctions; they become more proficient and natural in incorporating prostheses and other technical requirements into their patterns of daily living. The focus becomes one of achieving as normal a lifestyle as possible. Both the survivor and those who share daily living begin to trust in the future again.

However, daily living is not the same as it was before the cancer experience. The disease and its treatment have changed the survivor and those who share that daily living. For some, it has changed patterns of daily living. There are also some new, sometimes unexpected challenges in the long-term survival phase faced by the 5 million individuals in the United States who have experienced cancer and its treatment and the many millions more who share their daily life.

Medical Perspective

Medicine tends to define long-term survival statistically, in terms of the number of people diagnosed as having cancer who are alive (though not necessarily free of cancer) at 5- and 10-year periods. In the most recent statistics, the 5-year survival rate for all

---

* In organizing the content of this book, the survival phase is arbitrarily ended when the survivor dies of a disease other than cancer or experiences a recurrence of cancer. However, it is recognized that survival issues and strategies continue on into the crisis of recurrence and the chronic phase of advancing cancer.

sites, all ages, and all racial groups in the United States was actuarily estimated to be 40% (Myers and Gloeckler Ries, 1989). The 1989 Cancer Statistics reports in the United States a 5-year survival rate of 50% for whites and 37% for blacks† (Silverberg and Lubera, 1989). For all sites among adults, Myers and Gloeckler Ries (1989) predict a 28% chance of escaping death due to cancer at the end of 10 years.

Medicine is not a dominant player in cancer survivors' management of long-term survival. Interaction between the survivor and the physician tends to occur during the routinely scheduled physical examinations or at contacts based on concern about signs and symptoms of recurrence, delayed treatment effects, or health problems not related to cancer. Oncologists' perspective in the survival phase focuses on signs of recurrence, second malignant neoplasms (SMNs), and late iatrogenic sequelae. They, or the survivor's regular physician, also monitor and treat any difficulties that emerge from earlier treatment (e.g., stenosis of a colostomy, infections, lymphedema).

Generally, the patient's regular physician returns to a nononcologic focus, addressing issues of age-related health promotion and identifying and treating any other pathology that emerges. Obviously, medical diagnosis and treatment of cancer survivors must incorporate any relevant factors from the earlier malignancy or its treatment (e.g., considering the level and location of previous radiation exposure; taking blood pressures or blood samples from the arm that is not on the side of an earlier mastectomy and axillary node dissection; considering the status of immunosuppression).

An area of medical decision making concerning cancer survivors has to do with control of patient data. Release of documented information to third-party payers, insurance companies, or employers who pay for the survivor's health care is common. It is even advocated to "counter stereotypes" (Blum and Blum, 1988). Even when distribution of the information is not intended, given the accessibility of computerized data there is a risk of this information negatively affecting survivors' employment opportunities and insurance options. Physicians may not be aware that patients have a "bundle of rights" with respect to information in the patient record (Belair, 1989).

Some physicians acknowledge that their training has not prepared them to consider issues in managing daily living for long-term survivors other than medical problems (Kagan and Kagan, 1983; Vess et al, 1988). Thus, patients and their families report a "subtle sense of frustration and neglect" with physicians, should they seek assistance in managing problems and issues of long-term survival that are not directly involved with neoplasms or iatrogenic changes (Fisher, 1981). Cost containment efforts are resulting in heavier booking of physicians' schedules, so that even less time may be allowed for dealing with sensitive patient–family issues though the physician may have the skills and be comfortable in the interaction.

Nursing Perspective

As in the post-treatment phase, nursing contacts with survivors and their families tend to be limited in long-term survival unless there are problems requiring visits to a physician or unless the survivor participates in a nurse-led cancer support group or related volunteer activities. Occasionally, survivors will maintain contact with nurses who provided care during the treatment phase.

---

† Statistics for other ethnic groups were not given.

Because of the paucity of contacts, their time-limited nature, and the fact that the focus for health care may be directed to a different health problem, it is crucial that nurses maintain an awareness of the high-risk challenges and problems associated with being a cancer survivor. Only then can appropriate and efficient assessment and diagnosis be made to rule in or rule out problems of managing daily living effectively as a cancer survivor or as a person who closely shares the survivor's daily living.

Using the daily living–functional health status perspective, the areas for assessment, diagnosis, and treatment might include:

Living with the threats of recurrence and onset of late treatment side-effects

Difficulties in implementing changed life goals and priorities, and the effect on physical and mental health status

Managing interpersonal tasks linked to stigma or discrimination encountered, and associated dissatisfaction with role relationships

Managing daily living with reduced or altered external resources associated with residual financial burdens from the treatment, reduced job options, restricted insurance coverage, or withdrawal of former members of the survivor's personal network and failure to develop new personal resources

While nurses may not deal directly with many of the outside stressors (e.g., job options, insurance, financial burdens), they are diagnosing and treating the survivor and family members whose health and well-being are affected by these stressors (Holmes, 1978; Holmes and Masuda, 1973; Holmes and Rahe, 1968). Thus, acknowledgment of the presence of these seemingly non-nursing problem areas and support for effective use of internal and external resources to manage them is important. Political and community activism to improve the work and social climate for cancer survivors is an important contribution nurses can make that can subsequently prevent some survivors' problems and make more treatment options available.

Nature of Long-Term Survival

Long-term survival from cancer is not an experience that can exist in isolation. Instead, it forms a continuum with the experiences, outcomes, and responses of the earlier phases. Like Humpty Dumpty, neither the survivor nor those who closely shared the experience can be put back together and be the same as they were before. All have been changed in some way; both growth and losses may have occurred. The new challenges of daily living in the survival phase can require revised strategies using internal and external resources, which may have been diminished or changed in some way, or mobilization of new resources.

New and sometimes unexpected challenges in the survival phase appear in four different areas of daily life (Kagan and Kagan, 1983):

Professional life: Salary, health and life insurance, job and promotion opportunities, behavior of co-workers; or management of home and family responsibilities with altered capabilities or interest

Social life: Relationships with family, friends, and acquaintances; travel options; facilities for social gatherings and recreation

Sexual life: Belief in one's sexual desirability, satisfaction with interpersonal contacts in which sexuality or intimacy are factors

Private life: Management of one's inner experiences as a cancer survivor, self-concept, values, goals, priorities

The phenomena involved in living as a cancer survivor tend to cut across these four areas.

Threat of Recurrence or Second Malignant Neoplasms

Probably the greatest intrapersonal stressor is the "punishing worry" (Mullan, 1985) that cancer will recur or that SMNs will emerge. The etiologic factors that permitted the initiation and promotion of the initial neoplasm may still exist, making cancer survivors more vulnerable to second cancers (Greenberg et al, 1988). Chemotherapy, radiation, and compromised immunocompetence increase the risk (Fobair et al, 1986).

As the number of long-term survivors has increased and survival times have lengthened for some malignancies, the risks of iatrogenic cancers, both early and late, have been documented (Fobair et al, 1986; Greenburg et al, 1988). Documentation has shown the concern about recurrence or SMNs to be realistic and fully justifiable.

The number of long-term survivors of certain types of cancer (e.g., acute lymphocytic leukemias, Hodgkin's disease, non-Hodgkin's lymphomas, Wilms' tumor, and testicular carcinoma) is increasing (Silverberg and Lubera, 1989). Studies show that initial treatment of these cancers with radiation and chemotherapy increases the risk of SMNs significantly. For example, Hodgkin's disease survivors have an overall six-fold excess risk of second cancers (e.g., fatal leukemias) (Tucker et al, 1988), and a 20-fold risk of solid tumors 10 or more years after treatment (e.g., lung tumors; melanomas; stomach, bone, soft-tissue, and breast cancers) (Boivin et al, 1984; Tucker et al, 1988). Immunosuppression also seems to contribute to occurrence of tumors (Blattner and Hoover, 1985). Successfully treated childhood cancers (leukemias and some other cancers) have similar risks. Children who survive for 20 years have 10 times the risk of developing a SMN (Meadows et al, 1980). So time, rather than being a friend and decreasing the risks of second cancers, actually increases them.

Late Iatrogenic Problems

In addition to increasing the risk for second cancers, therapy can cause physiologic dysfunctions long after the treatment. While these are not common, they do constitute a risk and a concern. The dysfunctions associated with chemotherapy and radiation can occur from 1 to many years after treatment. Paresthesias and dysesthesias can emerge or continue as a chronic complaint. Additionally, the functional and structural changes created by surgical treatment persist; there are some risks associated with these as well (e.g., infections and skin breakdown associated with ostomies, stenosis, lymphedema distal to node dissections).

Chemotherapy

The possible late complications of chemotherapy include:

Second malignancies, impaired gonadal functioning, sterility, genetic defects in offspring (D'Angio 1983; Mulvihill and Byrne, 1989)

Pulmonary fibrosis (high to moderate risk with bleomycin sulfate, carmustine, and busulfan) (Bowden, 1984; Muggia et al, 1983; Wickham, 1986)

Brain atrophy following intrathecal methotrexate sodium as prophylactic treatment of central nervous system in acute lymphocytic leukemia in childhood (Brouwers et al, 1984; Ochs et al, 1980)

Radiation

Radiation also has associated complications.

Site of Treatment	Possible Late Effects
Bladder	Cystitis, contracted bladder
Bone and cartilage	Osteitis, joint dysfunction *In children:* Arrest of growth, shortening of bone
Bone marrow	Anemia
Bowel	Ulceration, fistula formation, adhesions, obstruction, malabsorption, enteritis (chronic diarrhea), proctitis (Kokal, 1986)
Breast	Fibrosis, loss of erotic sensations
Central nervous system	Myelopathy, leading to paresthesias in upper extremities or bowel and bladder dysfunction; vascular obliteration, leading to infarction and occlusion *In children:* Computed tomographic scan abnormalities, altered neurologic system findings (Brouwers et al, 1984); altered intellectual and attentional deficits manifested on psychologic testing (Lansky et al, 1986)
Esophagus	Fibrosis, stricture, ulceration
Eyes	Cataracts, optic nerve damage (ischemia), keratitis, retinal hemorrhage, dry eyes or excessive tearing, glaucoma
Heart	Fibrosis, pericarditis
Kidneys	Nephritis, renal failure
Liver	Hepatitis, cirrhosis
Lungs	Fibrosis, pneumonitis
Mouth	Dental caries, xerostomia (if parotid glands are irradiated), taste alterations, mucosal ulceration, osteoradionecrosis of mandible, trismus
Ovaries	Menstrual irregularity or menopause
Prostate area	Impotence
Skin	Hyperpigmentation or hypopigmentation, telangiectasis, atrophy, hair loss, subcutaneous fibrosis (usually after trauma)
Soft tissue	Fibrosis, necrosis, distal lymphedema
Stomach	Atrophy, ulcers, decreased emptying time
Testicle	Oligospermia or aspermia
Vagina	Stenosis, dryness

Long-Term Energy Loss and Depression

Energy loss tends to continue far longer than anticipated for many patients. It has been reported to be sufficient to interfere with vigorous, moderate, and, for some, even light activities (Cella and Tross, 1986; Fobair et al, 1986). In one study with a median time of 9 years after treatment, normal energy levels were found to return for all but about 37% in 12 to 16 months; the remainder suffered persistent low energy (Fobair et al, 1986). In another study with a median time of 2.5 years after treatment, 56% of the subjects reported failure to return to normal energy levels (Cella, 1983). Depression, advanced disease at the time of diagnosis, being older, and multiple treatment modalities including chemotherapy have been shown to be predictors of long-term energy loss (Fobair et al, 1986). While the subjects in these studies were survivors of Hodgkin's disease, it was suggested that similar factors may well apply to survivors of other forms of cancer as well (Fobair et al, 1986).

Studies of persons whose cancer was diagnosed and treated in their adult years showed that depression among long-term survivors was not much greater than that in the general population (Fobair et al, 1986; Heinrich and Coscarelli Schag, 1987; Kemeny et al, 1988; Tross et al, 1984). Among long-term survivors of childhood cancers, a higher-than-average incidence of depression occurred among those diagnosed and treated in midadolescence than in those diagnosed and treated at younger ages (Lansky et al, 1986). In the adults, a greater incidence of depression was found in the earlier years of survival (i.e., less than 3 years after treatment ended) (Fobair et al, 1986). Findings suggest that survivors have emotional resiliency and that emotional status returns to premorbid levels as duration of survival increases; however, the sense of mortality and vulnerability remains close to the surface (Fobair et al, 1986).

Self-Concept

The self-concept evolving in the extended survivorship phase has as its point of departure the preillness self-concept of the survivor. This serves as a baseline for each of the phases of the cancer experience. The survivor's self-concept is a product of combining the baseline self-concept with the effects of the experiences of the diagnostic, treatment, and post-treatment phases plus ongoing feedback from others, particularly during the post-treatment and survival phases. Where neither the tumor nor the treatment were aggressive, the premorbid self-concept—positive or negative—may emerge unscathed. On the other hand, where the threat to life associated with the pathology of the tumor has been great and where the treatment has been highly mutilative of structure and disruptive of functions, the assaults on even a highly positive self-concept can be tremendous. Thus, the tasks of daily living as a cancer survivor may well include healing for a bruised self-concept or therapy to upgrade a self-concept that is not adequate to the challenges of living life as a cancer survivor.

The healing and the transitions of return to more routine daily living in the post-treatment phase and the beginning of the extended survival phase offer several paths for changes in self-concept. For some, a return to the precancer self-concept occurs. These are the survivors who come to terms with or are unaffected by changes in appearance and function; they manage or have left behind the threats and stresses of the cancer experience. For example, one survivor whose self-concept was associated with her community work used her dysfunction as an advocate for the handicapped. When fatigue required her to use a wheelchair to conserve energy in order to accomplish her schedule of activities, she translated this into advocacy for wheelchair-accessible entrances to buildings and facilities. She barely noticed when her wig became somewhat askew. Survivors who cannot accommodate to the body changes and the life threat of the cancer experience face the tasks of survivorship with the additional burden and resource deficits associated with a lower self-concept.

For some survivors, conquering the challenges of the diagnostic and treatment phases is seen as offering a second chance at and a new appreciation for life (Quigley, 1989; Shanfield, 1980). They and their companions who shared the experience know how close death may have come during treatment, and have witnessed the journey back. It is an experience that can be talked about and validated by witnesses. Such battles of the body and the spirit, fought and won, sometimes create in the survivors a strong desire to seize an opportunity to be different, to accomplish goals that hadn't existed for them before (Blum and Blum, 1988). It may be that daily living had not fully tested their resources before and they now have found capabilities and strengths they had not previously recognized. The cancer experience then has become an impetus for growth, with attendant changes in self-concept.

Families and those who have shared the daily living before and throughout the cancer experience cannot help but be affected by the self-concept of the survivor. Spouses, children, and parents have built relationships over the years that were based on the survivor's premorbid self-concept. They have adjusted (or failed to adjust) to any transient changes in self-concept associated with the rigors of the diagnostic and treatment phases. In the survival phase, it would not be unusual for them to expect the survivor to revert to the premorbid self-concept and the comfort of established relationships based on this self-concept. Where changes in the survivor's self-concept occur, either an improvement or a lowering, these represent an additional challenge for family, friends, and co-workers to integrate into their relationships. These changes and the strategies of adaptation and nature of adjustment are areas for diagnosis and treatment when they impinge on the health of the survivor or others.

Sexuality

In the extended survival phase, sexuality represents one dimension of self-concept. It involves not only needs for sexual intimacy, but approaches to meeting affectional needs of patient and partner, role relationships, decision making about childbearing, and skills of accommodating structural and functional changes to achieve satisfaction in sexual activity. Like self-concept, sexuality for survivors and partners cannot be separated from the premorbid sense of sexuality, established relationships, or patterns in daily living involving affection, sexuality, and intimacy. For adults, patterns of sexuality and affection are a continuation, but often with significant modifications. For example, survivors and their partners report a continued desire for physical affectional behavior, but a decrease in desire for sexual intercourse. There are risks that one partner's needs are not the same as the other's, resulting in dissatisfaction and tension (Leiber et al, 1976; Wess et al, 1988). (See also Chapter 6, section on Sexuality.)

Problems associated with sexuality that arose during the treatment and post-treatment phases may not have been resolved by the time the survivor has reached the extended survival phase of the cancer experience. Persistent fatigue or depression can also affect sexual interest and performance (see previous section on Long-Term Energy Loss and Depression). The extensiveness of the treatment (e.g., breast segmentectomy versus mastectomy) affects body image and positive feelings of sexuality, and even the frequency of sexual relations (Kemeny et al, 1988). Some later side-effects of the treatment may create additional problems (e.g., ongoing changes in breast texture, further stenosis of the vagina, diarrhea, inadequate control of ostomies). Where facial reconstruction has not been done, for whatever reason, disfigurement may be a factor in sexuality. Laryngectomy and the resultant altered speech can also be a negative factor.

Sexuality in an Established Relationship

A history of an established, satisfying personal relationship between partners with open communication about needs and desires offers a positive prognosis for resolving any remaining sexual problems and regaining or maintaining satisfying expressions of affection and intimacy. However, where problems existed in the established relationship, or where strategies for resolving sexual difficulties have never been developed, the ongoing strains associated with altered appearance or sexual functioning can lay additional strains on fragile relationships. Even in relationships that have a sound foundation it does not pay to take satisfactions for granted; expressions of affection and intimacy may need to be adjusted as partners' needs and sources of satisfaction change.

One issue that may arise among younger cancer survivors and their partners is childbearing (Mulvihill and Byrne, 1989). For some, treatment has made conceiving or bearing a child impossible. For others, the capacity to conceive or bear children is only delayed. Chemotherapy with alkylating agents and radiation below the diaphragm create the greatest effect on fertility.

Two fears may arise concerning pregnancy and childbearing. One is the fear of long-term chromosomal damage that may create congenital abnormalities or increased incidence of cancers in the offspring. This fear would seem to be unfounded. Studies of survivors and the general population showed a 4% rate of major birth defects among cancer survivors, which is comparable to that of the general population, and no greater incidence of childhood cancers; however, there was an excess of fetal loss and low birth weight in offspring of women who had abdominal radiotherapy (Mulvihill and Byrne, 1989). With primary breast radiation a 2-year delay in childbearing is recommended. The second fear arises when the cancer survivor is the female partner. Here the concern may be that a pregnancy will increase the risk of reactivating the malignancy. Pregnancies occurring after treatment for breast cancer seemed to have no effect on survival; in fact, the patient may gain some protection from the pregnancy (Cooper and Butterfield, 1970; Peters, 1968).

For males whose reproductive capacity may be diminished by cancer treatment, sperm banking prior to treatment and artificial insemination when childbearing is desired is an option. Adoption is another alternative. However, some patients treated for cancer have reported subtle discrimination when they seek to adopt (Hassey, 1988).

Establishing New Relationships

For survivors who had no close sexual partner at the time of the cancer diagnosis and treatment, or who lost the partner during these phases, the challenges are different. Should these survivors wish to seek and develop relationships involving sexuality and intimacy, there are special challenges. One has to do with the survivor's own self concept of desirability, the ability to communicate sexual desirability to another person, and in some instances, the skill and resources to use cosmetics, clothing, prostheses, and so on to disguise any structural or functional defects. Going into situations with the purpose of dating may take more courage than it did before the cancer experience. Another challenge arises in deciding when and how to inform the person one is dating about one's history of cancer. Some survivors report being quite direct, and indicate that life is too short to waste time on persons who cannot accept a cancer survivor. Others are more tentative in their approach and handling of the responses. The visibility of any post-treatment structural or functional changes will be a factor, as will the survivor's own self-concept, confidence, and comfort with the post-treatment sexuality. An additional factor influencing new relationships is a wariness about setting future goals that may be implicit in long-term relationships.

Cancer-Related Interpersonal Difficulties

Interpersonal difficulties can involve the survivor and family members, employers, co-workers, or other social contacts. Survivors' perceptions of problems and their responses in these situations may arise from their own self-concept. Interpersonal difficulties may also be created by others' concept of cancer and cancer survivors.

These factors create several scenarios in the interaction of the survivor and others. The survivor may either seek normalcy in the relationships or be uncomfortable and feel alienated from others who have not had the cancer experience. People the survivor encounters may experience vulnerability (It could happen to me), or helplessness (I can't do anything to help this person), again generating feelings of discomfort with and alienation from the survivor. Effective survivorship in the area of interpersonal relationships may be based on the skills the survivor has in making others comfortable—telling one's cancer story as past history, putting cancer in its place, focusing on moving ahead with one's life. It may also involve understanding and sometimes accepting another person's discomforts, biases, or vicarious experiences with cancer and the resultant behavior when change is unlikely.

Myths about cancer and perceptions that a person who has had cancer is different from others can result in stigmatization for cancer survivors. The belief that cancer is contagious can cause others to avoid not only the cancer survivors, but also their primary care givers or close family members. Some parents have been known to keep their children from playing with the children of cancer survivors (Hoffman, 1989a; Trillin, 1981). Even spouses and family members may believe that the cancer is contagious and distance themselves physically (Fisher, 1981). Some children who fear the contagion of cancer have been known to physically distance themselves from the parent who is a cancer survivor and even avoid touching objects the survivor handles (Vess et al, 1988). A second myth that tends to stigmatize the survivor and result in strained relationships is the belief that cancer is a death sentence (Mellette, 1986). For example, a healthy but unemployed executive likened his employed colleagues' avoidance of him to behavior he and they had engaged in when they literally crossed the street to avoid having to talk with a person known to have a serious cancer (Fisher, 1981). The cancer experience can result in changes in the survivor's personal network, as family, friends, and acquaintances respond to their own fears and interpersonal discomforts (Bergholz, 1988; Taylor, 1988).

The social climate for survivors may be improving as we enter the 1990s. Well-known persons are publicly acknowledging their cancer experiences and managing their daily living with survival in full view. Survivors' organizations are springing up and are courting recognition on both national and local levels. With their numbers growing, cancer survivors are beginning to view themselves as a recognizable minority group and as people with high risks for discrimination. Like other minority groups, they work to both prevent and seek redress for discrimination based on the diagnosis of cancer or any disabilities associated with it. Local, regional, and national conferences and publications‡ of survivors' organizations create a resource for support and a pool of workers to lobby for fairness in conditions for cancer survivors. They focus on the management of daily living as a cancer survivor and provide information as well as support to the individual survivor. They also seek to mobilize resources for research to expand the body of knowledge about management of the challenges of cancer survivorship (Davis-Spingarn, 1988). The American Cancer Society has developed "The Cancer Survivors' Bill of Rights" (American Cancer Society, 1988). More survivors are "coming out of the closet" (Davis-Spingarn, 1988a) in cases when such admission would not seem to create unnecessary or unresolvable difficulties. Survivors see a need to help each other and to teach those who have not had the experience of cancer about its realities.

Challenges in the Workplace

Work and finances are major concerns to many cancer survivors. About 80% of adult cancer survivors return to work successfully after diagnosis of cancer and have approximately the same productive capacity as their co-workers (Hoffman, 1989). On the other hand, studies report that about a quarter of cancer survivors who are in the workplace or seeking to enter it experience some form of difficulty because of their cancer history. Reported problems include denial of new jobs, termination of employment, demotion or denial of promotion, unwanted transfer, changes in insurance benefits, isolation, hostility, and required medical examinations not related to job performance (Hoffman, 1989a). However, many of the studies have not reported on the survivor's actual capacity to fulfill the requirements of the job; thus, difficulties in the workplace may result from altered capacity to perform or from discrimination (Hoffman, 1989a). Low self-esteem and a tendency to complain have been identified as characteristics of survivors who reported negative experiences (Houts et al, 1980).

Returning to the Same Place of Employment

Survivors returning to previous jobs seem to have few problems if they can meet job requirements (Mellette and Franco, 1987). Years of positive work relationships tended to temper any difficult interactions during the transition time of returning to work during or after treatment (Staley et al, 1987). Changes in co-workers' behavior, including not knowing how to interact with the survivor, lack of understanding of what the survivor is experiencing, oversolicitude, and occasional stigmatization associated with misunderstandings about cancer and contagion, are examples of interpersonal difficulties. However, these are reported to dissipate as the survivor is again integrated into the work scene. Cancer survivorship does not "confer sainthood"; individuals who had premorbid employment work difficulties may well have similar difficulties after treatment (Mellette, 1985).

Mellette and Franco (1987), in their review of studies done in the 1970s, indicate

---

‡ See quarterly issues of the *NCCS Networker*, the newsletter for the National Coalition for Cancer Survivorship, for news, announcements of upcoming annual meetings or conventions, news on the cancer survival front, reviews of new books and videos, and announcements (e.g., National Survivors Day). Membership can be obtained by writing to NCCS, 323 Eighth Street S.W., Albuquerque, NM 87102. In 1989 individual dues were $20.00.

hat most employers retained employees who were treated for cancer and found them to perform satisfactorily. Problems the survivors face in returning to work in the same etting include changes in benefits, being transferred to another job, and, occasionally, being placed in physical isolation because of false beliefs in contagion of cancer (Mellette and Franco, 1987).

Seeking a New Job

Cancer survivors seeking work in both blue and white collar jobs are reported to have experienced rejections they believe were based on their cancer history (Mellette, 1985). The armed services reject applicants with a history of cancer.

Difficulties vary with the site of the disease. Breast cancer survivors experienced the least difficulty, while those with head and neck cancer experienced the most. However, the latter had a rather poor premorbid employment record as well (Mellette, 1985).

Where the post-treatment status does not present visible evidence of the cancer or the treatment, survivors may become increasingly wary of reporting their earlier cancers, particularly as survival time increases or when job rejections have occurred. Given the high and escalating costs of health insurance, employers may well be reluctant to hire persons who present known risks, quite aside from any personal biases and beliefs they have about cancer and the capabilities of survivors.

The importance of retaining insurance benefits and having secure employment is important to many cancer survivors. For these reasons they may remain in unsatisfying jobs when they would prefer to seek new and better job opportunities, and are qualified for them. This situation is called "job lock-in." It can be particularly devastating to young people seeking advancement opportunities or new experiences (Mellette, 1985).

Legal Redress for Job Discrimination

Where discrimination appears to be based on the worker's cancer history, legal redress is possible. The federal Rehabilitation Act of 1973 (with its 1974 amendment expanding the definition of handicapped persons to include those with a history of handicap or those perceived as being handicapped) and state statutes prohibiting employment discrimination offer possibilities for legal recourse. In 1989, new bills that would specifically aid cancer patients and survivors, among others with disabilities, were being introduced in Congress (Hoffman, 1989). In addition, the American Cancer Society-sponsored Cancer Employment Law Project of the Legal Aid Society in San Francisco has been providing help to some patients and researching state and federal laws that protect cancer survivors from discrimination. At present, few patients seem to be using legal forms of redress (Mellette and Franco, 1987).

Discrimination in Insurance Coverage

Obtaining or maintaining adequate, affordable health coverage is a serious challenge facing cancer survivors. Those who have had insurance can experience policy cancellations, changes in benefits, inflated premiums, and offering of only high-risk types of policies with high costs and major deductibles. Young adults reaching the end of their coverage as dependents on their parents' policies face major problems.

The best way to get health, disability, and life insurance is through employment. Employers are now required to continue company-based group coverage for up to 12 months after the person leaves employment because of illness. Additionally, in some states, some insurance companies such as Blue Cross have open enrollment periods when applicants cannot be turned away. Such policies may have a "previously existing" clause that limits coverage for preexisting conditions such as cancer, but it may be time-limited (e.g., 3 or 6 months) (Hunter, 1988). Organizations such as alumni associations or the American Association of Retired Persons (AARP) sometimes offer insurance benefits that might not otherwise be available. At least 15 states have high-risk pools or some plan for people who cannot get insurance in the open market. The premiums tend to be high. In 1989 those states included Connecticut, Florida, Illinois, Indiana, Iowa, Maine, Minnesota, Montana, Nebraska, New Mexico, North Dakota, Oregon, Tennessee, Washington, and Wisconsin. Information can be gained by contacting the state insurance commissioner. Insurance practices are being liberalized in relation to Hodgkin's disease because of its improved cure rate (Mellette and Franco, 1987). The National Insurance Consumer Organization (NICO), a nonprofit public interest advocacy and educational group, has printed information available giving tips on how to select an agent, what coverage to avoid, and so on. (Hunter, 1988). A list of publications can be obtained by sending a self-addressed stamped envelope to NICO, 121 North Payne Street, Alexandria, VA 22314.

Underlying Mechanisms

The cancer diagnosis and treatment phases are a time when the patient and family experience vulnerability and loss of control in many areas, large and small (Mack, 1984; Vess et al, 1988). The person cannot control the neoplastic process, the administration of the treatment, nor, to a great extent, the body's response to the treatment and its impact on daily living. These phases and the initial healing and transition of the post-treatment phase are now past. Quality of life in the extended survival phase may well depend on retaining, regaining, and maintaining a satisfying level of control in daily living—"keeping cancer in its place" (Flaherty, 1981). Taking control of oneself and one's daily living is not a passive process; rather, it is a matter of making daily choices and taking actions to live one's life in as fulfilling a way as possible (Mack, 1984). Taking control in daily living as a cancer survivor can, on occasion, be made easier and more effective when the survivor and an informed nurse pool their collective wisdom and experience in collaborative diagnosis of issues and problems in daily living followed by consideration of options for managing them.

Daily Living Factors

Activities in   Having a satisfying measure of control in a number of activities
Daily Living   in daily living is linked to effective management of cancer
                      survivorship. These activities include:

> Putting the cancer experience into one's past history rather than ruminating on it and being preoccupied with the risks of recurrence

Engaging in positive self-talk as needed to enhance self-concept, particularly on the "down" days

Incorporating self-care activities into daily routines (e.g., purchase, use, and maintenance of prostheses and supplies; skillful use of makeup, hairstyle, or clothing to disguise any scars or defects; efficient routines for ostomy care; diet and eating patterns to accommodate altered stomach capacity or to control bowel elimination)

Adjusting schedules and activities to accommodate any residual functional deficits (e.g., periods of low energy, loss of strength and endurance for a particular body part—such as the arm on the side of a mastectomy)

Incorporating protective behavior in activities that involve risk of infection (e.g., the arm and hand on the side of the mastectomy or node dissection, avoidance of close contact with people who have upper respiratory infections or influenza when one's immune system is compromised). (See Chapter 6, section on Vulnerability to Infection, under Nursing Diagnosis and Treatment.)

Engaging in self-monitoring at appropriate intervals (e.g., breast or testicular self-examination) (see Chapter 4)

Learning how to handle the uncomfortable responses of others to one's cancer history or residual defects (e.g., seeking to change their perceptions and feelings, avoiding or ignoring the responses when they cannot be changed)

Negotiating for adjustments in role responsibilities when residual deficits of cancer treatment do not permit fulfillment of usual or previous role expectations (e.g., job, homemaking, sexual behavior) or increasing requirements in daily living when functional status improves

Actively seeking and maintaining a pattern in daily living activities that provides frequent pleasure and feelings of fulfillment

Events in Daily Living

Some events will have particular significance and others may present particular difficulties for cancer survivors. These include (Bergholz, 1988):

Anniversaries of the date of the original cancer diagnosis (Quigley, 1989)

Return visits to the oncologist or other physician for routine checkups

Job interviews for new employment

Modifying or seeking redress for acts of discrimination

Learning of the recurrence of cancer or the death of other survivors

Joyous events, such as being given a "clean bill of health" after a visit to the oncologist for a routine checkup, getting the job one sought, finding rewarding new relationships, becoming a parent, or being able to help another cancer survivor

Demands in Daily Living

Demands in daily living for cancer survivors come from self, others, and possessions. These can create special requirements in the daily living of cancer survivors.

Self-expectations: Self-expectations that one will manage daily living and that one can find pleasures in life as a survivor—or the reverse, that one will face unsurmountable difficulties—seem to make a difference in survivors' quality of life. Engaging in positive self-talk, looking for small and large pleasures, and setting achievable goals according to one's priorities will require varying levels of a person's internal and external resources. Much will depend on the person's survival situation, post-treatment physical status, external resources, and native optimism or pessimism.

Expectations of others: As in the post-treatment phase, the expectations of others can be congruent with those of the survivor or they may create tensions because they are incompatible. When the latter occurs, the survivor's skills and energies are required to avoid, reframe, change, or ignore the expectations that create difficulties. (See Chapter 6, section on Role.)

Demands of possessions: The demands for attention and energy created by home, car, garden, or pets can be an asset or a problem for survivors. Where post-treatment fatigue persists and is severe, meeting the demands of possessions can be draining; stress can be created if the demands are not met. On the other hand, the day-to-day demands that possessions make can offer structure and comfort in daily living. Premorbid standards in housekeeping and home and car maintenance will be factors in the expectations for meeting demands in the survival stage. They can also influence the emotional response of guilt, anger, or satisfaction associated with meeting or not meeting these expectations. Effective survivorship may involve adjusting these expectations to a level that is compatible with existing energy and strength and with any new life goals and priorities that have been developed. It is well to be aware that changes in standards of maintenance from preillness levels can create tensions with family members who are comfortable with previous patterns.

Environment for Daily Living

The physical, microbial, and sensory elements of the environment each can contribute to or detract from the quality of life of the cancer survivor and family. The features of the environment likely to assume particular importance are related to the post-treatment physical and emotional status of the survivor.

Examples of physical aspects of the environment that may create added challenges include:

Features that require additional energy or form barriers to wheelchair use (e.g., stairs to frequently used facilities, long distances to public transportation or stores)

Stressors to which the survivor's post-treatment status cannot adapt (e.g., serious air pollution, lack of humidity)

Limited access to the bathroom

Lack of areas for privacy for some aspects of daily living, or the reverse—lack of areas for encountering others in ways that promote the meaningful sharing of daily living

The microbial environment will be significant for survivors whose immune systems continue to be compromised or those whose lymph nodes and channels have been disrupted (e.g., axillary node dissections). Facilities and equipment for maintaining cleanliness in food preparation, personal hygiene, the home environment, and laundry will be important. (See Chapter 6, section on Vulnerability to Infection.)

The survivor's needs for the sensory environment may be the same as before the cancer experience, but they can also be changed. Chronic paresthesias and dysesthesias, inability to dissipate worry about recurrence, concern about finances or relationships, and so on can create an internal sensory overload in which modulation of high levels of external stimulation may be desired. On the other hand, sensory underload, monotony, and lack of distraction or diversion can contribute to an unhealthy preoccupation with the cancer experience. There are good days and valley days in the cancer survival experience. Adjusting the sensory environment so that it is optimum at any given point in time is a responsibility of both the survivor and those who share the daily living. It requires perceptiveness and initiative from each.

Values and Priorities in Daily Living

It is not unusual for individuals who survive the diagnostic and treatment phases of the cancer experience to take a fresh look at life—what they want from it and what they want to give to it. Sometimes spouses, partners, and other close family members too engage in this type of reappraisal of life. Any change in values and priorities has the potential to change behavior and create repercussions in day-to-day relationships. Challenges and tensions can arise when individuals fail to communicate their revised views, goals, and plans for managing daily living to those who share that daily living (at home or work). Others presume that life is to go on as usual. For example, some male cancer survivors who have been career-oriented find that their families assume new importance and they wish to spend more time with them and participate in activities that they did not share before. This change in behavior may or may not be initially comfortable for individual family members or the family as a unit. They may well have built a lifestyle that accommodated an absent husband and father and be reluctant to change, yet feel guilty for not doing so.

It is not unusual for individuals who were passive in their premorbid approach to daily living to take a more assertive stance in implementing their values and goals as survivors. Again the change in style of daily living can be bewildering to companions until they become accustomed to the new person the survivor has become. While the communication of new values, goals, and plans cannot ensure agreement and comfort among those who share daily living with the survivor, at least it can reduce some of the surprises.

Functional Health Status

Given the challenges that accompany daily living as cancer survivors, there are special demands on their internal resources. In some instances family members, partners, or close companions also face new or altered demands on their internal resources.

Strength and Endurance

Strength and endurance can involve not only physical capacities, but also the survivor's spirit. Low energy that extends on into the survival phase obviously affects the way in which the physical, and sometimes the cognitive and emotional, requirements of daily living can be addressed. Loss of strength or function in a particular body part also can alter the way in which tasks are accomplished. Either of these changes in strength and endurance can require an examination of values and priorities. At times, ongoing deficits in functional capacities will require creative problem solving in order to produce a desired, or even an acceptable, quality of life.

There may be times when the emotional burdens of survivorship seem overwhelming. Only the strength of spirit to go on, to seek another form of support, to try again will sustain the survivor. For survivors or their family members who find greater strength in sharing, participation in local and national support groups may be a useful adjunct.

Cognition

Effective survivorship sometimes requires cognitive capacities involving knowledge and understanding from the lowest levels of recall to the highest levels of synthesis, application, and evaluation. The cancer survivor's required body of knowledge can include knowledge of:

Self: Premorbid self-concept, relationships, strengths, and limitations versus self in the survival phase—changes in self-concept, values, priorities, goals, and relationships with significant others

Cancer: Cancer as a treatable disease, cancer in remission, risk reduction for other cancers, strategies for health maintenance

Others' knowledge and responses concerning cancer and survivorship: Fears, myths, discomforts, needs, and so on of spouse or partner, other family members, companions, co-workers, employers, social acquaintances, needed in order to interpret their responses and, occasionally, to reframe the survivor's perception of the situation

Systems: The resources, needs, and biases of systems such as work, school, the medical system, and the armed forces, and the effects these factors can have on the survivors' participation in them

External resources: The resources, such as insurance companies, legal systems, community services, legislators, the media, cancer support groups, and written materials, that are available, and any constraints associated with cancer survivorship that may affect utilization of them

The survivor's use of knowledge in day-to-day interactions may involve setting a symbolic personal watchbird on one's shoulder to impersonally, neutrally observe situations and the interaction of oneself and others as a basis for data collection and problem solving. Another useful cognitive strategy is identifying what the other person's problem is and not making it the survivor's problem or responsibility.

Skills

Both psychomotor and interpersonal skills are needed for successful survivorship. Psychomotor skills are needed by some survivors to manage changes in structure and function plus any treatment technology in daily living activities in the home, at work, and in social situations. Interpersonal skills are needed to manage relationships that are strained or unsatisfactory because of the survivor's history of cancer or because of changes in structure and functioning. Skills are also needed in learning to use systems in ways to overcome barriers linked to one's history of cancer.

Desires

The desire to survive, to overcome, and to achieve life goals is a major resource in this phase. It is an internal resource that may be tested on a recurrent basis by changes in one's body, emotional states, difficult requirements in daily living, stresses associated with the behavior of others, and inadequacy or inappropriateness of external resources. While optimism and goal-directed behavior have not been consistently found to affect duration of survival (Cassileth et al, 1988), they do seem to bring other rewards (e.g., fewer job difficulties) (Houts et al, 1986).

Courage

Courage is a prerequisite for managing daily living as a cancer survivor. It takes courage to risk losses in telling others of one's cancer history. It takes courage to face, understand, and seek to overcome discriminations in daily living. It takes courage to "come out of the closet" and openly join survivors' groups; to volunteer to help other cancer patients, families, and survivors; to seek redress for discriminations; or to work for changes in attitudes, laws, services, and systems for survivors. Being a cancer survivor is not a game for sissies.

Challenges to Families' Internal Resources

Family members and care givers too can experience discrimination in employment and social situations. They too have lost control over some areas of their daily living, relationships, peace of mind, and some external resources. Sometimes they experience irretrievable losses in relationships, and support— the cancer survivor is not the same spouse/partner, parent, or child who shared daily living prior to the cancer experience. Financial resources for daily living can be severely compromised. Surviving as a person who closely shares the daily living of the cancer survivor demands many of the same internal and external resources as those needed by the cancer survivor (Podrasky, 1986).

Nursing Diagnosis and Treatment

Nurses, like physicians, do not play a major role in the survival phase. However, because nurses often have shared the bleakest moments in the earlier phases, they as individuals or as an occupational group can hold a special place in the trust and feelings of the patient and the family. Thus, even though the number and duration of encounters in the survival phase is limited, perceptiveness and resourcefulness on the part of the nurse in diagnosing actual or potential cancer survival problems, in legitimizing their existence, and in offering expert, current knowledge of strategies or resources can make a significant contribution to quality of life for survivors and their families.

Diagnostic Targets

The primary target available to the nurse for diagnosis and treatment is the survivor. Occasionally the nurse will encounter a spouse, partner, or other family member as a patient, and the issues of living with a cancer survivor may become relevant. In some instances, nurses might diagnose and seek to treat employers, schools, or systems that are engaging in inappropriate behavior toward the survivor or family member.

Risk Factors

Cancer survivors at greatest risk for not managing the challenges of extended survival are those who (Lazarus and Folkman, 1984; Mages et al, 1981; Quigley, 1989):

Had premorbid tendencies toward depression, pessimism, and passivity

Had advanced cancers or aggressive, multimodality treatment with greater residual structural changes and dysfunction

Are unable to put the cancer diagnosis and treatment into the past

Lack a strong personal network with open communication patterns and at least one confidante with whom to process the experiences, feelings, and strategies for managing survivorship

Experience difficulty in entering or returning to the workplace, discrimination, or job "lock-in"

Experience difficulty in obtaining health insurance or affordable health insurance

Have difficulties in negotiating adjustments in role responsibilities and role relationships to accommodate survival goals and post-treatment functional status with spouse or partner, family members, social or work groups

Have an unsatisfying sexual component in daily living or unmet affectional needs

Diagnostic
Areas

PATIENT

Ineffective management of or dissatisfaction with work situation* related to (R/T):

Inability to get a job because of cancer history, visible structural sequelae of treatment, or limitations in functioning (specify)

Discomfort with behavior of co-workers associated with survivor's cancer history (specify the behavior)

Discriminatory loss of benefits, lack of promotion, physical placement in work environment

Inability to maintain desired trajectory on career goals

Difficulty in obtaining needed health, disability, or life insurance R/T cancer history

Lack of a satisfying social life R/T:

Failure to replace friends and companions lost in the cancer experience

Lack of confidence in entering social settings because of appearance (specify) or risks of dysfunction (specify)

* This diagnostic area may also apply to the care givers of cancer survivors (Hoffman, 1989).

An empty premorbid social pattern that now leaves too much time to think about the cancer experience and its implications for the future

Ongoing difficulties (specify) or dissatisfaction in interpersonal relationships (specify which family members, friends, or acquaintances) R/T:

Others' discomfort (specify nature of it—e.g., belief in cancer's contagion or cancer as a death sentence, revulsion at appearance or other aspects of survivor, unwillingness to accept survivor's new goals or priorities in daily living) and the resultant behavior (specify—e.g., avoidance, superficiality, avoidance of talking about the cancer experience or talking about it when the survivor prefers not to, oversolicitousness and overprotectiveness, seeking to control the survivor)

Survivor's ongoing discomfort with own appearance or fear of embarrassment should there be a loss of control (specify function)

Inadequate skill in speech alternative (e.g., esophageal speech or speech devices) following laryngectomy

Lack of courage or skill to engage in problem solving to change the situation or to manage it

Lack of capacity to avoid, ignore, or reframe interpersonal situations that do not respond to survivor's problem-solving efforts

Difficulties with interpersonal relationships involving sexuality R/T:

Feeling undesirable because of cancer sequelae or the cancer history

Lacking courage to take risks in encountering or relating to others where sexuality is a factor

Uncertainty about or lack of skills in informing the other person that one is a cancer survivor

Ongoing physical discomfort with intercourse

Physical inability to engage in intercourse and lack of development of satisfying alternatives

Uncertainty about whether to have children

Concern that a fetus may have chromosomal damage because of the cancer treatment

Dissatisfaction with self-concept following treatment R/T:

Exacerbation of low premorbid self-concept

Verbal and nonverbal cues from others that contribute to current low self-esteem

Inability to afford reconstructive surgery or prostheses to improve appearance

Personal reluctance or constraints by others to obtain treatment or prosthetics to improve appearance

Lack of skill in use of makeup or clothing to minimize post-treatment changes, or lack of money to purchase them

Ongoing depression

Failure of energy level or ventilatory capacity to return to premorbid states

Inadequate control of ileostomy, colostomy, or ureterostomy

Discomfort or lack of skill with esophageal or electric speech

Rumination or preoccupation with risk of recurrence R/T inability to put cancer in its place

Difficulties in managing activities, events, and demands in daily living (specify) R/T:

Deficits in strength, endurance, or functional abilities (specify)

Deficits in willingness to take risks as they emerge in daily living

Excessive time needed to manage ostomy care or other treatment regimens

Ongoing egocentricity or preoccupation with the cancer experience

Difficulties in setting goals and priorities

Difficulties in implementing new goals, priorities, and life directions (specify) R/T:

Setting of difficult or unrealistic goals

Setting too short a time for goal achievement

Failure to communicate goals adequately to family, friends, co-workers, employers who are affected by the survivor's change in behavior and expectations

Lack of vision in knowing how to initiate the changes in lifestyle

Limitations in capacity to break the long-term goals into intermediate and short-term goals

Lack of skill in translating general priorities into immediate ones (this encounter, this hour's tasks, this day)

Lack of current energy to implement changes in behavior and to interact with others as needed to accomplish revised life goals and priorities

FAMILY

Difficulties in negotiating with the survivor concerning resumption of roles and functions R/T:

Closed or dysfunctional (e.g., double bind, in which the support person is made to feel wrong no matter what his or her response is) communication patterns in the family

Resentment when the survivor fails to resume previous role functions (Vess et al, 1988)

Unwillingness to relinquish the survivor's former roles and responsibilities, which they assumed during earlier cancer phases (Vess et al, 1988)

Difficulties in adjusting to the changes (specify) of the survival phase R/T established ineffective communication patterns (Vess et al, 1985)

Dissatisfactions with quality of life R/T inability to set limits on survivor's demands for attention or other manipulative behavior (Vess et al, 1988)

Inability of family members to resume normal lifestyles and meet their own needs R/T feeling guilty if all energies are not focused on the cancer survivor

Difficulties in funding basic needs R/T:

Residual and ongoing costs of the cancer care

Loss of sources of income

Manifestations

PATIENT

Increased deficits in self-esteem, lack of assertiveness in meeting the challenges of survivorship, pessimism about the future, chronic dissatisfaction with the behavior of others

Preoccupation with somatic cues and the risks of cancer recurrence

Failure to set goals and priorities that give meaning to life as a cancer survivor

Difficulties in personal accommodation to the residual deficits in function and structural changes

Dissatisfaction with role relationships in the home situation—feeling used because others do not understand the difficulties being experienced, or the reverse—feeling no longer needed because the family has taken over former roles and is reluctant to relinquish them

Dissatisfaction with physical and verbal displays of affection by spouse, partner, family members, friends (specify)

Lack or loss of sense of sexual desirability

Dissatisfaction with relationships that have a sexual dimension, involving spouse, partner, or others the survivor encounters or dates

Worry about or resignation to inability to find employment in a field in which the survivor has training, expertise, or capability

Concern about fulfilling job requirements (specify) because of residual functional deficits (specify)

Perception of discrimination in the work setting or in obtaining health insurance

Perceived lack of success in resolving interpersonal difficulties with others where survivor's cancer history is a factor

Inability to avoid, ignore, or reframe the responses of those whose behavior creates tensions and stress

FAMILY

Failure to set goals and priorities that give meaning to life as family of a cancer survivor

Closed communication patterns, in which members are aware of feelings and problems but are unable to discuss them

Allocation of changes in roles and responsibilities by default rather than doing it explicitly

Self-neglect (physical and emotional) from feeling it necessary to continue to focus all attention and effort on the cancer survivor

Inability to set limits when the cancer survivor makes demands for family resources (attention, presence, assistance) that are in excess of actual need or seeks to create guilt if family does not acquiesce

Prognostic Variables

A good prognosis for being an effective survivor is associated with:

Having had a treatment outcome that ensures a long enough interval of symptom-free status to establish a desired lifestyle

Having minimal residual structural or functional problems (Quigley, 1989)

Recovering an adequate energy level

Not experiencing prolonged post-treatment depression

Expecting less difficulty in coping, having a large network of family and friends, not being satisfied with one's life (Cassileth et al, 1988)

Having had a relatively positive premorbid self-concept and developing strategies to regain it even when there may be significant sequelae to the cancer experience

Having open communication patterns (Quigley, 1989)

Being able to set, communicate, and implement satisfying post-treatment life goals and priorities

Having or learning effective problem-solving skills as well as skills in mobilizing, using, and maintaining needed external resources

Having access to support persons or groups, when needed, to process the demands and skills of survivorship

Not experiencing discrimination, or having the courage, skill, and external resources to modify it when it occurs

Having knowledge of community and organizational resources for cancer survivors and the skills to use that knowledge in meeting ongoing needs

Complications

Failure to manage survivorship effectively can result in a deteriorating quality of life, alienation, loneliness, fear and worry about how the present and future can be managed, financial concerns, decreased self-esteem, or inability to work or to work in a satisfying way.

Extreme dissatisfaction with quality of life as a survivor can in turn result in self-neglect, poor eating, substance abuse, loss of will to live, and possibly suicide.

Treatment Guidelines

GENERAL GUIDELINES

The reality of taking control in one's life as a cancer survivor involves a deliberate decision to do so. It also involves some initial thought about priorities and goals in life. What is it that the person wants to experience? to accomplish? What is important now that may not have been important before? What is less important or no longer important? What are the areas in which control will be relatively easy in terms of self, others, and situations? What are the areas in which control may be more difficult? Regaining control over daily living with the challenges of survivorship and possibly with altered internal and external resources can be a major task.

Some survivors may work through these basic issues in a support group or with a counselor. Some will talk them through with a friend or family member. Still others may address these issues and make plans without use of external resources. The nurse can be useful in the latter stages of treatment or during encounters in the post-treatment phase in introducing the issues and strategies for approaching life and daily living after cancer treatment.

In addition to the general themes of gaining control and building a sound foundation by thinking through goals and priorities, there are more specific contingency treatment guidelines. Nurses can consider these treatment options should they encounter survivors presenting with these problems and issues.

PATIENT   *Preoccupation with risks of cancer recurrence*

Legitimize the reality that every cancer survivor retains some concerns about cancer recurrence—this is natural; however overconcern can reduce the quality of life.

Gather data on:

Premorbid mental status (e.g., any depressions, natural optimism versus pessimism)

Experiences with others who have had cancer and how this might realistically or unrealistically affect their concerns

Patterns in daily living in terms of activities that can distract or occupy the mind versus those that permit too much time for rumination and self-centeredness

Indicate that there is a need to talk about the cancer experience until it "makes sense" (i.e., is integrated into one's self-concept). Offer strategies that others have used (e.g., talking about it in support groups, individually with other cancer survivors, with a confidante, or with a counsellor). Suggest that it is important to choose the listener(s) and negotiate for a "sounding board" type of interaction so that one does not alienate needed support persons with repeated telling of one's cancer experiences.

Where cancer prognosis is good, provide reality-based information about the recurrence rates.

Where past experiences with others' cancers are inappropriately affecting expectations, offer correct information that differentiates survivor's situation from that of the others.

Explore options for altering patterns of daily living to increase the activities that interfere with self-preoccupation (e.g., helping others).

Focus on the survivor's strengths, desired goals, and responsibilities without deprecating his concerns.

Ongoing low energy

Suggest that survivor keep a journal of times of day or situations when energy is higher and lower as a basis for planning activities.

Propose that the survivor make three lists: one of activities and demands (self and others) in daily living that have high priority, a second of low-priority activities and demands, and a third of activities or experiences that would meet personal goals and provide personal pleasure. Suggest that the survivor use these lists and the journal on patterns of energy to consider revisions in daily living schedules and patterns that could result in a satisfying quality of life. (See also Chapter 6, sections on Fatigue and Role.)

Self-concept interfering with quality of life

Suggest that the survivor consider what his self-concept was prior to the onset of cancer and what has changed; what may have caused the change; what the desired self-concept is.

Gather data on what cues the survivor is receiving from others that are affecting self-concept either positively or negatively.

Suggest some self-talk that may support a more positive self-concept, such as:

Focus on realistic strengths, and resources that are available and how to use them to achieve desired outcomes rather than on the deficits and how they impede quality of life.

Instead of seeing oneself as a burden, consider what one can realistically give to others to improve their quality of life (e.g., affection, freedom to pursue their own goals, positive feedback for assistance given, time to listen to them, plus physical activities as the survivor's capacities permit).

Consider how to make the most of this moment in terms of quality of life. (If this is a new approach to the survivor, give some examples and then ask for others).

Where feedback from others is undermining a desired self-concept, recommend strategies for dealing with these people. The survivor can:

Try to alter any unfounded biases by providing correct information about current status, cancer, the situation, etc.

Deliberately alter behavior in ways that send messages to others that will not support their perception (e.g., if their feedback is that the survivor is a negative, complaining co-worker, be matter-of-fact or even joke about a difficulty; if they want to dwell on the cancer experience, indicate that it is past history and that the present and future are more important)

Avoid the person who disrupts the survivor's self-concept

Reframe or reinterpret the feedback; see the other persons' problems as their own; refuse to make them the survivor's problems

Difficulties in handling sexuality in established relationships

Indicate that the problems of intimacy that emerged during the treatment and post-treatment phase may continue or abate. Be aware of timelines for risks of new sequelae and gather data on relationships with partner at times when these changes may be occurring.

Suggest that strategies of giving pleasure to the survivor or the partner may become unsatisfying or painful, so it is wise to maintain an openness and an attitude that changes that are desired or needed by either party are probable, normal, and legitimate. Indicate that setting norms in advance of openly talking about these in a caring way is important. (See also Chapter 6, section on Sexuality, under Diagnostic Areas and Treatment Guidelines.)

Indicate that meeting affectional needs can be at least as important as meeting needs of intimacy (Vess et al, 1988). Suggest that both survivor and partner deliberately build patterns of affectional verbal and physical behaviors into daily living, either in addition to activities of intimacy or in lieu of them, as appropriate to the situation.

Recommend discussing questions about childbearing or the chromosomal status of a fetus with a gynecologic oncologist or geneticist.

Difficulties in handling sexuality in new encounters

Acknowledge to survivor that new encounters with a sexual orientation may take more courage than before. Suggest that the survivor identify the personal risks perceived in new encounters and consider strategies for reducing them.

Explore with survivor the issue of if or when to tell a person one is getting to know that one is a cancer survivor. Indicate that one strategy is that of "testing the wind": On a first or second date mention having visited a friend who was recently treated for (insert the kind of cancer the survivor has had), then observe the other person's reaction. Based on the reaction, the survivor can make decisions about whether, when, or how to reveal the survivor's cancer history. Indicate that some survivors see their time as being too precious to waste on people who cannot accept cancer survivorship and its sequelae— "Who needs them!" was one breast cancer survivor's comment.

Difficulties in developing satisfying interpersonal relationships in extended survival

Indicate that other survivors have reported on the importance of having at least one confidante with whom to process fears, goals, strategies, and events in daily living—to help to put the tasks of survivorship into perspective and to test new ideas and strategies.

Suggest recording experiences and emotions in a journal or diary to find objectivity, to keep fears from recirculating or building up in one's head, and to show patterns of change that might not otherwise be noticed.

Suggest identifying individuals in the personal network with whom relationships are unsatisfying, and identifying what the survivor would prefer to modify in each person's behavior. Ask the survivor to consider the idea that one cannot change another person, but that one can change oneself and what one gives others to respond to; for example:

> If the other person is giving pity and tolerance, not acceptance, is it because the survivor is sending "poor me" cues? It may be useful for the survivor to deliberately use more positive scripts, such as, "my cancer is past history" or "I manage quite well if I can get help with. . . . "

> If the other person is physically distancing, is it because of misunderstanding about contagion? A pamphlet discussing the causes of cancer might create changed understanding and alter the person's behavior.

Where the survivor has been active in changing life goals and priorities, or anticipates doing so, point out that others haven't had the same cancer experience and don't know it can affect the survivor's view of life. Suggest communicating explicitly the new goals and priorities to those who share daily living and then negotiating as to how they could be implemented most comfortably with others. Suggest that the parties together consider what changes in role behaviors and relationships may result. Recommend doing this early, rather than after problems arise.

Where the survivor is uncomfortable with oversolicitude or protectiveness, suggest that the survivor:

> Offer clear guidelines on capacities and limitations in daily living

> Negotiate mutually acceptable, valued types of help

> Negotiate survivor's behavior for communicating desires for help or desires for freedom to function independently

> Negotiate helper's behavior in offering help or expressing concern

Indicate that not all difficulties in interpersonal relationships are resolved by problem solving and that contingency plans for dealing with the persons who have their own problems are important. The survivor can:

> Avoid the person or situation

> "Consider the source" and ignore the disturbing behavior

> Understand the underlying dynamics of the other person's disturbing behavior

Choose deliberately not to make the other person's problem his own

Deficits in social aspects of daily living

Suggest that the survivor identify any losses and gains in the social network that have occurred during the cancer experience to date, then consider how it may be possible to add new people to the network, or to interact with those still in the network in ways that satisfy the social needs.

Where there is loss of confidence in meeting others because of the cancer history, suggest joining a cancer support group, in which others share the cancer experience (e.g., CanSurmount, International Association of Laryngectomees, United Ostomy Association, Make Today Count, National Coalition of Cancer Survivors, support groups associated with local treatment centers). Have lists of options, contact persons, and phone numbers available.

Discouragement in searching for work

Provide information about the following resources to get help: American Cancer Society brochure #4585—"Cancer, Your Job, Insurance and the Law"; local governmental anti-discrimination bodies; Legal Aid Society; Vocational Rehabilitation Services (Goldberg and Habeck, 1982).

Do not overemphasize problems of getting a job to the point of causing fear or unwillingness to try. Suggest the importance of seeking a job that is within the survivor's functional capacity.

Suggest contacting vocational rehabilitation service.

Suggest use of local support groups or National Coalition for Cancer Survivorship members as possible links to job opportunities.

As survival time lengthens, indicate that some survivors no longer mention their cancer history in job applications.

Difficulties in dealing with the return to work

Suggest to the survivor that some co-workers will not know how to respond and thus will be uncomfortable and unskilled in their interactions. Affirm that it is legitimate for the survivor to have some uneasiness about the reception of co-workers as well; however, many fears never materialize or are rather quickly dissipated.

Suggest that planning some contingency scripts may increase comfort in returning to work; for example:

"I never knew it could feel so good to be back to work."[*]

"Work certainly helps in putting the cancer experience behind me."

"I don't expect to have too many difficulties with the job, but I might have difficulty with this (specify). Is it OK with you if I occasionally ask for help?"

"It's good of you, Sam, to have taken this over for me. I know how much work you have to do and I'd like to pull my weight on the job as much as I can. Let me see if I can't manage. I'll let you know if I have any problems and maybe we can work something out that won't interfere with your workload too much."

"There's nothing like having had cancer to teach you more than you ever wanted to know about it. When I started out I actually thought that cancer was contagious."

"One of the other patients I met told me that cancer did not confer sainthood on survivors, so I expect I'll be my usual cantankerous self on some days. Just bear with me as you always have and I'll do the same for you on your off days."

Suggest that the survivor determine what behavior of the coworker or family member is creating the discomfort in work-related situations, then think through or talk through with a confidante the options for altering the situation. (See also treatment guidelines for "self-concept interfering with quality of life," above.)

Knowledge deficit concerning seeking redress for discrimination in benefits, promotion, and other work-related factors

Suggest that the survivor can:

Check first with the local unit of the American Cancer Society or the local office on discrimination for local regulations and procedures applicable to a cancer survivor's situation

Negotiate first with the company

If no satisfaction is forthcoming, refer case to the grievance committee of a union or an office of the federal Equal Employment Opportunity Commission. Indicate that it is important to check on deadlines that have to be met for reporting and taking action on such complaints. (If the commission does not act in time, it may be necessary to pursue legal action as an individual).

---

[*] Note that these suggestions apply not only to returning to the workplace outside of the home, but also to returning to roles within the home.

Refer the survivor to the local chapter of the American Cancer Society for information about lawyers who specialize or have experience in such matters.

Difficulties in obtaining insurance

Alert young adults reaching an age when their parents' policies will not cover them of the need to seek their own coverage.

Point out that employment is seen to be the best means of obtaining group insurance; if this is not available, encourage survivor to look for open enrollment periods or to consider fraternal groups, alumni associations, or the American Association of Retired Persons (AARP) for insurance options.

Suggest that the survivor seek information on open enrollment periods that may have only limited periods of lack of coverage for pre-existing conditions (e.g., 3 to 6 months).

Indicate that current information on insurance possibilities can be obtained by contacting the state insurance commissioner or the National Insurance Consumer Organization, 121 North Payne Street, Alexandria, VA 22314. The local offices of the American Cancer Society or the National Coalition for Cancer Survivorship can also be resources. (See also section on Discrimination in Insurance Coverage earlier in this chapter.)

Point out the risks of "cancer insurance policies"—there are many limitations and loopholes in these policies.

FAMILY   ### Difficulties with allocation of roles

Alert patient or family member to the issues and problems families have reported facing during the extended survival phase (see section on Diagnostic Areas, under Family, earlier in this chapter).

Suggest that the family consider their normal communication patterns in problem resolution and determine if this serves them well. Indicate that research has shown that families that openly address issues, feelings about them, and options for resolution tend to manage survivorship more effectively.

Continued centering of family members' lives around the survivor

Indicate that one of the problems the survivor faces is fear of being a burden on others, and that an antidote to this is family members resuming some normalcy to their lives.

Suggest that the ongoing health and well-being of family members is important to the well-being of the survivor; therefore, it is important that they maintain physical and emotional health by meeting their own needs appropriately.

Difficulty in limiting survivor's demands on family members and survivor's efforts to produce guilt

Legitimize limit setting and help family members to develop scripts and strategies that set limits in kind but firm ways.

Suggest that the survivor's desire to make family members feel guilty is no reason for them to take on this feeling.

Suggest that they explicitly identify the behavior the survivor is using to manipulate the family in order to recognize it for what it is.

Indicate that it is not helpful if family members make the survivor's problem their problem—the two should be separated and dealt with separately.

Difficulties in funding basic needs

Refer to treatment site social worker or American Cancer Society for information on possible options for refinancing health care debt to permit funds for basic needs of family members.

EVALUATION

Responses of survivors, their spouse or partner, and families to the challenges of extended survival can be evaluated in terms of their reported status of:

Appreciation for life, and goal and priority setting

Sharing of life goals and priorities with those who are affected by any changes in them

Self-concept, body image, sexuality

Ability to put the cancer diagnosis and treatment phases in the past and to place risk of cancer recurrence in the background so that it does not regularly interfere with daily living

Satisfaction with roles and role relationships with spouse or partner, with other family members, and in social and employment situations

Satisfaction with and skills in negotiating role responsibilities in home, work, and social life to accommodate life goals, priorities, and functional capabilities

Satisfaction with work situation

Effectiveness in responding to behavior of others that is affected by survivor's cancer history—status of attempts to change the behavior or strategies of avoiding, ignoring, or reframing it to minimize it as a stressor

Gratification of needs for affection and intimacy

Effectiveness and comfort in incorporation of self-care regimens, prostheses, makeup, and clothing to accommodate post-treatment status into daily living

Satisfaction with quality of life

Bibliography

American Cancer Society. The cancer survivors' bill of rights. Cancer News 1988; Summer:15.

Belair RR. Privacy alert [sic] sensitive health information goes to third parties: you have "bundle of rights" to your medical record. NCCS Networker 1989;3(1):4.

Bergholz E. Under the shadow of cancer. New York Times Magazine, p 73. December 11, 1988.

Blattner WA, Hoover RN. Cancer in the immunosuppressed host. In: De Vita VT Jr, Hellman S, Rosenberg SA, eds. Cancer: principles and practice of oncology. 2nd ed. Philadelphia: JB Lippincott, 1985.

Blum RH, Blum DS. Psychosocial care of the cancer patient: guidelines for the physician. Journal of Psychosocial Oncology 1988;6:119.

Boivin JF, Hutchison GB, Lyden M et al. Second primary cancers following treatment of Hodgkin's disease. Journal of the National Cancer Institute 1984;72:233.

Bowden DH. Unraveling pulmonary fibrosis: the bleomycin model. Lab Invest 1984;50:487.

Brouwers P, Riccardi R, Poplack D, Fedio P. Attentional deficits in long-term survivors of childhood acute lymphoblastic leukemia (ALL). Journal of Clinical Neurophysiology 1984;6:325.

Cassileth BR, Walsh WP, Lusk EJ. Psychosocial correlates of cancer survival: a subsequent report 3 to 8 years after cancer diagnosis. J Clin Oncol 1988;6:1753.

Cella D. Psychosocial adjustment over time to the successful treatment of early versus late stage Hodgkin's disease in young adult men. Ph.D. thesis. Loyola University, 1983.

Cella D, Tross S. Psychological adjustment to survival from Hodgkin's disease. J Consult Clin Psychol 1986;54:616.

Cooper DR, Butterfield J. Pregnancy subsequent to mastectomy for cancer of the breast. Ann Surg 1970;171:429.

D'Angio GJ. Early and delayed complications of therapy. Cancer 1983;51:2515.

Davis-Spingarn N. NCI devotes nine percent of budget to survivorship research, but plans to move forward. NCCS Networker 1988;2(3):3.

Davis-Spingarn N. The new breed of survivors. Cancer News 1988a; Summer:13.

Fisher RM. A patient's perspective on the human side of cancer. Proceedings of the American Cancer Society Third National Conference on Human Values and Cancer. Washington, DC, April 23–25, 1981.

Flaherty M. For Mara. Nursing Mirror, February 26, 1981.

Fobair P, Hoppe RT, Bloom J et al. Psychosocial problems among survivors of Hodgkin's disease. J Clin Oncol 1986;4:805.

Goldberg RT, Habeck R. Vocational rehabilitation of cancer clients: review and implications for the future. Rehabilitation Counseling Bulletin 1982;26:18.

Greenberg RS, Rustin ED, Clark WS. Risk of genitourinary malignancies after prostate cancer. Cancer 1988;61:396.

Hassey KM. Pregnancy and parenthood after treatment for breast cancer. Oncology Nursing Forum 1988;15:439.

Heinrich RL, Coscarelli Schag C. The psychosocial impact of cancer: cancer patients and health controls. Journal of Psychosocial Oncology 1987;5:75.

Hoffman B. Advocacy update: two bills would expand survivors' job rights. NCCS Networker 1989;3(1):1.

Hoffman B. Cancer survivors at work: job problems and illegal discrimination. Oncology Nursing Forum 1989a;16:39.

Holmes T. Life situations, emotions, and disease. Psychosomatics 1978;19:754.

Holmes T, Masuda M. Life change and illness susceptibility. In: Scott JP, Senay EC, eds. Separation depression: proceedings of American Association for Advancement of Science Symposium. 1973;94:161.

Holmes TH, Rahe RH. The social readjustment scale. J Psychosom Res 1968;11:213.

Houts PS, Lipton A, Harvey H, Martin B. Characteristics of persons who report negative work experiences following a diagnosis of cancer. Paper presented at the National Forum on Comprehensive Cancer Rehabilitation and its Vocational Implications. Williamsburg, VA. November, 1980.

Houts PS, Yasko JM, Kahn B et al. Unmet psychological needs of persons with cancer in Pennsylvania. Cancer 1986;58:2355.

Hunter R. Insurance for survivors? Difficult, tricky, not impossible. NCCS Networker 1988;2(3):5.

Kagan AR, Kagan JD. The quality of which life? Am J Clin Oncol 1983;6:117.

Kemeny MM, Wellisch DK, Schain WS. Psychosocial outcome in a randomized surgical trial for treatment of primary breast cancer. Cancer 1988;62:1231.

Koocher GP, O'Malley JE. The Damocles syndrome: psychosocial consequences of surviving childhood cancer. New York: McGraw-Hill, 1981.

Lansky SB, List MA, Ritter-Sterr C. Psychosocial consequences of cure. Cancer 1986;58(suppl):529.

Lazarus R, Folkman S. Situation factors influencing appraisal: person factors influencing appraisal. In: Lazarus R, Folkman S, eds. Coping and appraisal. New York: Springer, 1984.

Leiber L, Plumb M, Gertstenzang M, Holland J. The communication of affection between cancer patients and their spouses. Psychosom Med 1976;38:379.

Mack RM. Lessons from living with cancer. N Engl J Med 1984;311:1640.

Mages N, Castro J, Fobair P et al. Patterns of psychosocial response to cancer: can effective adaptation be predicted? Int J Radiat Oncol Biol Phys 1981;7:385.

Meadows AT, Krejmas NL, Belasco JB. The medical cost of cure: sequelae in survivors of childhood cancer. In: van Eys J, Sullivan M, eds. Status of the curability of childhood cancers. New York: Raven Press, 1980.

Mellette SJ. The cancer patient at work. CA 1985;35:360.

Mellette SJ. The semantics of cancer and disability. In: Proceedings of the Workshop on Employment, Insurance and the Patient with Cancer. New Orleans, American Cancer Society, 1986.

Mellette SJ, Franco PC. Psychosocial barriers to employment of cancer survivors. Journal of Psychosocial Oncology 1987;5:97.

Muggia FM, Louie AC, Sikic BI. Pulmonary toxicity of antitumor agents. Cancer Treat Rev 1983;10:221.

Mullan F. Seasons of survival: reflections of a physician with cancer. N Engl J Med 1985;315:270.

Mulvihill JJ, Byrne J. Genetic counseling of the cancer survivor. Seminars in Oncology Nursing 1989;5:29.

Myers MH, Gloeckler Ries LA. Cancer patient survival rates: SEER program results for 10 years of follow-up. CA 1989;39:21.

Ochs JJ, Berger P, Brecher ML et al. Computed tomography brain scans in children with acute lymphocytic leukemia receiving methotrexate alone as central nervous system prophylaxis. Cancer 1980;45:2274.

Peters MV. The effect of pregnancy in breast cancer. In: Forest APM, Kunkler PB, eds. Prognostic factors in breast cancer. Baltimore: Williams & Wilkins, 1968.

Podrasky PA. The family perspective of the cured patient. Cancer 1986;58:522.

Quigley K. The adult cancer survivor: psychosocial consequences of cure. Seminars in Oncology Nursing 1989;5:63.

Shanfield SB. On surviving cancer: psychological considerations. Compr Psychiatry 1980;21:128.

Silverberg E, Lubera JA. Cancer statistics, 1989. CA 1989;39:3.

Staley JC, Kagle JD, Hatfield AK. Cancer patients and their co-workers: a study. Soc Work in Health Care 1987;13:101.

Taylor S. Ten issues that cancer patients have to teach. Surviving: A Cancer Patient Newsletter. Department of Radiology, Stanford University Medical Center, 1988; Jan-Feb:2.

Trillin AS. Of dragons and garden peas: a cancer patient talks to doctors. N Engl J Med 1981;304:699.

Tross S, Holland JC, Bosl G, Geller N. A controlled study of psychosocial sequelae in cured survivors of testicular neoplasms (Abstract C-287). Proceedings of the American Society of Clinical Oncologists 1984;25:74.

Tucker MA, Coleman CN, Cox RS et al. Risk of second cancers after treatment for Hodgkin's disease. N Engl J Med 1988;318:76.

Vess JD, Moreland JR, Schwebel AI. An empirical assessment of effects of cancer on family role functioning. Journal of Psychosocial Oncology 1985;3:1.

Vess JD, Moreland JR, Schwebel AI, Krant E. Psychosocial needs of cancer patients: learning from patients and their spouses. Journal of Psychosocial Oncology 1988;6:31.

Wickham R. Pulmonary toxicity secondary to cancer treatment. Oncology Nursing Forum 1986;13:69.

9

Living With Cancer's Recurrence

Cancer recurrence is the crisis feared by any person who has had an initial remission or experienced years of survival after treatment for cancer. The onset of persistent fatigue or anorexia or the appearance of suspicious symptoms can trigger a resurgence of fear of recurrence. The physician's report of an abnormal blood count or other findings can bring an abrupt end to the relative security of the survival phase.

Some individuals find the recurrence less traumatic than the original diagnosis. These tend to be people with localized tumors and few symptoms, or those who were "waiting for the other shoe to drop"—who never let themselves believe that they were free of the disease (Weisman and Worden, 1985–1986; Worden, 1989). The greater proportion of people find that recurrence is more traumatic.

Occasionally, survivors who experience a recurrence receive treatment and again remain in remission for extended periods. Or, with low-grade superficial skin cancers, recurrences may be expected and nonthreatening. For most survivors, however, recurrence represents the shift from cancer as an acute, cured disease to one that has become chronic, one that will be ultimately fatal unless another fatal pathology intervenes. Recurrence thus can represent a greater crisis than the original diagnosis (Chekryn, 1984).

The chronic phase of the cancer may be very short or may extend for years. Its progression may assume a variety of patterns, as shown in Figure 9-1. Figure 9-1A shows a rapid, steady decline in functioning from recurrence to death. Figure 9-1B shows cancer as a chronic disease, with treatment creating long plateaus of functional stability that may last from months to years; however, with each relapse functional status is lower than before. Figure 9-1C illustrates a pattern of more frequent relapses and shorter remissions. In this pattern the treatment causes serious loss of functioning; the patient survives, but at a lower level of functional capacity.

Treatment has now extended life expectancy in many cancer survivors even as the neoplastic process continues. However, given the life threat associated with the presence of cancer, many patients and families continue to see it in terms of cure or death, rather than as a chronic disease with remissions and exacerbations. For these people,

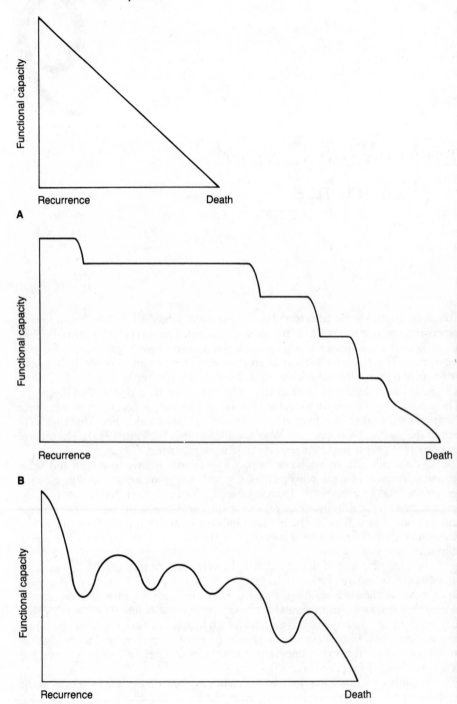

Figure 9-1. *Patterns of progressive dysfunction with cancer recurrence.*

each remission represents an opportunity for hope that the cancer has again been cured and each renewal of neoplastic activity is an occasion for despair. For patients and families who are unable to accept cancer as a partially controlled chronic disease, life in the recurrence phase becomes a roller coaster ride between repeated highs of hope and lows of despair. Others, at least intellectually, accept the chronicity of their cancer and the current limitations of medical therapy. They hope for the best possible outcomes of their therapy, but remain aware of the constraints (Vess et al, 1988).

Life in the recurrence phase involves elements of each of the preceding phases as well as the next phase, that of advancing disease.* The patient and family have the memories of their previous cancer experiences as they again participate in diagnostic activities, give informed consent to treatment or choose not to undergo further treatment, and, if treatment is chosen, go through additional treatment and post-treatment adjustments. The challenges of the survival phase can still be present in their daily lives.

With recurrence there are two significant differences from the original diagnosis and treatment. The patient and family are familiar with many of the experiences; this may bring either greater confidence in participating or greater dread. Second, the initial treatment was usually infused with hope of a cure. With recurrence, hope is either tempered by realistic knowledge of prognosis or inordinately buoyed up by the defense of denial. The emotional climate as well as the internal and external resources for managing the requirements of daily living in the recurrence phase can be quite altered from those that shaped responses in the initial cancer experiences. The patient and family tend to know what support systems are needed and available, but resources may be attenuated by the earlier demands of the prior phases of the cancer experience.

Medical Perspective

The medical focus when cancer recurs is to determine whether the recurrence is local, regional, or distantly metastasized and to accurately locate the lesions (Kupchella and Burton 1987). Surgery is not as widely used in recurrence. It may be used to palliate or prevent problems (e.g., removing a local or single metastatic lesion, relieving an obstruction, preventing a pathologic fracture in a weight-bearing bone). More often radiation, chemotherapy, and hormone therapy are used to shrink tumors, relieve symptoms, and produce remissions.

The medical task of providing accurate information about risks, benefits, and quality of life during and after treatment of recurrence is probably even more important to the patient's and family's decision making now than it was in the initial treatment (Houts et al, 1984). Patients and families now truly must balance predicted duration of life associated with different treatment options against the physical, emotional, and monetary costs and the quality of life offered by each. There is a physician responsibility to balance hope with reality, to assure patients that their current decisions regarding treatment are not irrevocable, and that continuity of physician care and support will be provided (Blum and Blum, 1988).

At some point during recurrence the physician is faced with the task of indicating

---

* This chapter will deal with recurrence only in terms of its crises and the special decision making and adaptations it requires. The reader is referred to earlier chapters for problems associated with new diagnostic tests, treatment of the recurrence, post-treatment aspects, and ongoing survival issues, and to the next chapter for daily living problems and dysfunctions associated with advancing disease and dying.

that there is no more treatment of the neoplastic process that can offer any benefit. The patient hears such statements as, "There is nothing more we can do for you"; "We can't give you any more radiation or chemotherapy"; or "You have failed the treatment." Patients and families often lose faith in orthodox medicine at this point, and seek hope through unproven alternative treatments. Physicians are then faced with the task of dealing with patient decisions that they believe can cause the patient and family needless expense and possible bodily harm (Cassileth and Browne, 1988; Jarvis, 1986). Physicians are urged to bring up the subject of alternative treatment, since patients may be afraid or unwilling to do so, but also to discourage its use by providing a technical critique, and, finally, to express willingness to continue to provide needed care even if the patient and family reject their advice (Blum and Blum, 1988).

Philosophies can vary among physicians (and nurses) about the aggressiveness with which recurrent cancer should be treated. For some, cancer is an enemy to be battled aggressively as long as possible. Others look to quality of life and situational factors as well as control of the neoplastic processes. Given this variability, there is a possibility of incongruence between the physician's goals and those of the patient and family. Because of the life-threatening nature of the situation and the dependence of the patient on the physician for symptom control, seeking a good and comfortable fit between the physician and the patient and family can be important. In most health care situations it is possible to find an oncologist or other physician whose philosophy of treatment fits comfortably with that of the patient.

Nursing Perspective

The nursing perspective in recurrence is somewhat similar to that of the initial diagnostic stage. Many of the daily living tasks of the recurrence phase are comparable to those in the diagnostic phase; however, some of the variables that affect patient and family participation are not.

Tasks of Daily Living in the Recurrence Phase

As in the diagnostic phase, there are specific tasks in daily living to be accomplished. These include:

Development of strategies for coping with waiting for tests and test results

Management of uncertainty, anger, self-protective behavior, and anticipatory grieving as these affect decision making and participation in daily living

Assimilation of the diagnosis of recurrence with local, regional, or distant metastatic spread and recognition of the aggressiveness of the tumor, with understanding of the implications this knowledge has for treatment options, living with chronic disease, survival time, and quality of life

Management of daily living in the presence of emerging signs and symptoms

Decision making about courses of action to take as this is affected by:

The capacity to take in and process information

Memories of previous treatment experiences

The treatment philosophy of the physician

Patient and family goals and priorities

Societal values and sanctioning forces

Decision making about sharing the information of the recurrence and its implications

Managing the crisis of the recurrence and remission patterns within family relationships and with resources that may already have been altered by the earlier cancer experience

Factors Making the Tasks in the Recurrence Phase Different

The nursing perspective is influenced by two major factors that can affect the patient's and family's approach to the crisis of recurrence. First, for most, recurrence represents a greater threat than the initial diagnosis because of its implications for an ultimately poor prognosis. A second variable that makes the recurrence experience different from the initial diagnosis is that the patient and family have already experienced and managed some variant of the diagnostic and treatment phases of the cancer experience. It would be inappropriate for nurses to stereotype patient responses based on either of these variables. However, they are important factors to assess and consider in terms of diagnosis and treatment of patient and family functioning and daily living during the recurrence phase.

Nature of Living With Cancer Recurrence and Underlying Mechanisms

Several common themes emerge in the responses of patients and families to the experience of cancer recurrence. Many patients and families genuinely expected a cure or were led to expect cure or remission (e.g., by the surgeon's remark after the operation, 'It looks like we got it all"). They are then surprised, shocked, and angry to learn that the earlier treatment was not successful. They may feel that it is unjust that they are being assaulted again after having gone through the previous cancer experience. There is a resurgence of uncertainty and fear about the future, about survival, and about the family's well-being. Denial is not a strong strategy (Weisman and Worden, 1985–1986). There may be the response of grieving (crying, self-preoccupation, and agitation) or passive acceptance; but conversely, there can also be an approach of hope, rational confrontation, and a readiness to take action (Chekryn, 1984; Weisman, 1979).

Changing Goals

During the initial treatment phase and during uneventful extended survival, the goal has been living with cured cancer or with cancer in remission. With recurrence, that valued goal is no longer possible. Circumstances have changed, and the new goal in daily living is control of a progressive chronic disease for as long as possible or desirable. This loss of a significant goal in life is likely to be accompanied by a grieving process, with features of anger, sadness, a feeling of betrayal, and energy loss. Some patients and families continue to expect and work for the goal of cure. Many other patients and families are able to replace the goal of cure with other goals more compatible with their altered health situation, such as living effectively with long-term chronic disease or making the remaining time available to them as rewarding and effective as possible.

Changing the Timeframe and Energy for Goals in Daily Living

Two other phenomena occur in the recurrence phase. These involve the change in the timeframe of personal goals in daily living and the vigor with which they are pursued.

When there is hope, patients and families believe in their goals and put their heart and energy into pursuing them. With the betrayal of recurrence and subsequent relapses, belief collapses. Patients and families say, "It takes everything out of you." Hope and vigor are replaced by sadness and loss of physical and emotional energy.

For many patients, long-term planning is replaced by shorter-term goals. Goals may also have a tentative, "if it's possible" quality. Given the capricious course of many cancers (Slaby, 1988), there is a need to balance the needs of the todays with the uncertainties of the tomorrows (Mack, 1984). Eventually, most patients and families tend to live with day-to-day goals; however, there are others who never make the adjustment. In some parts of the recurrence phase it becomes difficult to predict the patient's health status beyond a very short period; thus goals are set and adjustments are made on an ongoing basis, depending on the functional health status of the patient at that particular time. For some there is new attention to making each moment and each day count in small but important ways.

The Emotional Roller Coaster

As was shown in Figure 9-1, the patterns of remission and relapse in the neoplastic process can vary remarkably. For some the diagnosis of recurrence is followed rapidly by end-stage disease and death. Many other patients experience again the assaults of the therapy, with all its discomforts and difficulties, followed by periods of relative well-being (Schmale, 1976; Scott et al, 1983).

The Lazarus Syndrome

Where the therapy creates life-threatening situations followed by remarkable recoveries, the patient and the family both experience the Lazarus syndrome (from the Biblical story of Lazarus being returned to life after death). The anticipatory grieving begins as death and separation seem inevitable, then the patient recovers and the grieving process is interrupted. These patterns of preparing emotionally for separations, beginning to separate, and then having to reestablish bonding can be devastating to patients and families. They know that eventually the disease will create the ultimate separation of death, yet the need for genuine affection and emotional support continues.

The personal adjustments involved in preparation for separation and then in reestablishment of relationships take time. These intensely emotion-laden transition periods create vulnerability for both patient and family members as they individually or together struggle to integrate and manage the experiences in the light of:

Their beliefs and values about their responsibilities for caring

Their capacities for providing that caring

The other demands and priorities in daily living

The realities in the situation

Feelings of anger, resentment, frustration, and guilt are not uncommon. The emotional roller coaster pattern may be made easier if the participants can learn before they actually experience it about the tasks of separation and reestablishment of relationships in the recurrence phase, the realistic time periods needed to make these transitions, and the genuine difficulty of reversing one's orientation in terms of separation versus return. Both patient and family members will still experience the pain and difficulties involved, but it may bring comfort to know that what they are experiencing and the ways in which they are responding are shared by many others—that these are legitimate, expected responses in the situation.

Fear of Abandonment

One of the fears that accompanies recurrence is the fear of being abandoned by support persons. Nurses have noticed that some physicians tend to be less involved and spend less time with patients for whom medical treatment of the neoplastic processes is no longer effective. Their documentation becomes more cryptic, and is limited to basic signs and symptoms. Patients fear any deterioration in the physician's concern and support for them. They also fear emotional and physical distancing of their family members and care givers should the burdens of their signs and symptoms, prognosis, and care become greater or more prolonged than others can manage. Patients often realize that life goes on for others and that the course of the cancer will prevent their being a part of it.

Testing the Support System

Patients who are uncertain or uncomfortable with dependency on others for understanding and support may engage in testing behavior that alienates others. The behavior often assaults the significant other in a vulnerable spot, somewhat like kicking a post in a weak-looking spot to see that it will hold before leaning on it (Gates, 1988). Emotions such as anger, rage, fear, and helplessness that the patient cannot bear alone are transferred to the other person through *double bind* communication. This is a pattern of communication in which the support person is made to feel wrong no matter what the response is. For example, if the support person acts concerned about the patient's symptoms or difficulties, the patient becomes upset because the behavior is seen as oversolicitous or smothering. On the other hand, if the person then backs off and does not seem as concerned, the patient complains of neglect, of being unloved, or an unwanted burden. It can be very difficult to recognize this behavior as the request for help it is rather than as an assault (Gates, 1988). Unless the dynamics of the communication pattern can be understood by both parties, distancing tends to occur and the abandonment the patient feared can become a reality.

Vulnerability of Health Care Providers

Health care providers too are in a different situation during the recurrence phase Patients and families lose confidence in the health care system and particularly in the physicians (Blum and Blum, 1988; Cassileth and Browne, 1988). Physicians may fee more frustrated and vulnerable in their efforts to help the patient (Hersh, 1982). At a time when patients and families are struggling with their own needs for security they may sense a tentativeness in support from physicians when the goals of care shift from cure to seeking to restrain neoplastic growth or to palliate.

On the other hand, because recurrence presents ever greater challenges to the management of daily living, nurses become increasingly involved with management o symptoms and with assisting in the control of requirements in daily living. Diagnosing and treating the emotional and physical challenges of daily living in the recurrence phase requires special expertise, perceptiveness, and stamina among nursing clinicians

Decisions About Treatment

With cancer recurrence comes a new demand to consider the medical treatment options available for trying to manage the neoplastic activity. No longer is the choice for cure or death, but for some degree of neoplastic control or palliation in a chronic disease Sometimes treatment is a way of keeping fear at bay.

Previous Experience as a Factor

One might predict that because patients with recurrence have had previous experi ence with the cancer and have previously given "informed consent" for treatment they would be more knowledgeable about the disease and its treatment when it recurs. Studie have shown that many "experienced" cancer patients are not more knowledgeable than others about the disease and treatment (Heinrich and Coscarelli Schag, 1987; Taylor e al, 1984). Theories to explain this lack of knowledge propose that:

> Not knowing or not remembering information serves an adaptive purpose by which the patien can focus on nondisease-related issues and manage daily living more effectively (Heinrich and Coscarelli Schag, 1987)

> Retaining illness-related information as a coping skill has no adaptive value (Taylor et al, 1984

> Controlling information one chooses to acknowledge is the least effective method of managing aversive events, especially when the outcome cannot be controlled (Thompson, 1981)

Thus it is not appropriate to presume that the patient or family has acquired o retained knowledge on which to base decisions. They have, however, had experience with varying forms of treatment, and these may influence their decisions about choosing to experience them again.

The shock of the diagnosis of recurrence may have the same "shut down" effect on the capacity to take in information as did the original diagnosis (see Chapter 5).

Relationship With the Physician as a Factor

The patient's and family's relationship with the physician can also be a factor in making treatment decisions in the recurrence phase. Anger at and loss of confidence in the medical profession due to failure to control the disease during initial treatment ma lead to mistrust of recommendations for another round of treatments. Differences in values between the physician and the patient about giving priority to treating the neoplasms versus focusing on maintaining symptom control and quality of life can be another factor compounding the difficulties in negotiating mutually satisfactory treatment decisions. Physician responses to patient choices of no treatment or use of unorthodox treatment can further shape the relationships and decision making. The patient's and family's vulnerability, given the prognosis and ultimate dependency on the medical profession for symptom control, may make them reluctant to be assertive in promoting their own wishes and goals in cancer treatment; they may fear medical abandonment if they disagree with the physician. Given all these factors, the decision making about treatment in the recurrence phase would seem to be more complex than in initial treatment.

Societal Values

Societal and religious group values can be forces that shape patient or family decisions about treatment when cure is no longer possible. These values vary more widely at the beginning of the 1990s than they did in the past, with strong emotions in both extremes. Some groups value maintaining life under all circumstances, and vigorously sanction any behavior that would shorten it. Other groups, such as the Hemlock Society, believe in the right of terminally ill persons to choose the time and manner of their death (Saunders and Valente, 1988). Surveys show that members of society are considering quality of life as a factor and are more accepting of the person's right to control conditions that lead to death (Droogas et al, 1982; Engelhardt, 1986).

In recent years the concept of rational suicide has evolved. This involves a self-inflicted, self-intended death by a person who has clear mental processes not impaired by psychologic illness or severe emotional distress, and who recognizes the consequences of the act (Saunders and Valente, 1988; Siegel and Turkel, 1984). Some members of society, and even of the patient's health care team, might interpret a decision not to engage in further treatment to control the neoplasm as a form of rational suicide, since the action may hasten death.

The societal values that weigh most heavily on the patient or family can influence the decision about participating in further treatment. They can also affect the emotional consequences of the decision. For instance, the patient who rejects treatment may feel guilt if this is viewed as a form of suicide, and the patient who participates in treatment may feel guilt if significant others promote unorthodox forms of therapy or see the acceptance of medical treatment as a violation of religious beliefs and faith. Families too can have mixed emotions over supporting further treatment or ceasing therapy.

Incongruence in Values and Goals

There may be greater occasion for incongruence and conflict between the values of the patient, the family, and health care providers when the treatment goal is no longer cure. For example, the patient may wish to have no further treatment, the family may have unfinished business and be unwilling to let the disease take its course, and the physician may be one who sees cancer and death as the enemy to be held at bay as long as possible. Or, the patient may value extending life as long as possible, while the family may have other priorities for expenditure of family resources. Sometimes families have not recovered financially from the costs of initial treatment, and the costs of ongoing treatment may create despair. Long held, basic values as well as values associated with the requirements and allocation of family resources for present daily living can play an important role in decision making about treatment of recurrent cancer. These values may exert an influence of their own, independent of the concrete elements of the decision having to do with the responsiveness of the tumor cells to treatment and the availability of treatment options.

Decisions About Discontinuing Tumor-Control Treatment

As the recurrence phase progresses and neoplastic processes are inexorably advancing, eventually decisions have to be made to shift efforts from control of the cancer to control of the symptoms. There may come a time when the decision will involve whether to continue medical palliative treatments that are not only making the person somewhat more functional and comfortable, but are maintaining life (e.g., travelling 50 miles to the clinic for blood product transfusions three times per week). Some patients, families, and physicians fight death to the very last moment. Others make (and remake) the decision to discontinue treatment fairly early in the recurrence phase.

With the decision to discontinue cancer control-oriented therapy may come a basic change in the perspective from which daily living is viewed. Ideally, the perspective shifts from setting goals and priorities associated with living with the chronic condition of recurrent cancer to setting goals and priorities associated with living with dying. The focus is no longer on controlling the disease process, but on symptom control and achieving the goals and priorities of one's life on a day-to-day basis and for the life span that remains. This can involve putting one's business, monetary, and legal matters in order; resolving unfinished family business; preparing spouse and children to manage in the patient's absence; sorting through memories and mementos and sharing them with others; accomplishing goals that had been previously postponed; enjoying pleasures that had previously been given lower priority; and so on. Many patients and families undertake the task of finding meaning in the experience of living with and dying of cancer. On the other hand, some patients are not able to engage in any of these transitional tasks and leave their affairs untended.

Nursing Diagnosis and Treatment

This chapter has focused on one dimension of the recurrence phase—accommodation to the experience of the cancer's reappearance and the implications of recurrence for the patient and others who are closely involved. However, life does not divide itself so distinctly. Dealing with the tasks of incorporating recurrence into daily living presents some particular issues and problems; these are addressed separately in this chapter. Thus, nursing diagnoses and treatment from this chapter may stand alone. However, they may accompany *or be integrated with* diagnoses and treatment plans from other chapters, because in recurrence the patient may once again experience problems associated with daily living in the diagnostic, treatment, and post-treatment phases, and continue to face the ongoing challenges of the survival phase. Where the disease is advanced, the diagnoses and treatment covered in Chapter 10 should also be considered.

New variables will affect the patient and family as they move into the recurrence ɔhase. Diagnoses and treatment developed in the earlier phases should be modified to ɲcorporate the variables associated with response to recurrence. Additionally, diagɲoses and treatment plans may be more transient, as they are adjusted to accommodate ɭuctuations in patient and family perceptions and behavior in this transition phase.

Diagnostic Targets	The patient and family are primary targets for diagnosis and treatment. However, the doctor and other health providers may also need to be diagnosed when their philosophy of care or behavior prevents the patient and family from dealing with recurrence according to their own values, goals, and needs.
Risk Factors	Individuals who are likely to have difficulty in coping with recurrence include those who (Worden, 1989):

Believed that they were cured and thus feel surprised and betrayed at the reappearance of the disease

Have rapidly advancing disease and disability

Have difficulty in dealing with cancer as a chronic disease with opportunities for but also constraints on its control

Blame self or others for the return of the cancer

Suffer from preexisting mental health problems, such as alcoholism, are depressed, or are pessimistic

Live alone or lack a functioning supportive family and personal network

Use double bind communication patterns to test the genuineness of significant others' willingness to share the experience of recurrence (Gates, 1988)

Lack trust and confidence in the physician and health care system

Have poor coping skills and tend to repeat ineffective behaviors

Have concurrent problems (financial, work, family)

Lack religious affiliations

Are preoccupied and concerned about dying and death

Diagnostic Areas

PATIENT

Impaired capacities for managing roles, tasks, and decision making in daily living related to (R/T):

Acute grieving over loss of "cured" status

Persistent depression, hopelessness, and helplessness, leading to (L/T) apathy, withdrawal from roles and responsibilities, and inability to make decisions

Loss of emotional and physical support from key significant others (e.g., spouse, children, physician, nurses) R/T incongruence in goals, priorities, or choices about treatment

Fear of abandonment by health care personnel R/T decision to accept only palliative treatment, no treatment, or unproven alternative treatment

Vacillation between unrealistic hope and deep despair R/T unrealistic expectations about treatment's effectiveness in controlling the cancer and cancer as a chronic disease

Dissatisfaction with relationships with others (specify) R/T:

Limited ability to make life goals and priorities known and accepted by others

Inability to negotiate satisfactory role relationships

Sensing that others are beginning to engage in separation or distancing behavior

Demands on others that exceed or impair their capacity to respond

Use of disguised, indirect, or double bind communication patterns instead of direct, open ones in expressing feelings or needs

Difficulties in making informed decisions about medical treatment of recurrence R/T:

Being in the denial stage of grieving

Intellectual "shut down"

Inability to understand the nature of the pathology and the treatment options

Conflicting goals between patient, physician, and family

Wanting to undertake alternative treatments that are physiologically harmful or use up restricted financial resources

Fear of alienating and subsequently being abandoned by physician if physician's preferred treatment is not accepted

Choice of physiologically harmful or financially draining alternative treatment methods R/T:

Continuing belief that the cancer is curable

Fear of dying

Inability to integrate the prognosis into self-concept and the future

Search for a more supportive environment

FAMILY

Emotional separation from the patient R/T:

Difficulties in managing the separations and reestablishment of relationships associated with patient relapses and improvement (Lazarus syndrome)

Inability to accept patient's life goals and priorities

Resentment, anger, or guilt over the priorities in expenditure of family energy, time, or money R/T demands of cancer as a chronic disease

Dissatisfaction with patient's attitude or behavior R/T family member's denial of prognosis or the difficulties the patient is experiencing

Ineffectiveness in handling patient's testing and double bind communication R/T lack of understanding that it reflects the intensity of the patient's anger and helplessness, L/T progressive distancing (Gates, 1988)

Dissatisfaction with role responsibilities and relationships R/T:

Patient's variable functional capacities for or interest in taking on essential tasks and roles in day-to-day living

Unwillingness or inability of patient or family members to establish norms and strategies for ongoing negotiations about needs, tasks, and role relationships

Manifestations

PATIENT

See Chapter 5 for patient and family manifestations associated with the diagnosis of recurrence of the cancer.

Manifestations that the patient is not meeting the challenges of daily life effectively include reported or observed:

Fear, anger, or denial of cancer's return

Blaming of self or others for cancer's recurrence

Inability to participate in decision making about treatment options

Concern about financing of continued health care

Prolonged hopelessness or helplessness

Withdrawal from roles and responsibilities even when physical capacity to carry them out is present

Anger at or dissatisfaction with physician or other health care providers

Inability to accept or understand the nature of pathology involved in recurrence and the goals of treatment

Inability to accept cancer as a chronic disease with constraints on treatment's effectiveness

Setting of goals for treatment or health care that are incompatible with the treatment philosophy of the physician and other health care providers

Discomfort with differences in desires for treatment between patient and family members

Dissatisfaction with treatment recommended by physician

Participation in harmful alternative treatments

Discomfort with dependence on health care system and family, and fear of abandonment

Vulnerability to the influence of other individuals or groups not directly involved with treatment decisions who seek to promote their own beliefs or wishes to the patient

Difficulty in altering life goals to make them compatible with chronic disease or limited life span

Difficulties in negotiating roles and relationships with family (see also Chapter 6, sections on Role and Sexuality, under Manifestations)

Use of disguised, attacking, or double bind communication with significant others in expressing feelings or needs

Feelings of loneliness and alienation from others

Lack of a confidante or support group with whom to share the experiences of recurrence

Making of excessive or inappropriate demands on family members or care givers, or use of manipulative behavior to gain compliance

FAMILY

Manifestations of the family's ineffective management of daily living with recurrence of cancer include reported or observed:

Fear, anger, or denial at cancer's recurrence

Blame of patient or others for cancer's recurrence

Dissatisfaction with the patient's treatment goals, or with physician's recommendations

Resentment, anger, or guilt over prolongation of expenditure of family resources on patient's health situation

Inability to set limits on patient's demands

Inability to interpret patient's disguised requests for help and understanding

Distancing from patient

Physical and emotional fatigue

Absence of any effective respite

Lack of one or more confidantes or of a usable support group

Ineffective negotiations to manage tasks and role relationships in daily living between patient and other family members

Prognostic Variables

A good prognosis for coping with daily living effectively during the experience of recurrence is associated with:

Limited duration of denial of the significance of the recurrence ("impact denial") (Worden, 1989)

Functional capacities (e.g., energy, cognition, freedom from severe symptoms) that permit participation in addressing the tasks of daily living with recurrence

Presence of a functional support system and comfortable effective communication patterns for the patient and family

Congruence in treatment philosophy and goals between physician and patient (and family)

Adequacy of financial, health insurance, and other external resources

Absence of blaming self or others for recurrence

Possession of effective coping or problem-solving skills

Capacity to set goals and priorities that deal with a noncure situation

Complications

Failure to effectively manage grief work over the loss of cure as a goal, failure to make satisfactory decisions about treatment, and lack of maintenance of relationships with family and care givers can result in a greater sense of loneliness and fear of abandonment as the disease progresses, less physical well-being, a shortened life span, and suicide.

Treatment Guidelines†

Disrupted functioning R/T acute or prolonged grieving over cancer recurrence

Gather data on onset of grief reaction, response to initial cancer diagnosis, and any history of premorbid depression.

Where there is history of chronic affective disorders or prolonged dysfunctional grieving after the initial cancer diagnosis, check with physician for possible medication or referral for therapy.

Where the acute grief reaction is in response to the diagnosis of recurrence:

Listen, if patient or family wants to talk about the experience and what is happening. If circumstances do not permit dis-

---

† Many of the treatment guidelines are applicable to family members as well as patients.

cussion with the nurse, suggest that there is comfort in talking about the concerns and the feelings being experienced with someone who is a good listener. Suggest that the patient or family member can set the tone of the interaction with a guideline such as, "I need someone to talk to about what is happening, not so much for advice or even sympathy—but just a caring listener."

Legitimize the symptoms and dysfunction being experienced. Point out that grief is an uncomfortable but common response to the stress and that it tends to moderate within a period of a few weeks.

Suggest that it may help for the patient to accept the body's temporary responses to the stress and delay or adjust activities or decisions until the initial acute reaction has moderated.

Discuss strategies for making family (or others involved) aware of the need for accommodation—or perhaps mutual accommodation—in daily living to manage the tasks and relationships in the face of each person's grief-related dysfunctions.

Difficulties in making treatment decisions

Gather data on:

The patient's knowledge of the cancer, its previous treatment, and any expectations about treatment for recurrence. (Don't presume knowledge or expertise based on past experience or informed consent.)

Experiences associated with past treatment that may affect attitudes toward treatment options with the recurrence

Important goals and priorities at this point

Interest in and information about alternative forms of treatment

See Chapter 5 under Treatment Guidelines for management of informed choice with problems of denial, "shut down," inability to understand pathology and treatment options, and fear of abandonment.

Help the patient to look at contingencies (e.g., If you choose this, what will you do?; If this happens, what will you do?; or What is the worst that can happen if you. . . . ? What is the best that can happen if you. . . . ?).

When the patient shows definite interest in or is actually engaged in alternative therapy:

Maintain a neutral attitude

Offer concerns about the burdens of the treatment, the risks and the benefits

Conflict in physician and patient philosophies on treatment of recurrence

If the patient has difficulty in negotiating with the physician, provide the physician with nursing data on patient's goals and wishes in treatment. Determine physician's comfort with them. Suggest to the patient strategies for negotiating treatment decisions.

If there seem to be irreconcilable differences, indicate to the patient that individual physicians differ in their approaches to treatment of recurrences and that a second opinion is quite ethical. If asked, provide the names of several physicians whose known philosophy of treatment is congruent with patient goals.

Conflict in nurse and patient philosophies on approaches to health care with recurrence

Interact with the patient to determine the information and important values used in arriving at health care decisions. Look for gaps in information, misinformation, and values or goals that shaped the decisions. (Learning about how the patient reached the decisions may enable the nurse to more comfortably and therapeutically provide care within this framework).

Engage in self-examination to determine your commitment to meeting the patient's needs and wishes despite philosophical differences. Ask yourself, If I were this patient, what would I want and need from the nurses?

Where one or more nurses who provide care to the patient are creating added stress because they disapprove of patient or family decisions, if possible, reassign the patient to nurses who can offer nursing care in a genuinely nonjudgmental manner. If staffing does not permit reassignment, initiate nursing conferences to explore and prescribe options for therapeutic interaction between the patient and the nursing staff, despite their differences.

Incongruence of patient and family wishes regarding treatment

Gather data on the positions of the patient and family members regarding issues in the family situation that relate to treatment decisions. (Note that there may be hidden agendas such as unfinished personal business with the patient; desire to allocate family resources of time, energy, caring, and money to other members of the family or other goals; difficulty in tolerating prolongation of the uncertainty of the course of the disease, and so on.)

Identify personal and family beliefs that strongly influence a choice for or against further therapy (e.g., medical treatment shows an insufficient faith in God; one must use all of the technology that is available in the fight for life; declining treatment is a form of suicide and suicide is a sin; the cancer is a form of punishment for earlier sins and therefore must be endured; a cure may be found if we hang on long enough).

Where underlying issues or problems can be addressed separately, so that they need not be covert influences on the decision about treatment, help the participants to consider this possibility. (See treatment of "unfinished personal business" in Chapter 11, section on Separations.) Suggest that they not permit other people's problems with the situation to become the patient's or family's problem.

Dissatisfactions with roles and role relationships

Identify roles and relationships in which patient or family members have concerns.

Legitimize these concerns and comment on their wisdom in trying to deal with them rather than allowing them to develop.

Listen for complaints from patient (e.g., "They just don't understand") or significant others (e.g., "No matter what I do it's always wrong"). This may represent an inability of the patient to communicate intense feelings of anger about the situation or testing of the caring of significant others. Ask the patient about concerns (do not use the word "problems") and feelings. Ask if and how these feelings are shared with others. Explore strategies for being more direct in talking about them.

> *With significant others*, talk about how everyone tests support systems, but cancer patients do so more than others. To explain the patient's attacking behavior, use the analogy of kicking the post where it looks weakest before leaning on it. Indicate that it is easier to share physical difficulties than emotional ones, so seeking support for emotional difficulties may take an indirect approach. Suggest that they try to translate attacking or double bind communications into requests for help. Indicate that it is often best to return to normal give-and-take in relationships rather than to be too nice or too understanding, since unreleased anger will emerge in passive ways or result in distancing (Gates, 1988).

Point out that in recurrence, both the patient's and family's physical and emotional resources for managing roles and relationships can vary, so it is important to expect variability, negotiate as needed, and keep options open.

See also Chapter 6, sections on Role and Sexuality, under Treatment Guidelines.

Discomfort with emotional or physical distancing of significant others

Indicate that:

> Feeling alone and isolated in one's situation is a frequent occurrence for both patients and family members when cancer recurs

Communication about uncertainty and loneliness is difficult, so the cues may be given in disguised form (e.g., an angry "You don't love me anymore" may really mean, "I am worried that you don't care about me now that my cancer has come back")

Worry can either bring people closer together or isolate them

Help patient and significant others to develop scripts for communicating experiences, feelings, and needs more directly and for helping the other person to do so

Fear of abandonment by health care providers if the recommended treatment is not accepted

Suggest that the patient and family maintain contact with the family physician as well as the oncologist and that they share their concerns about continuity of care and symptom management.

Indicate that they may wish to express their concern about loss of continuity of treatment and symptom management to the physician.

Unrealistic expectations about control of the cancer

Gather data about the patient's (and family's) expectations about the pattern the cancer and treatment may take.

If the expectations are unrealistic, provide information in a nonthreatening way, using the patient's or family member's own words to explain treatment goals and the patterns the cancer tends to take (e.g., "When a tumor comes back it is more like a chronic condition, particularly now, when we have treatment available to give some control. It is somewhat the way we treat heart disease. The treatments don't make either of the diseases go away completely, but they do help to manage them, often very well").

Helplessness

Ask the patient (or family member, if this is the person who is experiencing the symptoms) to identify specific, concrete areas of concern (not "problems"), and issues in daily living that he or she worries about.

Model breaking the problems into smaller, manageable areas and together brainstorm options for managing them. Include "dumb" suggestions as well as practical ones. For example: the mother doesn't have enough energy to keep the living room neat. Options: hire a maid; live in fewer rooms; make a family agreement that each person must pick up or put away anything he takes out or else clean the whole room; pick up and clean during hours when energy is highest; assign tasks on a rotating basis to each member of the family; schedule a "clean the house" date and plan a treat when the work is done, etc. Suggest that the patient or the patient and family brainstorm strategies for managing difficulties as they occur (Worden, 1986).

Point out to the patient that gaining a sense of control in some areas of one's life helps one to live with other areas that are less open to control; thus, actively taking control, even in small, concrete areas is a health-promoting behavior.

Hopelessness

When patient communication begins to reflect a transition in the focus of hope and goals, assist with the redefinition by using strategies of paraphrasing and clarification. (Note that the patient may wish to do this in private in order to protect loved ones.)

Help the patient to clarify goals and the shifts being made in hopes and goals (Dufault and Martocchio, 1985).

Where needed, support the validity and achievability of new goals and help in identifying strategies for achievement of the new goals.

Difficulty in managing the Lazarus syndrome

Prepare family members (and if appropriate, the patient) for the strains that relapse and remissions place on the relationships between family members and the patient (Schmale, 1976; Scott et al, 1983). Indicate that preparing for separation from a loved one when life is threatened and then reestablishing the bonds as recovery occurs is a difficult, painful task that is not instantaneous, but requires time. Help participants to become aware that individuals may make adjustments at a different pace, so that they may be "out of sync" with each other in their adjustments and therefore in their needs.

Indicate the importance of expressions and gestures of affection to both patient and family members during these times of stress.

Legitimize feelings that may produce guilt in family members. If the care giver or family member wishes that the patient could die and that everyone could be released from this suffering, the nurse might respond, "Sometimes loving and caring is wishing that the loved one would not have to suffer any more." If the family member says that he can't tolerate the situation any longer, the nurse might respond, "Do your feelings make you want to leave?" If the person the patient is depending on actually moves to leave the patient, the nurse may use a somewhat confrontational strategy, such as, "When do you think that you might be back?" or "What do you want me to tell _____ (the patient)?"

Suggest that talking about the situation to a confidante may lend perspective to the experience and facilitate acceptance of the associated discomforts.

Where the patient is having difficulty adjusting goals from living with dying to living with remission again, indicate that this is difficult and requires some time. Help the patient to understand that family members are sharing these transitions and that the depth of their caring is reflected in the difficulties they too have. Suggest that sharing their individual difficulties may make the burdens easier for each one to bear.

Evaluation   Evaluation of patient and family response to the experience of recurrence may be made in terms of the status of:

Adaptation to knowledge of recurrence, its prognosis, and implications

Capacity to engage in informed decision making regarding treatment

Adaptation to altered life goals and priorities

Satisfaction with decision making and relationships with physician

Adaptation to trajectory of disease in recurrence (e.g., remission–relapses, downward trajectory)

Effectiveness of and satisfaction with communication patterns and relationships with family and other support persons

Adequacy of external resources (e.g., health insurance, finances, support network, housing, transportation) to manage costs and requirements in daily living in the recurrence phase

Bibliography

Blum RH, Blum DS. Psychosocial care of the cancer patient: guidelines for the physician. Journal of Psychosocial Oncology 1988;6:119.

Cassileth BR, Browne H. Unorthodox cancer medicine. In: Psychosocial issues and cancer. New York: American Cancer Society, 1988.

Chekryn J. Cancer recurrence: personal meaning, communication, and marital adjustment. Cancer Nurs 1984;7:491.

Droogas A, Siller R, O'Connell AN. Effects of personal and situational factors on attitudes toward suicide. Omega 1982;13:127.

DuFault K, Martocchio BC. Hope: its spheres and dimensions. Nurs Clin North Am 1985;20:379.

Engelhardt HT. Suicide and the cancer patient. CA 1986;36:106.

Gates CC. The "most significant-other" in the care of the breast cancer patient. In: Psychosocial issues and cancer. New York: American Cancer Society, 1988.

Heinrich RL, Coscarelli Schag C. The psychosocial impact of cancer: cancer patients and healthy controls. Journal of Psychosocial Oncology 1987;5:75.

Hersh SP. Psychosocial aspects of patients with cancer. In: DeVita VT, Hellman S, Rosenberg SA, eds. Cancer: principles and practice of oncology. Philadelphia: JB Lippincott, 1982:264.

Houts PS, Lipton A, Harvey HA et al. Nonmedical costs to patients and their families associated with outpatient chemotherapy. Cancer 1984;53:2388.

Jarvis W. Helping your patients deal with questionable cancer treatments. CA 1986;36:293.

Upchella CE, Burton RM. Cellular biology of cancer. In: Groenwald SL, ed. Cancer nursing: principles and practices. Monterey, CA, Jones & Bartlett, 1987.

Mack RM. Lessons from living with cancer. N Engl J Med 1984;311:1640.

Saunders JM, Valente SM. Cancer and suicide. Oncology Nursing Forum 1988;15:575.

Schmale AH. Psychological reactions to recurrences, metastases, or disseminated cancers. Int J Radiat Oncol Biol Phys 1976;1:515.

Scott DW, Goode WL, Arlin ZZ. The psychodynamics of multiple remissions in a patient with acute nonlymphoblastic leukemia. Cancer Nurs 1983;6:201.

Siegel K, Turkel P. Rational suicide and the terminally ill cancer patient. Omega 1984;15:263.

Slaby AE. Cancer's impact on care givers. Adv Psychosom Med 1988;18:135.

Taylor SE, Lichtman RR, Wood JV. Attributions, beliefs about control and adjustment to breast cancer. J Pers Soc Psychol 1984;46:489.

Thompson SC. A complex response to a simple question: will it hurt less if I can control it? Psychol Bull 1981;90:89.

Vess JD, Moreland JR, Schwebel AI, Kraut E. Psychosocial needs of cancer patients: learning from patients and their spouses. Journal of Psychosocial Oncology 1988;6:31.

Weisman A. Coping with cancer. New York: McGraw-Hill, 1979.

Weisman AD, Worden JW. The emotional impact of recurrent cancer. Journal of Psychosocial Oncology 1985–86;3:5.

Worden W. Cognitive therapy with cancer patients. In: Freeman A, Greenwood V, eds. Cognitive therapy: applications in psychiatric and medical settings. New York: Human Sciences Press, 1986.

Worden W. Coping with cancer: psychosocial interventions for health care professionals: A cognitive–behavioral approach. Presented at the American Cancer Society, Washington Division Workshop, Seattle, WA, April 28, 1989.

10

Living With Advancing Disease

Advanced cancers are those neoplastic processes that have metastasized and/or are no longer fully controlled by antineoplastic treatment. They produce increasing symptoms and dysfunctions. Palliation rather than cure becomes the focus of medical treatment. In this chapter, advancing cancer will be considered in terms of some of the common problems associated with its progressive encroachment on the patterns of daily living and functional capacities of patients, their families, and care givers to manage the changing requirements of daily living.

Many of the phenomena described in earlier chapters will be addressed again in this chapter. However, these same phenomena develop different features when cancer has become a chronic or end-stage disease:

Anorexia	can become	cachexia
Fatigue	becomes	asthenia
Intermittent pain	can become	unremitting, progressive moderate to severe pain
Time-limited nausea and vomiting	can become	gradual inability to retain any food or fluids
Episodes of dyspnea	can become	longer, more severe dyspneic episodes with shortening intervals of "normal" breathing
Temporary changes in cognition or level of consciousness	can become	confusion, or progressive decline in level of consciousness to stupor and coma
Hope of cure	changes to	a growing understanding of the inability of med eradicate the ca control of symp achievement of pleasurable exp living

Not only are the symptoms more progressive, but they usually occur in combinations whose interaction augments dysfunction and distress. Further, the patient's growing dependence on family members and care givers alters their daily living and taxes their functional capacities. Thus, the diagnosis and treatment of significant family members and care givers becomes crucial.

In this chapter, the *differences* in the nature of the phenomena and underlying mechanisms associated with the chronic stage of cancer as compared to the initial treatment stage serve as the foundation and basis for nursing diagnosis and management of altered capacities and challenges in daily living.* Common major phenomena occurring in this phase of the cancer experience will be addressed in separate sections, since each has a distinct knowledge base and affects daily living and functional capacities in particular ways. However, in the actual patient situation, the clinician is urged to look at:

The cumulative effects of the multiple phenomena on daily living

The ways in which dysfunction from any given phenomenon will affect another and alter functional capacities (e.g., asthenia affects mobility, skin integrity, self-care, socializing, eating, drinking, and toileting patterns; nausea and vomiting affect pain and limit routes for analgesia; the stage of grieving over losses of function, lifestyle, and separations affects participation in daily living and any treatment activities)

Nursing diagnoses and treatment plans should reflect an integration of knowledge about the way in which individual phenomena are occurring and interacting in the patient's situation. They also will incorporate the combined impact on the patient's or family's capacities to manage daily living.

Daily living during the terminal phase of the cancer experience presents other challenges for both the patient and the family. These include issues surrounding the role of the dying person, symptom progression, monotony in daily living, separations, unfinished business, knowledge deficits about dying and death, and powerlessness.

Living With Asthenia

Fatigue is a common symptom associated with cancer and its treatment (see Chapter 6, section on Fatigue). However, with advancing cancer it takes on a new more dysfunctional dimension, *asthenia.* Here serious mental and physical fatigue are compounded by generalized progressive weakness (Bruera and MacDonald, 1988). This condition occurs in more than two thirds of patients with advanced cancer. Asthenia increasingly erodes the patient's capacity for independence and self-care in daily living and creates concomitant problems that affect both patient and care giver well-being.

Medical Perspective

The cause of asthenia for most cancer patients is unknown. However, physicians do seek to diagnose and treat possible etiologic factors such as infections, anemia, metabolic abnormalities, malnutrition, drug or treatment side-effects, depression, and the cancer

---

recognized that cancer may have reached the advanced stage at the point of initial diagnosis, and that *treatment may be palliative from the beginning for some patients.

itself. Where the cancer itself seems to be a major factor, corticosteroids have been found to bring some improvement for about 3 weeks. The amphetamine methylphenidate hydrochloride (Ritalin hydrochloride) offers some patients improvement in activity and has an antagonizing effect on the side-effects of narcotics (Bruera and MacDonald, 1988).

Nursing Perspective

The nursing perspective addresses issues in daily living associated with helping patients and families to maintain effective daily living for all participants while tailoring daily living requirements to match decreasing physical and mental strength and endurance. One goal is to maintain the dignity and self-worth of patients as they become more dependent by planning for pleasurable experiences and achievement of patient goals even as strength and endurance deteriorate. Another is to maintain the physical and emotional well-being of those who are providing the care and maintaining the home environment. A third goal is to maintain positive relationships between patient and family or care givers in a situation in which many strains are common.

Nature of Asthenia

The fatigue and weakness occurring in the asthenia syndrome are thought to be the result of structural and functional abnormalities in the muscles. The condition is a multicausal syndrome; however, a substance or group of substances produced by the neoplastic processes is a probable factor (Theologides, 1986).

Asthenia does not exist in isolation, but is usually one of a constellation of symptoms (e.g., pain, nausea, anorexia, sleep disruption), each one contributing to the other and eroding the patient's physical, cognitive, and emotional functional capacities. Each patient's symptom complex must be considered as a gestalt in providing nursing care to the patient and family in a presenting situation. However, each separate symptom affects particular dimensions of daily living and functioning and requires specific consideration before the nurse can integrate it into the whole of the care plan. Thus, asthenia will be considered as a distinct phenomenon in this section.

Asthenia as a Message to the Patient and Family

The incidence and progression of asthenia provide undeniable evidence to the patient and family of the progression of the cancer, though some patients seek to ignore the signals and plan ahead for their lives as if they could function as before. For most patients the fatigue and weakness will not only disrupt physical and cognitive aspects of daily living, eventually involving the most basic of activities (e.g., turning in bed, having a bowel movement, planning, speaking), but will also create further discouragement and despair.

During initial treatment there is hope that treatment will relieve the tumor-related fatigue and that iatrogenic fatigue will dissipate upon the completion of treatment. In advancing disease the patient may hope that tomorrow will be better, but aside from remissions, the long-term outlook is for a downward trajectory. This difference in perspective affects the associated issues in daily living.

Areas in Daily Living Affected by Asthenia

The presence and progression of asthenia in the presenting situation of the patient with advanced cancer and the family create certain issues that need to be addressed. They will need to develop strategies to:

Prioritize and manage requirements of daily living with progressively less capacity for self-care by the patient

Meet the patient's physical, cognitive, and emotional needs

Recruit support persons to supplement or take over tasks the patient is no longer capable of doing

Anticipate or address problems associated with the patient's transition to dependence and the changing role relationships between patient, family members, care givers, and any others who are affected

Assure that patient and family members recognize their individual and collective goals and incorporate them into the planning and prioritization of daily living, so that even when energy levels are extremely low some goal-related pleasurable experiences continue to be provided for each of the participants on a regular basis

Give attention to care givers' physical and emotional problems that are associated with managing additional burdens over the full course of the patient's illness

Underlying Mechanisms

Pathophysiologic Factors

In advancing cancer the pathophysiology of asthenia is still a dilemma. Concomitant disorders such as anemia, infections, metabolic disturbances, drugs, radiation, and depression can contribute to it, and patients are improved when these conditions are successfully treated. However, the presence of the cancer seems to be a principal factor (Theologides, 1986). Malnutrition has been shown to produce a major loss in muscle mass that contributes to weakness; however, at present, there is no subjective improvement in asthenia with nutritional treatment (Bruera and MacDonald, 1988). People with advanced cancer, even when nutrition is not seemingly disrupted, can experience muscle abnormalities (Theologides, 1986; Wesdorp, Krause, Von Myenfeldt, 1983). Muscle changes involve atrophy of type II muscle fibers (Warmolts et al, 1975) decreased maximal strength, decreased relaxation velocity, and increased muscle fatigue in involuntary muscles (Bruera et al, 1987); and increased production of lactic acid (Holroyde et al, 1979).

Cachexia

One concomitant condition in many advancing cancers is the phenomenon of cachexia. Normally, the body acts to conserve energy when caloric intake is reduced, and an increased desire for food accompanies increased energy expenditure. Thus, a balance is maintained within a narrow range (Kaempfer and Lindsey, 1986). In cachexia a paradox arises, wherein increased energy requirements in the body are accompanied by a loss of the normal urge to take in more food (De Wys, 1982; Lindsey, 1986; Morrison, 1976). Even nutritional support may not relieve the resultant body wasting (Bruera and MacDonald, 1988b).

Pathology-Based Increased Demands for Energy

Beyond the basic increase in energy expenditure seemingly associated with the neoplastic processes (Buera et al, 1987; Bruera and MacDonald, 1988a; Norton and Brennan, 1980; Theologides, 1982), other concurrent conditions may also increase the demands on the person's energy resources. Some of these conditions include dyspnea, coughing, fever, insomnia, diarrhea, urinary frequency, vomiting, pain, and hiccups.

Daily Living Factors

Most elements of daily living, including activities, events, accommodating to demands of self, others, and possessions, accommodating to barriers in the environment, and even implementing one's beliefs and values, require expenditure of energy or are affected by energy level. As fatigue and weakness increase, the activities, events, and demands are initially trimmed, the living environment is modified to accommodate, and priorities are revised and pared down.

Eventually, the patient is no longer able to manage daily living without the physical assistance of others. The demands on self and others change, and role relationships are altered, sometimes even reversed (e.g., the dependent child may become the care giver, the homemaker may have to become both breadwinner and homemaker, the authority figure may become subject to others' authority). In addition to role reversals, there is often role expansion on the part of family members and care givers as they take on tasks that they have never assumed before and may fear or prefer not to undertake now. There is high potential for role incompetence, role strains, and role conflict for the patient and those who share the daily living.

Values and beliefs can be subtle but significant factors in the adjusting of daily living to accommodate the decline in the patient's self-care capacities and the assumption of responsibilities by others. Values and beliefs may determine who is expected to assume responsibility for the care; typically the care givers are the patient's spouse (Stetz, 1989), partner or housemate, children—particularly daughters or daughters-in-law (Brody, 1981, 1985), or sisters. Earlier family experiences can shape values that affect relationships between care giver and patient, such as when the patient was an abusing parent and the abused child is now the care giver (Copstead and Patterson, 1986). Family beliefs about providing care to the patient will affect both their behavior and emotional responses as the patient's strength and endurance decline. These beliefs may involve the assignment of family resources and priorities (e.g., placing greater priority on meeting the needs of the younger generation and sacrificing the needs of the older member of the family), the definition of caring, and placement of obligation for providing patient care.

Another area for value consideration involves activities or experiences the patient enjoys. By carefully considering valued activities and experiences it is possible to determine which must be abandoned, but also which can be preserved, and strategies for continuing them as long as possible (Billings, 1985). It is important for the primary care giver to engage in these same evaluations and for equal consideration to be given to this person's need for regular pleasurable experiences.

Functional Health Status

**Strength,
Endurance,
and
Cognition**

Asthenia affects internal resources of physical strength and endurance. Grooming and care of the immediate environment may deteriorate as bathing, shampooing, and laundry become too much of an effort. Shopping may become more difficult. Eventually, the patient may find it takes too much energy even to prepare meals, and so resort to snacking on convenience foods. As the asthenia progresses, cognition is affected and the patient becomes less able to plan for energy-saving strategies (e.g., doing two or three things that need to be done in the kitchen on one trip, or placing needed objects within easy reach). If going to the bathroom is seen as difficult, fluids may be restricted to minimize the number of trips. As strength and endurance wane further, speech may be affected. The patient becomes more quiet, and uses energy-sparing scanning speech patterns, omitting nonessential words, using half sentences, and shifting rapidly from one subject to another (e.g., "need tissues... forgot to let dog out") (Molbo, 1986).

Patterns in fatigue and weakness may vary. Patients may experience a sudden unexpected onset of incapacitating exhaustion that may take hours or days to abate (Molbo, 1986). Such experiences may make patients reluctant to leave home for fear of experiencing an attack and being unable to get help in returning home. Sudden exhaustion may also make them unable to manage basic activities in daily living because needed assistance may not be available.

It is also critical to take into consideration the strength and endurance of the primary care givers. This is particularly true where the care giver is an older person, or one who also has physical or emotional health problems. Even though they may be motivated to provide the patient's care, they may not have the capacity to provide the assistance the patient needs. It is not unusual to see primary care providers neglect their own health in order to care for the patient.

**Knowledge and
Skill**

Several areas of knowledge and skill are involved in managing daily living with progressive fatigue and weakness. These involve energy conservation strategies, accurate interpretation of communications involved in helping relationships, and recruitment and maintenance of support systems.

An important area of both knowledge and skill involves energy conservation strategies tailored to the specific daily living situation and environment of the patient *and care givers* (e.g., grouping tasks, allocating physical activities to periods of higher energy in the day or doing them on "good days," and planning rest periods). Approaches to nutrition also can have an impact on the physical and emotional energy of patient and care giver.

Associated energy conservation skills may involve developing schedules that accommodate energy constraints, providing energy-sparing physical assistance in moving or in treatments, making the living environment more compact and convenient, and mobilizing resources that permit genuine respite for the care giver on a predictable basis.

A commonly encountered problem that creates a nontherapeutic climate and unnecessary demands on physical and emotional energy is the daily conflict between care giver and patient about eating. Urging food on the unintentionally anorexic patient may create distress and energy demands for both parties and do nothing to improve the patient's nutritional and physiologic status (Billings, 1985).

Knowledge of available external resources in the social network and community and the skill to utilize them is also important to patient and family. One skill that can be legitimized and learned is that of communicating specifically when seeking assistance from others (e.g., "It is so nice of you to offer to help. What we really need at this point is some of your famous chicken vegetable soup in one-cup servings that we can keep in the freezer" or "I need to set up an appointment with the dentist. Would you be willing to stay with Fred for 2 hours if I show you what care he will need?")

To maintain optimum functioning between the dependent patient and those who provide care over the weeks and months of the illness, it is important to know what communication patterns are used by each and what difficulties each party is experiencing as the patient's asthenia and dependency progresses (e.g., the patient who is angry about being dependent may disguise requests for assistance so that accurate interpretation is difficult, or the care giver may wait to be asked to give assistance for fear of intruding on the patient). While understanding the dynamics of the behavior may not reduce the discomforts the patient and family experience, it may legitimize these experiences and feelings and help to put them into perspective. The associated skills will involve accurate interpretation of the dynamics underlying another person's behavior, values clarification, role negotiations, setting limits, and engaging in behavior to achieve role competence and comfort.

Burnout

Burnout is a high-risk condition among those who share the daily living of advanced cancer patients, not only the family and personal care givers, but professional health care personnel as well (Slaby, 1988). The lack of control, uncertainty about course of events, constant physical and emotional demands in the situation, and inadequate opportunities to replenish one's resources create a situation in which burnout can occur. When it does occur, the individual or family experiences physical and emotional depletion, caring changes to apathy, involvement changes to distancing, and the person becomes self-protective, feels helplessness and hopelessness, and has a less positive self-concept and a negative outlook (Pines et al, 1981; Slaby, 1988). If it is feasible to moderate the demands in daily living that lead to burnout and to provide adequate support, it may be possible to prevent, delay, or minimize burnout among care givers and thus provide the patient with a more functional support system.

Mood

The patient's asthenia, particularly when it is associated with cachexia, correlates with depression. The patient may become apathetic, dysphoric, and more socially isolated (Noyes and Kathol, 1986). In turn, these patient moods may make it more difficult for care givers to participate in the patient's care comfortably and effectively.

Uncertainty, anticipatory grieving, the Lazarus syndrome, and role strains or conflicts can affect the moods of family members and care givers. Those who are closest to the patient and who care the most are most likely to be affected. In turn, family moods can affect the well-being of the patient (Leahey and Wright, 1987). Living with progressive life-threatening disease tends to cause each participant to become increasingly sensitive to the moods of others. Setting norms and strategies for regularly sharing what is happening may make these experiences easier to bear.

Desire and Courage

With the asthenia, it becomes increasingly difficult for the patient to initiate plans and activities. There may not be enough energy to think of activities or accept invitations, much less recruit and negotiate for needed assistance. Daily living can eventually become a plodding, circumscribed existence with too much time for solitary reflection (Billings, 1985; Molbo, 1986). Becoming tired from a pleasurable activity can be worthwhile, and getting assistance in mobilizing the special equipment needed to make excursions possible can be seen as challenge, not a deterrent (Billings, 1985).

Families and care givers too may face deficits in motivation as the patient's needs for care require an increasing investment of the family's resources. Uncertainty about what is to come, including the duration of the demands, can drain motivation. The previous history of the relationship and background characteristics will also have an effect (Copstead and Patterson, 1986; Stetz, 1989). Positive, caring relationships and open communications may result in a continuation of this pattern in the present situation, while unresolved difficulties or dysfunctional communication can make for ongoing uncomfortable and difficult care giving and receiving.

Courage to try new approaches, to face up to encounters, or to arrange for participation in events by either the patient or the family member may wane as the period of care giving lengthens. Courage may also be required to seek assistance from others if this is a new experience for the patient or care givers.

External Resources

External support for the patient and family is crucial to their well-being when progressive asthenia is occurring. External resources that can make a difference in daily living include:

Personal networks that can be counted on to provide respite and encouragement, to serve as a sounding board, and to bring variety to the days

Services and supplies in the community that are available to the patient and family to improve mobility, safety, convenience, and comfort (e.g., equipment for loan from the American Cancer Society)

Financial resources to purchase services and buy or rent equipment to reduce energy requirements and increase safety as the patient becomes weaker

Available, usable transportation for both patient and family members to accomplish routine tasks in daily living, have an outing or attend an event, or travel to the clinic or hospital

Communication devices to increase the sense of security for both patient and family and to bring others closer (e.g., telephone, intercom, linkages to a local hospital)

Nursing Diagnosis and Treatment

Where the presenting problems of the patient with advanced cancer include asthenia, nursing diagnosis and treatment must focus on both the patient and care givers as parts of an interactive system. The environment and external resources, as these affect energy expenditure and morale, are also critical elements for consideration.

It is rare for asthenia to exist in isolation. Other symptoms coexist and compound the difficulties. In the end the individual patient and care giver diagnoses may best integrate the problems; however, it is important to maintain an awareness of critical issues of daily living and functioning associated with the asthenia itself.

Diagnostic Targets

The patient, care givers, those who share daily living, and those who are affected by the patient's eroding energy (including pets) are targets for nursing diagnosis.

Risk Factors

PATIENT

Risk factors that affect the capacity to manage the requirements of daily living include:

The severity and progression of asthenia

Presence of other energy-demanding symptoms (e.g., coughing, hiccuping, vomiting, pain, muscle cramps, dyspnea, or diarrhea or urinary frequency, which make frequent trips to the bathroom or commode necessary)

Being depressed

Living alone

Having inconsistent, unpredictable care providers and personal support network

Lack of funds to purchase services

Inconvenient shopping facilities

Inadequate transportation resources

Lack of telephone or other communication devices

A home environment with stairs or barriers to bathroom, kitchen, and laundry

Having role responsibilities involving the care of dependent others (e.g., young children, a disabled spouse)

Having difficulty in asking for or accepting assistance from others

Engaging in manipulative, guilt-producing behavior as a means of seeking to have one's physical and emotional needs met

FAMILY, CARE GIVERS

Care givers and family members may be anticipated to have difficulty in managing their own daily living effectively and offering the most usable assistance to the patient if they:

Have their own health problems and physical or emotional dysfunctions

Are healthy but elderly and lack the physical strength and endurance or skills to give needed physical assistance

Lack equipment to compensate for the patient's inability to be mobile and engage in self-care

Have unresolved past interpersonal difficulties with the patient

Have other crucial role responsibilities that diminish time or energy for meeting patient's needs

Have communication patterns that preclude sharing of feelings or purposeful negotiation of changes in role or activities

Resent the care giving requirements

Have difficulty in adjusting anticipatory grieving when the patient experiences remissions and relapses

Believe that the patient really isn't trying as hard as might be expected

Are unable to correctly interpret disguised communication or understand the basis for the patient's behavior

Feel manipulated

Diagnostic Areas

PATIENT

Dehydration related to (R/T) voluntary reduction in fluid intake to decrease trips to the bathroom or commode

Snacking on convenience foods R/T inadequate energy to prepare or eat nutritionally sound meals

Social isolation R/T:

> Limited capacity to carry on conversations in person or on the telephone

> Reluctance to have others see deterioration in personal grooming and home maintenance

> Reduced capacity to leave the home to attend social events or to visit others

> Inadequate energy for going out or conversing with others

> Fear of episodes of sudden exhaustion

> Alienation of others through manipulative or guilt-producing behavior as strategy for seeking to meet physical or emotional needs

Inability to engage in *——————— (*self-care, cooking, care of home environment, laundry, shopping, trips to doctor, care of financial matters, care of pets—specify areas) R/T:

> Asthenia or functional disability (specify)

> Environmental barriers (specify)

> Cognitive exhaustion, leading to (L/T) inability to plan ahead

> Lack of equipment or supplies (specify)

Inability to maintain skin integrity R/T weakness-associated immobility

Anxiety, distress, anger R/T inability to maintain self-care and environment

Inadequate assistance with requirements of daily living R/T:

> Lack of family or personal network who can and will give assistance

> Lack of community resources or lack of knowledge about community resources

> Unwillingness to tell others about the situation

> Reluctance to ask for or accept offered help

> Difficulty in communicating specific needs to those who offer assistance

Unpredictability and inconsistency of assistance

Difficulty in maintaining positive relationships with care givers (see Chapter 9, Testing the Support System and Diagnostic Areas)

Reduced pleasure in life R/T lack of courage to participate in events or seek assistance

Frustration R/T lack of family or care giver understanding about difficulties or dysfunctions (specify) being experienced

Risk of falls R/T weakness

Difficulty in chewing and eating R/T weakness

Distress over noxious odors R/T inability to maintain hygiene, bathing, oral hygiene, or toileting or to change the bed or do laundry

Inability to continue care of dependent other(s) (specify—children, spouse, parent, pet) R/T progressive asthenia

FAMILY

Inadequate assistance with patient's daily living requirements R/T:

Lack of knowledge about patient's needs

Lack of physical strength and endurance to assist patient

Failure to understand patient's disguised requests for assistance or testing of the support system

Unresolved interpersonal issues with the patient or past history that makes providing care difficult

Other role responsibilities and demands that take priority over patient's needs

Lack of desire to be involved

Burnout R/T:

Physical and mental exhaustion from the unremitting demands of the patient care situation and other requirements in daily living

Lack of genuine respite on a regular, predictable basis

Lack of a confidante with whom to regularly process the emotional or cognitive elements of the care giving task

Inability to set limits on patient's demands or manipulation for emotional or physical attention

Lack of knowledge or ability to recruit assistance from other family members, social groups, or community agencies

Manifestations   See Chapter 6, section on Fatigue, under Manifestations

Difficulties in managing the requirements of daily living with progressive physical and mental fatigue and weakness are reported by and observed in both the patient and those who share the daily living. Anticipation of a downward trajectory in strength and endurance can be expected to affect both patient and care giver perceptions about the situation.

PATIENT   Reported:

Being increasingly tired, feeling "shaky," never feeling rested, progressive weakness, unsteadiness, fear of falling

Being too tired to fix food or to eat

Not caring about activities that used to be important (e.g., personal grooming, visiting with friends or family, caring for a pet)

Worrying about how to manage the basic requirements in daily living (e.g., shopping for food, cashing checks, paying bills, doing laundry, cooking, changing the bed)

Concern about how long it will be possible to maintain role responsibilities involving the care of others

Reducing fluid intake to decrease trips to the bathroom or commode

Sudden unpredicted episodes of utter exhaustion when "the bottom suddenly drops out," requiring hours or days to improve; reluctance to leave home for fear of such an episode

Distress at the deterioration of home maintenance, undone laundry, the inability to control noxious odors. (As asthenia progresses, distress may change to ignoring or not caring about deterioration in self-care or the immediate environment.)

Worry about who will provide the care when self-care is no longer possible; anger at being forced to be dependent on others; frustration and anger that others are not being perceptive of the patient's needs and responding to them; or concern about "being a burden"

Reduced capacity to think and plan for managing requirements of daily living

Falls

Remaining in bed an increasing amount of time

Observed:

Deterioration in patient appearance (looks less well put together than before); patient no longer gets dressed; clothing or bedding are changed less often

Skin breakdown in perineal, perianal, or pressure areas

Home environment is less clean and orderly (e.g., soiled clothing, sheets, towels piling up in bedroom; dishes unwashed; spoiled food in refrigerator; bathroom dirty)

Bills unopened or unpaid

Timidity about participating in events, accepting invitations, or seeking help from family, friends, or agencies

Quieter; communicates in scanning speech (i.e., omits words, makes half sentences, shifts from one topic to another)

Urine concentrated, has constipated stools

Unsteady gait; moves slowly; falls

Complains about inadequacy of care givers, family, and friends in meeting needs, or worries aloud about being a burden to others "as things get worse"

FAMILY   Reported:

Worrying about not being available to the patient because of job or other family responsibilities or travel distances

Worrying about their physical capacities to provide the assistance the patient needs

Difficulty in care giving due to earlier problems in the relationship with the patient (e.g., unresolved quarrels, childhood abuse or neglect)

Lack of adequate respite from the demands of the situation: "John hasn't slept well for weeks and neither have I. It's a 24 hour a day, seven day a week job."

Burnout

Dissatisfaction with patient behavior: patient isn't trying hard enough to get better, won't eat, won't help himself; patient is reluctant to permit them to help; patient's behavior is demanding, manipulative, or guilt-producing, making it difficult to give help with a positive attitude

Observed:

Depersonalization of the care—focusing on the tasks rather than on the patient, talking about the patient as if he or she were not there

Complaining about the patient: "Dad isn't trying to help himself"; "Mary is never satisfied no matter how much I do or how I try"; "No matter what I do it's wrong."

Neglect of their own well-being in the interest of providing care to the patient—loss of weight, failure to schedule doctor's appointments, refusal of invitations to go out even when other care givers are available

Physical incapability of assisting the patient

Unavailability for the tasks and times when they are needed

Prognostic Variables

A good prognosis for managing the requirements of daily living despite progressive asthenia is associated with:

An adequate, consistent group of care providers who are physically able to give assistance and who are available to the patient and primary care giver

Open, effective communication between the patient and care providers; credibility of the patient

Ability of the patient to communicate needs specifically and directly (not using disguised behavior) and to accept assistance with some concern for the care provider's well-being

Some risk-taking ability on the part of the patient in terms of maintaining a social life as long as possible

Scheduled, predictable, adequate respite for the primary care giver

Capacity of care givers to set limits on patient behavior in a caring way, based on a valid understanding of what the patient is experiencing and responding to

Complications

Failure to manage daily living with progressive asthenia can result in unnecessary suffering, social isolation, more rapid physical deterioration, depression, and possibly suicide.

Treatment Guidelines

See Chapter 6, section on Fatigue, under Treatment Guidelines

PATIENT

Inadequate fluid and food intake

Gather data on the pattern of fluid and food intake, the basis for any voluntary restrictions on food or fluids, and any physical difficulties in shopping for food, food preparation, or eating.

If seemingly purposeful fluid or food restriction[†] is based on incorrect knowledge (e.g., saving energy by decreasing the number of trips to the toilet or commode), provide correct information about the risks of restricting fluids (e.g., urinary tract infections, constipation, dehydration, and electrolyte imbalance).

If the patient cannot shop or prepare meals and does not have a care provider to do it, explore options of Meals on Wheels, chore services, or recruiting a volunteer to help.

[†] Change in food and fluid intake may be an early sign that the patient is making a transition to the terminal cancer stage.

Discuss option of keeping a supply of preferred fluids and nutritious snacks at chairside and bedside.

Suggest preparation of larger amounts of foods on "good days" and storage in the freezer of extra portions in single-portion servings (or meal-size portions to feed the family) for days when energy is lower.

If the patient has family or friends who are asking how they might help, suggest that the patient or care giver have in mind the specific needs for food, the portion sizes needed, and the days when they will be needed.

Lack of assistance with daily living requirements

Gather data on the tasks in daily living that are becoming difficult and the kind of assistance and equipment that would be preferable or acceptable, possible sources of assistance and any constraints in recruiting them, and any personal difficulties associated with accepting help from others.

Help the patient to talk about any difficulties in seeking or accepting help. Explore strategies, scripts, and approaches that would be more comfortable (e.g., the use of humor or mild self-deprecation). Suggest, or help the patient (or care giver) to develop, a repertoire of scripts (e.g., "I've been such an independent soul that it's hard to have to ask others to help out").

Where the patient has no personal network, provide information, refer, or assist in making contact with an individual or an agency that can provide assistance, given the patient's financial status. Consider specific elements, such as pharmacies that deliver or volunteers who will shop for those who cannot.

Where the patient (or primary care giver) does have assistance among family and friends, suggest that the patient list the people and the kinds of assistance each one might be interested in and capable of doing, then negotiate for assistance. For example, the patient might say to a neighbor, "Mary, it has become so difficult for me to shop for food these days. If I were to make a list and give you the money, would you be willing to pick up some groceries for me at the same time that you do your shopping each week?"

Suggest that the patient develop scripts and behaviors that will make it easier for the patient to retain desired control and to foster shared role expectations (e.g., "At present I am able to do... and I would prefer to do it myself. I do need help with.... My strength changes from week to week so we may need to make adjustments fairly frequently" or "It's hard to turn over control of one's daily living to someone else. It would make it easier if we could plan together").

Environmental factors deterring self-care

Suggest creating a more compact environment. Suggest placing frequently used objects and equipment in close and convenient locations and developing a "personal center" that clusters needed materials, telephone, pictures, cherished objects, radio, television, and books conveniently near the chair or sofa where the patient rests in the daytime. Create a similar environment at the bedside.

Suggest obtaining hampers with tight lids for storing soiled clothing and disposing of used dressings, for ease in keeping the immediate environment neater and minimizing odors.

Skin breakdown

Inform care giver that when asthenia progresses to the point where mobility is impaired and toileting hygiene becomes difficult, assistance is needed to prevent or manage skin breakdown.

Suggest controlling the time the patient remains in one position. Direct patient (using a mirror) or care giver to check skin in pressure areas for reactive erythema after a change in position. If erythema fades in less than 20 minutes the duration of the position is OK. If the fading takes longer than 20 minutes, instruct the patient to change position more frequently. If erythema does not fade, keep area pressure-free until it does. Instruct the patient to provide intermittent pressure relief by shifting weight, adjusting the position of the back in a recliner, and lifting weight off the ischial tuberosities.

Use pressure-distributing surfaces (e.g., air mattress, water mattress, air-fluidized bed, airflow bed, or high-density foam mattress cover). (Note that pressure-relieving surfaces further reduce independent movement.) Protect heel or malleolus by placing a rolled bath blanket or towel under the heel cord when the patient is lying supine or above the malleolus when in a side-lying position. For extended sitting in a chair, instruct patient to use a 4-inch foam cushion if there is some standing or walking time, or a "low-profile" wheelchair cushion. Donuts are contraindicated for skin pressure relief (Heard, 1988).

Use moistened wipes or toilet tissues to gently but thoroughly cleanse the perineal or perianal area following urination or bowel movements, then pat dry and apply ointment to the area if reddened or painful.

Social isolation

See also Chapter 6, section on Fatigue, treatment guidelines for disrupted interpersonal relationships related to fatigue.

Suggest to patient and care giver that they determine the times of highest energy and greatest comfort and try to arrange for visits or excursions at these times. Encourage the patient (and care giver) to make excursions, attend events, and have friends in, even if it means having some "tired days" afterward.

Help patient and care giver to develop scripts to assist visitors to be comfortable with the patient's current status (e.g., "I tire very easily, so I talk less, but it is so good to have you come and bring me news of what is going on in your world"). Recommend that the care giver (or patient) let the visitor know how long a visit the patient can tolerate (e.g., "Fred can manage to visit for about 20 minutes these days").

Suggest to patient and care giver the need to negotiate with a family member or friend to serve as a confidante who will listen and be a sounding board as the patient or care giver processes current experiences or considers new strategies for more effective management of the upcoming requirements of daily living. Note that either telephone or face-to-face contacts will serve, but keeping the content of conversations confidential is crucial. If the patient or care giver is uncomfortable with taking the initiative each time, suggest letting the confidante know, so that it is the confidante who initiates the call, or suggest that a regular schedule of contacts be made (e.g., a phone call each morning, or every other day, or on Thursdays).

Where the patient's manipulative or guilt-producing behavior is alienating others, point out to the care provider that this is a symptom of feelings of helplessness and loss of control. Suggest that the care giver respond by seeking to give the patient more control (e.g., suggesting that the patient propose new routines or set the times for medications, treatments, or activities), by setting limits on manipulative behavior, and by interpreting the behavior as a symptom (like a cough or a bruise) over which the patient has no control rather than as a personal attack. Where possible, help the patient to develop some different scripts that will be more effective in gaining the desired attention and control.

Frustration with others' lack of understanding of patient's difficulties and dysfunctions

Determine the areas in which there is misunderstanding and patient frustration.

Explore options for scripts whereby the patient can describe more specifically the difficulties being experienced. With patient permission, legitimize these difficulties and dysfunctions by providing medical data on the patient's current physical status to the care giver or a family member.

Risk of falls

Identify the risk of falls to the patient and care giver.

Recommend arranging the environment (rugs, electrical or phone cords, furniture) and providing adequate lighting (including night lights) to minimize risks.

Suggest use of cane or walker, raised toilet seat, hand bars beside toilet and tub, bedside commode, etc. as needed. Identify resources for obtaining them.

Difficulty in eating and chewing

Suggest selecting foods and preparing them in such a way as to reduce energy needed for chewing (e.g., using softer fruits, vegetables, and cereals; preparing meats by braising—meat balls, stews, pot roasts, fricassees; serving fish or shellfish; cooking vegetables longer).

Suggest scheduling more frequent, smaller meals, but arrange that one or more involves eating with the family or with a friend (if it is usual for the family to share the patient's daily living or friends are available).

Limitations in capacity to control noxious odors

Assist patient or care giver to control odors from bacterial growth in moist necrotic tissues by teaching them how to cleanse the area with soap and water, a normal saline solution, or an antiseptic agent such as chlorhexidine gluconate 4% emulsion (Hibiclens) or 1% aqueous solution (Hibitane). Encourage use of an odor barrier such as an ostomy bag or odor-absorbent dressings. Advise that oil of orange or peppermint added to the dressings may cover some odors (Billings, 1985). Instruct patient or care giver to apply Ostozyme spray to skin areas where bacterial, urinary, or fecal materials are causing skin breakdown and odors (Ritter, 1982).

Suggest using tightly closed hampers for storing soiled linen and clothing until it can be laundered and for disposing of soiled dressings or disposable pads. A covered diaper bucket with a deodorizing solution may be helpful for particularly soiled clothing, incontinent pads, or small pieces of linen.

Frequent oral hygiene, diluted mouth washes (to minimize drying), and mints can help reduce fetid breath.

Partial baths between full baths or showers and use of deodorants and lotions may limit body odors and improve a feeling of freshness.

Placing scented soap or sachets among sleeping garments or undergarments, or setting them about the room may add a fresh scent for the patient.

Charcoal (available for fish tanks or barbecues) set in a dish at the chairside and bedside may absorb some odors.

Provide for circulation of air (windows, fans, air conditioners) to lessen intensity of odors.

Use solid or spray room deodorizers.

Use disposable pads or launderable pads with a piece of plastic underneath for incontinence or drainage. Change frequently and dispose of them as indicated above.

Inadequate capacity to continue to provide care for dependents

See Chapter 6, section on Role, under Treatment Guidelines.

Lack of courage to participate in activities or seek assistance

Determine what the patient considers to be the risk in participating in a given activity or in asking for help.

Suggest that the patient consider what would be the three worst
things that could happen if the activity were undertaken and
what would be the three best outcomes, then think about any
strategies that could minimize the risks (e.g., changing the
timing of the activity, locating rest stops, using a wheelchair,
planning scripts and behaviors, rehearsing).

Be perceptive when the reluctant patient does take some risks
and be warm in acknowledging the behavior.

FAMILY, CARE   *Lack of knowledge about patient's needs for assistance and care*
GIVERS
Determine care giver's perception of patient's status, trajectory,
and needs for assistance. Where they are inaccurate, provide
accurate information using nonthreatening language (e.g.,
"Right now Phyllis is feeling quite tired, particularly in the
afternoons. This is not unusual for a person with her type of
cancer. If someone is able to stand by, she should be able to take
a shower by herself and dress herself. She probably can wash her
dishes, but changing the bed, doing the laundry, and going
alone to the store are probably beyond her strength and endurance. We anticipate that gradually she will feel less able to
care for herself, but being such an independent person, asking
for or even accepting help is going to be hard for her").

Difficulty in interpreting patient's disguised requests for assistance

Determine the behavior of the patient that is difficult for the
care giver to understand or accept.

Discuss the dynamics of unaccustomed dependency and helplessness and the strategies helpless people use to vent their anger
at their situation and seek to gain some measure of control.
Indicate that the behavior is a symptom of the patient's stress
rather than a deliberate attack or "put down" of the care giver.

Suggest that the care giver initiate a discussion of the situation
the patient is in (e.g., "It must be hard to feel so *————
(*weak, tired, uncomfortable, miserable) and be unable to do
things the way you want—I don't know how you manage!"),
and allow time for the patient to respond. Later the care giver
can offer options that allow the patient to determine the help
desired (e.g., "I want to help and to make it as easy and
comfortable as possible for you to accept my help. Why don't we
talk about how we can work together most comfortably?").

When the patient engages in disguised requests for assistance, suggest that the care giver take a deep breath to maintain personal control and then neutrally translate it into a direct request (e.g., "Do you mean that you would like me to...?").

Unresolved personal issues with the patient

If the care giver gives evidence of having extreme difficulty in relating to the patient or behaves in an impersonal, mechanical manner, it may be possible to gather data on factors that contribute to the difficulties.

If the situation creating difficulties can be resolved, suggest that doing this will make care giving much less difficult. If the difficulties do not lend themselves to resolution, suggest that the care giver attempt to perceive the person receiving care as a patient and provide care the way it would be given if the patient were a stranger, not a relative or friend.

Lack of strength, knowledge, or skill to provide care

Determine the match between the patient's needs for physical assistance and the care giver's physical capacity to provide this assistance. If the care giver is not strong enough, arrange for equipment (e.g., lifts, trapezes, wheel chairs) or additional professional or volunteer assistance with tasks that are beyond the care giver's capacity.

Where there are deficits in knowledge or skill, provide verbal and written or pictorial information about such activities as transfer, lifting, toileting, mouth care, bathing, dressings, skin care, positioning, medications, and so on.

Arrange for a home visit by a nurse to set up the activities in the actual situation in which the care will be delivered.

Competing role requirements and demands in daily living

Explore with the care giver the additional demands in daily living and any adjustments that are possible. Legitimize the difficulties being experienced. Suggest prioritizing other demands, getting assistance with them, and getting assistance with the patient's care needs. Try to allay any guilt feelings associated with the role conflicts by indicating that their experience unfortunately is not too unusual.

Discuss the situation with the patient (if the care giver wishes this). Explore possibilities for meeting the patient's needs that will lessen the conflicts that the care giver is genuinely experiencing. Maintain an awareness that the patient may feel ambivalent about being a burden to the family, but at the same time need to feel loved and cared about. Approach both dimensions in working through ways of making both care giver and patient feel relatively comfortable with the choices. Indicate the importance of keeping the options open as the situation for each one changes.

Lack of desire to provide the care

Determine the reason for the lack of desire to be involved in providing patient care (e.g., fear of the patient dying, discomfort with treatment and care needed, own health problems).

Explore any options for meeting the care giver's needs and those of the patient. Allow time for care giver to adjust to the possibilities. Suggest that the care giver and patient have private time to talk over the situation. Explain to the patient that often it is the person who cares the most who has the greatest difficulty in providing the care.

Burnout (Note: patient may also experience burnout)

Gather data on the pattern of ongoing responsibilities of the person, the health status (including physical and mental energy), areas in daily living over which the person has control and those where there is lack of control, stress awareness, the concerns or worries (including behavior of others that is difficult to understand or handle), personal goals and priorities, the actual status of the person's support network, availability of a confidante, and opportunities for genuine, planned, scheduled respite.

Legitimize the importance of the care giver's self-protection in maintaining physical and emotional well-being on an ongoing basis. Help the care givers and family members to see the consequences for the patient and for themselves if they neglect their own well-being.

Point out that it is common for family members and care givers to feel that it is wrong to experience pleasure and enjoyment in life when the patient is suffering. Talk in terms of the functions that emotional release and enjoyment play in maintaining well-being so that it is possible to continue to give emotional support to the patient over time. Give "permission" to significant others to engage in activities and behaviors that provide care for themselves.

Explain that one factor contributing to burnout is a sense of loss of control over life (see Chapter 9, treatment guidelines for helplessness). Suggest that they think about what is really possible and how this fits with the goals they have—contrasting what should or might be done with what feasibly can be done, given the resources and the circumstances (Weisman, 1981).

Explore the options for obtaining regular, planned, scheduled respite that is of long enough duration to permit actual replenishment of resources. This may mean having an afternoon off, going out for dinner, or having an uninterrupted night's sleep. Note that many patients who fear being a burden may be less troubled if significant others are able to continue other aspects of their lives (Vess et al, 1988).

Discuss the importance of being able to talk about stresses, difficulties, successes, guilt, anger, worries, and so on to a nonjudgmental listener. Point out that the act of talking about the situation sometimes tends to place it into perspective.

Evaluation

Evaluation of the patient's management of daily living with progressive asthenia will include consideration of the status of:

Food procurement, food preparation, and eating

Fluid intake

Management of basic requirements in daily living (e.g., personal hygiene and grooming, toileting, laundry, care of home environment, management of financial matters)

Skin integrity

Pattern of social interaction and satisfaction with it

Capacity to recruit and maintain adequate assistance

Management of transition to increasing dependence

Relationships with care givers and family

Feelings of being cared for and cared about

For care givers and family members who participate in the patient's daily living, effectiveness in living with the additional responsibilities of caring for a patient with progressive asthenia may be evaluated in terms of the status of:

Incorporating new care giving responsibilities into usual requirements of daily living

Ongoing physical and emotional capacity to provide the assistance needed by the patient

Competence and comfort with the care giving tasks

Insight into the dynamics of the relationship of patient to care giver and the effectiveness of their communication patterns

Respite or burnout

Relationship between care giver and family members

Living With Eating and Feeding Problems

Malnutrition and weight loss are present in the majority of patients with advanced cancer and are most prevalent and severe in those who are terminally ill (DeWys, 1986; Bruera and MacDonald, 1988). Loss of desire to eat; difficulties in eating created by past

. treatment, new tumor growth, or further treatment; and nausea and vomiting can reemerge with advancing cancer (see Chapter 6, sections on these topics). Diminishing hope, the progressing cancer, the associated malnutrition, and, often, cachexia tend to create escalating food-related problems in daily living for the patient and those who seek to maintain the patient's nutrition and well-being.

Medical Perspective

Anorexia and weight loss in patients with advancing cancer are usually the result of remote tumor effects, but they can also be associated with other conditions (e.g., biochemical abnormalities, medications, antineoplastic treatment, uremia, dehydration, pain, or constipation) (Grosvenor et al, 1989). Differential diagnosis of the causes of the problem is very important because it may be possible to improve the appetite and nutrition through treatment of the causes.

Where other factors have been ruled out and the malnutrition is attributed to tumor effects, a major medical concern is the decision of how best to maintain the patient's hydration and nutritional status (Nixon, 1986). Malnourished patients do not respond as well to chemotherapy and radiation and have a decreased survival time (DeWys et al, 1980). They also are less active in their daily living. On the other hand, studies have shown that aggressive nutritional therapy does not alter tumor response, toxicity, or survival (Evans et al, 1986; Koretz, 1984). Research with animals has shown that aggressive nutritional therapy can significantly increase tumor growth; however, there are no comparable findings with humans (Torosian and Daly, 1986).

While treating the malnutrition may be difficult, an even more difficult treatment decision may be that of discontinuing aggressive treatment of dehydration and malnutrition when it offers no further benefit and may even prolong patient suffering. Decisions about how to treat dehydration alone present some dilemmas. Table 10-1 identifies patient benefits and hardships associated with dehydration in patients who have reached terminal stages. Medical decisions about prescribing nutritional, fluid, and electrolyte therapy involve both physiologic and ethical–legal issues (Lynn and Childress, 1983; Micetich et al, 1983).

Nursing Perspective

Eating and drinking are integral parts of established patterns of daily living. Food and water have symbolic significance that goes beyond their contribution to nutrition and hydration. They are seen as being essential in expressing caring to a vulnerable human being (Caspar, 1988). Thus, a chronic and progressive loss of desire and ability to eat becomes a pervasive and sensitive problem for patients and for those who care for and about them.

Nursing's focus for diagnosis and treatment includes the patient and care givers or family members. Areas of concern where the patient is the focus include:

Access to foods and fluids that the patient prefers and can ingest

Control issues involving who decides when, what, and how much the patient should try to eat or drink

Table 10-1.   Benefits and Hardships of Dehydration in Terminally Ill Cancer Patients

Effects of Dehydration	Benefits	Hardships
Decreased urine output	Less need for bedpan, urinal, commode, or catheter; less incontinence	
Decreased gastrointestinal fluid	Fewer bouts of vomiting	
Decreased pulmonary secretions	Reduced coughing and congestion	Continued cough reflex
Decreased pharyngeal secretions	Relief from choking and drowning sensations with dysphagia	Continued apprehension that choking may continue
Decreased total volume of body fluids	Decreased peripheral and pulmonary edema	
Reduction in edematous layer around tumor	Relief from pressure and tumor mass	
Increased concentration of electrolytes	Natural anesthetic agent for central nervous system—drowsiness, lethargy, decreased awareness of suffering	Increased neuromuscular irritability, cardiac arrhythmia, muscle twitching, restlessness, nausea, disorientation
Decreased moisture in mucous membranes		Discomfort from dry mouth, cracked lips, other mucosal membranes; food debris and dried sputum may coat oral cavity
Mucosal surface barrier impaired		Increased risk of viral, bacterial, or monilial infection

(Billings, 1985; Dolan, 1983; Zerwekh, 1983)

Management of food and fluid intake in as effective, comfortable, and satisfying a way possible in the presence of anorexia, difficulties in ingesting food, or nausea and vomiting

Management of interaction with care givers whose goals in feeding or feeding behavior create difficulties for the patient

Continued options for social interaction involving food, if this has been a previous pattern and is currently desired

Areas of concern where the care giver or family members are involved include:

Seeking to feed the patient as a means of supporting denial of the patient's prognosis

Knowledge deficits about the way in which the patient's advancing neoplasms physiologically and psychologically affect eating and body response to nutrients

Equating loving with feeding and believing that the patient's reciprocal love or appreciation of the food provider is evidenced by eating the food that is provided

Frustration of the food preparer when the patient persistently refuses or is unable to eat or drink the food and fluids provided

Nature of Eating and Feeding Problems

The major challenges in the eating problems of the patient with advancing cancer has to do with provision of food and fluids in ways that are most conducive to the patient's well-being and comfort as the desire and capacity to eat decline. (See Chapter 6, sections on Loss of Desire to Eat; Nausea, Vomiting, and Retching; and Difficulties in Eating for discussion of other eating-related problems.)

With advancing cancer other factors begin to play a significant role in food- and eating-related decisions, behavior, and associated relationships occurring among patient, family, and health care providers. At least three categories of phenomena may be involved in the eating, feeding, and nutritional problems encountered. These are the goals of each of the participants (e.g., physician, patient, family, and care giver), the ethical beliefs or values that shape the perspectives of the participants, and the behaviors that each party exhibits.

Goals for Nutrition-Related Activities

Each of the participants involved in the patient's nutritional and hydration status will have either implicit or explicit goals as a basis for behavior. The participants' goals may or may not be congruent with each other.

It is possible that all of the participants may be seeking to achieve positive nutritional goals. For example, the physician may be seeking to constrain the neoplastic processes with further treatment and to provide concurrent aggressive nutritional therapy with the goal of assuring the greatest therapeutic effect. Nurses may choose to use idealized desired outcomes from standard care plans. They will then write nursing orders and engage in activities to seek to attain such a goal. Families may still be in the denial stage of responding to knowledge of the cancer's progression, and want the patient to eat in order to support their implicit goal of denial. Patients may actively seek to maintain optimum nutrition because it offers the best hope of achieving their goal of cure or longer survival. Where participants hold congruent goals for extending survival as in these examples, efforts to promote optimum nutrition would have consistent support.

Congruence in participant goals in a reverse situation may also occur. The physician may have made the clinical judgment that the pathology has reached a point where aggressive nutritional therapy is no longer beneficial and decided to use nutrition and hydration only as palliative measures (Billings, 1985; Bruera and MacDonald, 1988). Nurses may have set goals of providing pleasure and comfort associated with food and fluids and chosen to accommodate patient desires of limiting intake. The patient may find that life is filled with such suffering that the goal of prolonging survival is no longer desirable. The family too may have come to accept the patient's prognosis and may not wish to extend survival when the quality of the patient's life has so deteriorated. Again there could be agreement about the goals and strategies where comfort is the primary goal.

It is not unusual, however, for the participants to bring differing and incongruent goals to the issue of nutrition. Some participants may be opting for aggressive nutritional therapy, while others may feel that this approach is no longer appropriate. Nurses are often faced with diagnosing and mediating in these situations.

Ethics and Beliefs

Because food and fluids are such an integral and ordinary part of daily living there are societal norms, values, and beliefs that surround them and affect any deliberate manipulation of them. Food and fluids have symbolic meaning quite apart from the nutritional elements. Particular ethical considerations thus may shape decisions about providing food and fluid to patients as their capacity to ingest food and fluid declines. Legal considerations may also enter into deliberations about provision of nutrients and fluids to patients who are no longer able to credibly communicate their own wishes in the matter.

Ethical or legal considerations that may affect health care provider behavior include beliefs that health care professionals are obliged to (Lynn and Childress, 1983):

Provide ordinary or proportionate care (as compared to extraordinary or disproportionate care)

Continue treatments once they are started

Avoid being the unambiguous cause of the patient's death

Provide symbolically significant treatment

Avoid futile treatments or those that bring additional suffering without commensurate benefit

Health care providers can give varying interpretations and weight to these ethical factors and may combine them with pathophysiologic elements in the patient situation to derive varying decisions about nutritional and hydration therapy.

Family and patient beliefs about patients' rights and responsibilities can vary widely also (see Chapter 9, Societal Values and Incongruence in Values and Goals). Whereas antineoplastic treatment is primarily under the control of the physician and may be seen as extraordinary treatment, the decision to continue to eat and drink or not to do so is primarily under the control of the patient, unless altered mentation or levels of consciousness interfere. Questions may arise as to whether the patient has the right to give in to the anorexia, the difficulty in eating, or the nausea and vomiting, or whether there is an obligation to continue to ingest food and fluids despite the symptoms. Family members and care givers may struggle with their sense of obligation to feed the patient, their empathy for the eating difficulties the patient is experiencing, and beliefs about individual rights to retain control of daily living.

Feeding Behavior

The behavior of others toward the patient in the area of providing food and the interaction about eating may be a reflection of beliefs, knowledge about the patient's status, degree of acceptance of the prognosis, and the status of unresolved or resolved personal business with the patient.

Families who have unresolved problems with the patient, who are not ready to accept the prognosis, or who need and hope to extend the survival time may place great emphasis on food preparation and urging the patient to eat. For example, a woman with metastatic brain lesions was close to discharge. She was somewhat confused. Her son, who was becoming increasingly uneasy and stressed about taking his mother home, told her nurse that his mother wanted some watermelon to eat, and became very angry when it was not delivered quickly enough. It was unclear to the nurse whether the mother did indeed want watermelon, or whether it was the son's desire for the mother to eat it.

Families and care givers who have resolved these issues may find it easier to show love and caring by providing the patient with foods and fluids they know the patient likes at times when the patient is most comfortable with eating and drinking. It may bother them that the patient does not eat, but they accept, nonjudgmentally, the patient's eating or not eating.

Families may or may not understand the effect of the neoplasms on the patient's difficulties. They may vary in their abilities to translate knowledge into food preparation and understanding of patient behavior surrounding food and fluids.

Where family dynamics are dysfunctional, food and feeding behavior may trace its origins to quite different problem areas that have little or nothing to do with nutrition. The feeding behavior may be only a symptom of other problems. (See also Chapter 2, Families and the Experience of Cancer.)

Underlying Mechanisms

Pathophysiologic Factors

There are many contributing factors in malnutrition and eating problems among patients with advancing cancer; however, the relative significance of each has not yet been established (Bruera and MacDonald, 1988). Weight loss is primarily attributed to decreased caloric intake combined with increased utilization of calories by the tumor and altered metabolism (Bruera and MacDonald, 1988). (See also Chapter 6, section on Loss of Desire to Eat, under Pathophysiologic and Iatrogenic Factors, and this chapter, section on Asthenia, under Cachexia.)

Decreased intake of food and fluids can be associated with a variety of factors (Heber et al, 1986). Altered taste, pain, and severe depression will cause a patient to eat less (Baines, 1988). Anorexia and food aversion in advancing cancer has been linked to neurotransmitter abnormalities or tumor effects (Bernstein, 1986; Beutler and Cerami, 1986; Bruera et al, 1986; DeWys, 1979). The "squashed stomach syndrome" caused by hepatomegaly, tumor involvement of the stomach lining, esophageal or pyloroduodenal obstruction, intestinal obstruction, uremia, electrolyte abnormalities, and, occasionally, increased intracranial pressure are other possible contributing factors (Baines, 1988; Bruera and MacDonald, 1988; Twycross and Lack, 1984). Delayed gastric emptying time (190 minutes compared to 70 minutes for control subjects) possibly associated with a syndrome of autonomic insufficiency may also contribute to eating problems (Bruera et al, 1987). Previous experiences of vomiting after eating may create anxiety and reluctance to eat. Initiation of an analgesic regimen involving morphine and some other opiates can cause nausea for about a week (Baines, 1988).

Daily Living Factors

So many aspects of daily living are linked to food and drink that persistent, serious aberrations in eating and drinking patterns cause disruptions and discomfort for the patient and any who share food-related activities. When these eating problems are combined with the progression of a life-threatening disease or knowledge of the patient's prognosis, the difficulties each participant faces are multiplied.

Activities and Events in Daily Living	Any food- or eating-related activity or event in daily living involving the patient, care giver, family, friends, business associates, or social contacts can be an area for nursing attention.

Shopping for food may be a problem for the patient who lacks energy, interest in food, transportation, money, or someone to help out on bad days. It can be a problem for the care giver who is no longer able to leave the patient, or who has "tried everything" and no longer knows what foods and fluids to buy that may tempt the anorexic patient.

Food preparation becomes an increasing problem for the patient who has anorexia, food aversions, nausea and vomiting, or asthenia. It can become an increasing source of frustration to the care giver when the food prepared is continually rejected by the patient.

Social and business occasions involving eating may be difficult for the patient and others to manage as eating difficulties become more severe.

Demands in Daily Living

Self-expectations regarding control of eating and the demands of others may well create interpersonal difficulties. Care givers and families, concerned about the patient's well-being, may urge food and fluids on the patient and the patient may resist and resent their behavior. The family may feel that the patient is not trying hard enough. On the other hand, the patient may feel neglected or unloved if family members or care givers do not make sufficient effort to provide preferred foods or empathize with eating difficulties. For example, the housemate of a terminally ill man was trying to postpone the reality of his companion's impending death and was vigorously pressuring the patient to drink nutritional supplements. The patient asked the nurse not to take the empty cans away, saying somewhat angrily, "I've got to have those to prove to him that I did it." The interaction was a continuation of a confrontational pattern that was apparently comfortably characteristic of their 30-year relationship.

Health care professionals' demands for compliance with a nutritional regimen may be congruent or incongruent with the patient's or family's wishes. The patient's unwillingness to accept or inability to carry out the prescribed nutritional regimen can create feelings of anger or guilt and concerns about abandonment, feelings that can compound the patient's worry and suffering.

Environment for Daily Living

Ease of access to food storage and food preparation areas is important for the patient with advancing cancer. Having a freezer and microwave so that food can be prepared on good days or donated by others and stored in single-serving portions, then heated with a minimum of odors is a major asset. (See also Chapter 6, sections on Loss of Desire to Eat; Difficulties in

Eating; and Nausea, Vomiting, and Retching, under Environment for Daily Living.) Access to stores to purchase foods is also
an important consideration.

**Values and
Beliefs**

Traditional values and cherished patterns of socialization surrounding food and eating patterns are considerations as the
patient's desire and capacity to eat decline. Variations in eating
patterns could include: the patient is a solitary person who has
always eaten alone; the family situation was one in which the
mother prepared the meals and everyone shared one or two
meals each day; the extended family always gathered for a shared
meal on Sundays or special holidays; or both parents worked and
shared shopping and cooking duties and members comfortably
ate singly or together, however it was convenient. Each pattern
and the strength of valuing it will affect expectations and
behavior when the eating problems of advancing cancer occur.

Beliefs about the role that food plays in health and illness may
also be a factor influencing behavior. For example, a belief in the
old saying, "Feed a cold and starve a fever," could result in
withholding food when the immunosuppressed person has an
infection and needs extra calories, not fewer calories. Ethnic
beliefs about "hot" versus "cold" foods will influence dietary
patterns. Belief in the curative powers of unproven dietary
therapies (e.g., macrobiotic diets) will also be a factor for some
patients and families.

Functional Health Status

**Strength and
Endurance**

Physical strength and endurance will be major factors in the
patient's capacity to procure and prepare food, and even to
chew and swallow it. This will be true of the care giver or food
preparer as well, particularly in continuing to function effectively when the patient has persisting difficulty in eating food
that is prepared.

Cognition

The patient's capacity to think about food, nutrients, and fluid
and to plan ahead for purchases and meal preparation may be
impaired by asthenia and, eventually, clouded mentation. The
care giver's capacity to understand the patient's pathophysiology and its effects on eating and nutrition, and then to apply
that understanding to both food preparation and interaction
with the patient about eating will be areas for assessment and
possible diagnosis.

Skills

Skills in food preparation and creativity in serving in ways that
tempt a jaded appetite will be important, whether the patient is
preparing the food or the care giver is doing so. Skills in
controlling the cooking odors can also be important.

Another area for both patient and care giver skill is their interpersonal patterns as these relate to food and eating. The caring and nurturing aspects embedded in food and eating add dimensions and complications to the interaction. Perceptiveness and sensitivity are required on the part of both the giver of the food and the receiver. Each has needs to be recognized and met and goals to be achieved in the transaction.

Mood Depression, particularly severe depression, is linked to malnutrition. Depression affects the energy for and interest in food preparation as well as eating. Frustration, anger, or depression in the care giver could also have a negative effect on the patient's eating behavior.

Communi- The capacity to communicate about food preferences, diffi-
cation culties, or reluctance to eat is important as a functional capacity for the patient. In the care giver or family member skills associated with communication about food and fluid will center on the ability to draw out information on the patient's current status relative to eating and to convey concern and interest in the patient's eating behavior without nagging.

Nursing Diagnosis and Treatment

Considerations of nursing diagnosis and treatment in the Chapter 6 sections on Loss of Desire to Eat; Difficulty in Eating; and Nausea, Vomiting, and Retching are applicable to comparable problems where the patient and family are facing advancing cancer; these topics are not repeated in this section. The differences between diagnosis and treatment of eating and feeding problems in the initial diagnosis stage versus in advanced cancer lie in the meaning assigned to the symptoms and food-related behavior. The patient's symptoms and behavior associated with eating persistently remind both patient and family of the progressive nature of the neoplastic processes and the ultimate outcome—death for the patient and loss of a loved one for the family.

In this chapter the approach to eating problems will presume a foundation and inclusion of the content of eating-related sections in Chapter 6. It will focus on the adaptations to eating problems associated with the progression of the cancer and its meaning to the patient and family.

Diagnostic The diagnostic targets include the patient who is experiencing
Targets eating difficulties, family members who share daily living and eating experiences with the patient, health care professionals, work associates (some patients wish to or must continue to work as long as possible to maintain health insurance and income), friends, and social contacts. Note: The nurse may gather data on nonpatient diagnostic targets through the patient or family and may treat them directly or through the patient; however, the diagnostic target is still the other person(s) rather than the patient.

Risk Factors

Patients who are at greatest risk of not effectively managing daily living in the face of eating problems associated with advancing cancer are those who:

Live alone

Lack a consistent, functional, caring support network that is present in "valley times" as well as good times

Have severe or multiple pathophysiologic deterrents to eating (e.g., head and neck cancer, persistent vomiting, fungating wounds or fistulas creating noxious odors for patient and those who share the eating experience)

Have severe asthenia affecting physical and mental capacities

Experience inadequately controlled pain

Are seriously depressed

Want to die

Lack services to assist in procuring or preparing food

Lack money for food or dietary supplements

Have unresolved control or value issues with health care professionals or personal care givers regarding food and eating

Engage in passive–aggressive behavior patterns toward the care givers

Family members or care givers at greatest risk for experiencing difficulties in managing problems in daily living associated with the patient's eating behavior are those who:

Are in the denial stage regarding acceptance of the patient's advancing cancer and its meaning

Have unresolved problems from earlier times and are using eating and feeding issues as a focus for their difficulties

Have not resolved the issue of whether the patient has the right to control his or her eating behavior

Feel that the patient is "not trying hard enough," does not understand the difficulties the food provider is having in the situation, or is creating intentional difficulties for the care giver

Are repulsed by the patient's appearance, dysfunctions, or odors

Are unskilled or unimaginative in food preparation

Are easily frustrated or depressed by the patient's behavior

Have other major responsibilities that limit time and energy for focusing on the patient's eating problems

Are experiencing burnout

Lack transportation or assistance for obtaining food, particularly if the patient cannot be left alone

Diagnostic Areas

PATIENT

Iatrogenic physiologic complications (specify) R/T seeking of cure through an unproven, non-nutritious diet (specify nature of diet)

Food intake less than patient's desire to eat R/T:

Capacity to eat is incongruent with the patient's goal and belief that maintaining optimum nutrition will hold cancer at bay

Unavailability of food that patient can ingest (e.g., wrong consistency, tastes bad to the patient)

Lack of person to procure, prepare, and serve the food

Loneliness at mealtime

Unpleasant experiences with eating (specify) R/T:

Unresolved control issue over eating between patient and health care providers, personal care givers, or family members (specify)

Obvious distancing of family or companions in eating situations

Being served unappetizing, unattractive foods or foods that do not take taste distortions into account

Being made to feel guilty about eating behavior

Feeder ignoring patient's preferred patterns of eating

Care giver or family member using eating as a vehicle for venting feelings associated with unresolved issues

Insensitivity of others to the patient's needs for attention or affection associated with feeding

Impaired caloric and fluid intake R/T:

Progressive asthenia limiting capacity to shop, prepare food, serve food, chew food (specify)

Impaired mentation or lower level of consciousness (specify nature and status of dysfunction)

Severe depression

Inadequately managed pain

Fear of inducing another bout of vomiting

Desire to reduce needs to urinate or defecate

Lack of assistance with shopping, food preparation, serving, or feeding

Lack of knowledge, skill, or equipment to prepare food in a manner that it can be ingested

Belief that restricting nutrients will slow tumor growth

Desire to shorten survival time

FAMILY, CARE GIVERS

Inappropriate expectations about patient's eating behavior R/T:

Being in the denial stage of adjusting to the patient's advancing cancer

Belief that feeding symbolizes loving and that the patient's eating symbolizes gratitude or reciprocation of that loving

Belief that a particular diet will cure the cancer

Lack of knowledge about the patient's changing pathophysiology and its effect on desire to eat, responses to taste and odors, symptoms, and capacity to eat

Unresolved decisions about whether the patient has the right to control eating behavior or has obligations to comply with expectations of others

Frustration, anger, guilt, depression (specify) R/T:

Continuing inability to prepare food or fluids that the patient will accept

Patient's persistent "unwillingness" to eat or drink food prepared by others

Patient's "not trying hard enough to eat"

Patient's persistent complaints about the nature or quality of the food

Patient's requests for specific foods and subsequent rejection of them

Patient's failure to express appreciation for the efforts of others to provide appetizing food (even though it may remain uneaten)

Loss of traditional or valued eating patterns with the patient R/T associated sights, sounds, or odors, L/T guilt over causing patient additional suffering at seeming to reject the patient, or loss of family members' satisfaction with meals

Sadness R/T the meaning of the waning capacity to eat and drink

Manifestations

PATIENT

Weight loss, cachexia, and inanition may well be inevitable manifestations of the particular neoplastic process the patient is experiencing; however, they may also occur sooner or more extensively than the status of the organic disease would suggest if food and eating issues are poorly managed on a daily basis.

Reported:

> "I make myself eat. I need to remain in good shape. You never know when they will come up with a new treatment that will cure my cancer."

> Trying a new diet regimen believed to cure cancer

> Lack of strength and endurance to shop for and prepare food

> Forcing self to eat, food tasting bad, constant low-grade nausea, intolerance of food odors, early satiety

> Responding "I eat enough" when queried about eating patterns is often a cue that dietary patterns have changed to a less nutritious status (Molbo, 1986).

> Resentment of others nagging about patient's eating patterns; desire to control own eating

> Resentment or hurt that others are not sufficiently concerned about eating problems

> Inadequately managed pain interfering with food preparation or eating

> Fatigue and weakness decreasing strength and endurance for chewing, self-feeding

> Increasing dysphagia, regurgitation

> Distaste for texture of minced or pureed foods

> "Getting up to go to the bathroom is so tiring and painful that I'm not drinking as much."

> "Having a bowel movement is both exhausting and painful. I'm eating less so it doesn't happen so often."

> "I think something would taste good, but when it's ready I just can't eat it."

> Concern or anger at food preparer's emotional response to patient's inability to eat food that is offered

> Undesired social isolation associated with eating

> "Life isn't worth the effort of eating."

Observed:

> Eating and drinking decreasing amounts or beginning to refuse all nutrients (Note: This may be an early symptom of transition to the terminal stage.)

> Decreased urinary output; constipation and less frequent stools (rule out opioids or other medications as constipation-producing factors)

Dry mouth and cracked lips

Experiencing unrelieved pain at mealtimes

Vomiting after eating

Few foods and fluids in refrigerator, freezer, or cupboards

Eating alone

Disfigurements, dysfunctions, or noxious odors that tend to cause others to maintain a distance, particularly in eating-related activities

Complaining or abusing others about food preparation

FAMILY, CARE
GIVERS

Reported:

"If John will just eat properly and do what the doctor says, I'm sure everything will be just fine."

"We're going to eat right and lick this thing."

"Mary is just not trying to eat."

"He thinks it's just his life, but his difficulties affect us too."

"No matter what I buy or how I fix the food, she complains and won't eat it. I don't know what to do. I get mad and then I feel guilty."

"When I see Harry not eating and just wasting away before my eyes, I go off by myself and cry."

"It's getting so I can't leave her alone even long enough to go to the grocery store."

"What with staying up with him at night and caring for him in the daytime, I'm getting so tired myself that I don't want to eat, much less try to fix food for both of us."

"He's ready to go. He's so miserable that I don't blame him for not trying to eat or drink anything anymore. I've quit urging him—I offer, but I don't push anymore."

"I know dad's lonely and used to eating with the family, but his coughing and choking and spitting and that odor—they're so awful, who could eat?"

Observed:

Avoiding using the word cancer or the patient's neoplastic diagnosis

Urging the patient to eat as a means of maintaining health

Telling the patient that he or she has an obligation to himself, the children, or the family to comply with a nutritional regimen to maintain weight and strength

Getting angry and nagging, fussing, begging, or crying when

the patient does not eat and drink as much as they think is appropriate

Avoiding being around the patient at mealtimes

Preparing foods that are unappealing, poorly prepared, unattractively served, give off strong food odors, or are difficult for the patient to chew, swallow, or digest given the particular neoplastic pathology

Failure to report ineffective pain management regimens or failure to set a schedule that provides the patient with a degree of pain control at mealtimes

Prognostic Variables

A good prognosis for managing daily living in a way that is effective and satisfying for the patient and those involved may be associated with having:

Access to appropriate food and fluids

Clear and congruent nutritional goals among participants

Congruence among participants about whether the patient or others should have control over the patient's eating behavior

Support persons willing and skilled in shopping, preparing, and serving food when the need arises

Sensitivity to the personal needs and symbolism involved in both the giving and receiving of food and fluids, and appropriate acting on these perceptions

Effective pain and other symptom management

Control of noxious odors

Adaptations to permit continuation of valued meal patterns (socialization) as long as possible

Congruence of goals and actions that take into account patient comfort and well-being in dealing with nutrition and hydration in the terminal stage

Complications

Failure to manage the tasks and relationships in daily living associated with nutrition and hydration as cancer advances can result in premature loss of weight, strength, energy, and capacity; loss of interest in activity; shorter survival time; greater discomfort; dry mouth (De Conno et al, 1989); constipation; and increasingly strained, uncomfortable relationships among participants.

Treatment Guidelines

Decision or encouragement to follow high-risk, unproven diet

Determine whether patient or others have decided on the diet.

Identify the nutritional elements that are lacking in the diet and the body changes associated with deficits in these nutrients.

Indicate that activity levels (and therefore, presumably, strength and energy levels) have been found to be higher in people who can maintain optimum nutrition.

Provide written information on an optimum diet and any adaptations that may need to be made because of patient's pathophysiology.

Purposeful dietary or fluid restrictions

Note that not eating and drinking may be the first manifestation of transition into the terminal phase of cancer rather than a deliberate patient decision.

If it is unlikely that the patient is becoming terminally ill, seek data on the rationale for the patient's restricting nutrients or fluids (e.g., to decrease trips to the bathroom to urinate [fatigue or pain], to decrease the need to defecate [fatigue or pain], to "starve the tumor," to decrease survival time because of poor quality of life or being a burden on the family). If the latter reason is suspected, approach the issue gently (e.g., "You're not eating or drinking much these days, Nancy. Are things getting you down?").

If the rationale is to decrease urination or defecation, provide information about the body's need for fluids for many processes, and indicate that other discomforts resulting from fluid restrictions may outweigh the effort it takes to make trips to the bathroom or get up on the commode. Also indicate that stools become dryer when less fluid is available and that elimination then requires greater energy and can cause greater anal–perianal pain than if the stools have more moisture in them.

If the purpose is to "starve the tumor" and slow its growth, indicate that there is no research in human beings at this time to show that this actually takes place.

If the patient is seeking to shorten survival time, seek to determine the problems in symptom management or in managing daily living that are creating the discouragement, or the expectation of future events that is frightening. Determine whether greater control of symptoms and in problem solving about daily living may create an improved quality of life.

Inability to ingest the amount of calories and fluids desired

Determine the patient's caloric and fluid goals and the rationale for the desired goals (Horton, 1988).

Provide written information about ways to increase calories in the diet in foods the patient can ingest (e.g., increasing fats [by increasing intake of whole milk, cooked eggs, high-fat cheeses, real ice cream, butter or margarine, and oils] and sugars in foods and fluids, eating 10% to 15% of one's diet in fruits and vegetables rather than a lower amount; eating dried fruits; eating meats that are marbled with fat [if the taste of meat is tolerated], and adding diet supplements). Suggest eating smaller but more frequent meals, but also point out that early satiety and a slower emptying time for the stomach are not uncommon. Suggest taking fluids between meals rather than with meals. Indicate that eating fairly rapidly is a possible way of ingesting more food before the brain signals satiety.

Lack of equipment to provide the most effective meals with advancing cancer

Check on the availability of a small microwave oven, a freezer section in the refrigerator, and a miniature food chopper for the person who is having difficulty in chewing or swallowing. If these are not available, check on the possibility of purchasing them, receiving them as gifts, or borrowing them.

Indicate to the patient that it is helpful to be able to prepare foods on good days and store them in single portions in the freezer in microwavable dishes or plastic for days that are not so good, or to be given single portions of food for freezing. If the person is having trouble with cooking odors, suggest the use of the microwave to defrost and heat food as a means of limiting food odors. Indicate that it is also useful for cooking foods so that they are soft enough to be easy to chew.

Indicate that a miniature food chopper is useful in making meats or vegetables easy to chew, and that the size of the pieces can be varied according to the person's needs. Chop *after* cooking.

Lack of physical strength, endurance, or mentation to procure or prepare food

Determine the current patient status, pattern, and trajectory of strength, energy, and mentation.

If energy levels show a circadian pattern, explore the possibility of shopping or preparing food during the "up" times or days for use during times of low energy.

If energy or mentation have dropped to the point where self-care in meals is no longer possible, gather data on patient perceptions of personal network assistance options. Offer other ideas such as Meals on Wheels or referral for assistance (e.g., shopping volunteers, chore services).

Inadequate symptom management

See section on Chronic Pain and Suffering in this chapter.

Where analgesics such as morphine sulfate seem to be causing gastric stasis, or nonsteroidal anti-inflammatory drugs are causing gastric irritation, check with physician for prescription of metoclopramide hydrochloride to induce gastric emptying for the former or an H2 agonist for the latter (Baines, 1988).

Determine who is bothered by the vomiting (e.g., the patient may prefer to vomit once or twice a day rather than have a nasogastric tube inserted, but the family may be bothered). If the family has the difficulty, help them to manage their distress by discussing the patient's choices and showing them what equipment (receptacles of adequate size with covers, damp washcloths or towels, mouthwash, and breath mints) should be available to efficiently manage the vomiting (Moseley, 1985).

Note that when vomiting has followed eating several times, the patient may be wary of eating again, and the expectation of vomiting may not resolve quickly. Recommend trying small meals of foods not involved in previous vomiting episodes, and using relaxation techniques. (See also Chapter 6, section on Nausea, Vomiting, and Retching.)

Suggest that laxatives, enemas, or suppositories, increased fluid intake, and increased fiber in the diet (if it is not contraindicated) may help relieve constipation, as may controlling pain prior to defecation (Moseley, 1985). (See also Chapter 6, section on Constipation.)

Feeding issue used as a support mechanism for family denial of patient's situation

When the care giver or family members are using the feeding of the patient as a means of supporting their denial, explain the patient's constraints on eating and assimilating food in words that do not use the terms cancer or tumors (e.g., "John's not eating as much these days is he? I think that you'd like to see him eating more, but our experience has shown us that at times the stomach feels full more quickly and also takes longer to empty. Then the person just isn't able to eat as much and doesn't feel hungry, no matter how good the food is. It might be helpful to John if you fix lighter foods and fluids that you know he likes. Offer him small portions on a salad plate instead of a dinner plate and put his drinks in a smaller glass or cup. It will also help if he can rest for about 30 minutes before it's time to eat and if he is not having any discomfort at mealtimes").

Knowledge deficit of impact of advancing neoplastic processes on eating and nutritional status

Determine the symptoms the patient is having that interfere with shopping or food preparation (e.g., altered taste, anorexia, early satiety, feeling full long after the meal, nausea, vomiting, pain, asthenia).

Explain to patient (or care giver, if knowledge deficit is impairing this person's functioning or comfort) in nonthreatening language the basis for the symptoms (e.g., "Jim is feeling full after eating just a little because his liver is a bit bigger and it is taking up space the stomach had—so there's less room for the food"; "Pat is nauseated this week because we just started her on a new medication for her discomfort. It is not uncommon for this drug to cause nausea for about a week or so"; or "For some unknown reason the food tends to remain in the stomach longer than normal—that's the reason you feel full for so long after you've eaten").

Lack of skill or creativeness in food preparation

Arrange a contact between patient, care giver, and nutritionist to discuss information and ideas about food options, given the patient's present and predicted eating difficulties.

If the care provider is assuming a new role in preparing food, suggest asking a person who has these skills to give some lessons in the store and home on shopping for and preparing the types of foods the patient will need and be able to ingest.

If the patient's likes or capabilities limit the range of foods, suggest that the care giver consider small variations (e.g., if the patient eats one kind of melon, try other varieties; if only bland juices are tolerated, consider varieties among the nectars, such as apricot, peach, pear, or guava; if energy for chewing is limited and the taste of meat is tolerated, try ground meats cooked a long time, as in meat balls, or pot roasts, stews, or chicken pies).

Suggest requesting family and friends who have offered to help to cook foods the patient will tolerate or enjoy and package them in single-size servings.

Conflicts concerning control: self-determination versus compliance

Determine the areas of eating in which unresolved issues of control exist, and what the previous patterns of control between the patient and those involved has been. Determine the kinds of difficulties and discomforts the control issues are currently posing to the patient and to others.

Explain to care providers and family members that the timing and amount of eating may be beyond the patient's control—that discomfort, nausea, early satiety, and prolonged fullness arise from tumor effects, and that willpower or wanting to please may not be enough to overcome the body changes.

Explore alternative ways of expressing caring other than trying get the patient to eat and drink. Point out the risk of backlash or of increasing suffering through the addition of guilt feelings. Suggest offering food or fluids in a neutral way at times when the patient seems comfortable, but being accepting if there is a refusal and dropping the subject.

Talk with the patient about responses to the controlling behavior of others in the area of eating. Suggest the development of scripts that communicate both the desire to accommodate and the difficulties (e.g., "I know it bothers you when I can't eat, and I'd like to—if only to make you feel better, but I just can't eat right now. Perhaps later it will be better"), or scripts that indicate that the patient is taking control (e.g., "I'm not able to eat now. I'll save it until I can. Let's not talk about food right now. I'd rather hear about....").

When the patient and family are facing the situation of dehydration associated with terminal illness, indicate that they have the option of accepting or refusing intravenous fluids (Gargaro, 1980). Explain the advantages and difficulties associated with dehydration and with hydration (see Table 10-1). Discuss whether they want to communicate the patient's and family's wishes to the physician or have the nurse speak for them (Zerwekh, 1983).

See also Figure 11-1, "physician directives" or "living will" for communication of patient–family wishes regarding parenteral or enteral nutrition and support of hydration in the terminal phase.

Miscommunication about eating related to lack of understanding of the symbolic aspects of food

If patient and care giver or family members have emotionally laden disagreements about food-related situations but are focusing on the nutritional value of food alone, help them to understand the dynamics of their miscommunications by introducing the idea of food giving more than nutrients to the one who receives the food and also giving something to the one who provides it. Suggest that the patient and those who provide food talk about what food and eating have personally meant to them—what each one has wanted from people who provided them with food and what each wanted from those they fed when they were food providers. Ask them to consider if any of these needs or wishes apply in the present situation: What does the patient need or want from the food provider? What does the food provider want or need from the patient? Is it possible for each to give this to the other? What behavior or strategies would be needed? How can love, caring, or affection be communicated in food-related situations?

Social isolation

Determine patient desires for companionship associated with eating, current experiences, who is or could be available, and patient signs, symptoms, or other deterrents that might make others reluctant to share eating experiences.

If the patient is in the hospital, schedule treatments (e.g., suctioning, dressing changes, ostomy care, oral hygiene, analgesia, and rest periods) so that the patient is as functional, odor- and symptom-free, and rested as possible for planned shared eating experiences. If in the home, suggest that the patient or care giver attempt a similar approach to care.

If the patient is having difficulties in eating, suggest that perhaps only one part of the meal (e.g., a dessert that is easily managed) be shared, or that the patient be present at the whole meal but not attempt to eat everything.

Encourage companions who plan to share a meal with the patient to set an explicit goal of providing pleasure to the patient in the encounter and to consider, in advance, strategies for doing this.

If the patient lacks the energy to eat and participate extensively in the conversation, discuss with care giver or family members strategies for including the patient without requiring too much from him. Alert them to the risk of patient loneliness within the group if others talk "around" the patient. Discuss the option of one-to-one meals on trays at the patient's chair or bedside with conversation and companionable silence employed as the patient's status dictates.

Where unresolved personal issues create tensions and lack of genuine companionship in sharing meals, indicate that different approaches could be considered: participants can acknowledge the limited time remaining in which to resolve unfinished business and work through the difficulties to find understanding and forgiveness for actual or perceived wrongs or misunderstandings, or shared meals can be considered a time of truce in which participants agree to seek to create a pleasant social occasion that will bring pleasure to the patient and other participants.

See also Chapter 6, section on Difficulties in Eating, under Treatment Guidelines.

Frustration and burnout of the food preparer-care giver

See in Chapter 6, section on Difficulties in Eating, treatment guidelines for dissatisfaction with the lack of positive feedback from the situation; discouragement and feeling of wanting to give up; and frustration with the monotony of preparing the same foods in the same way day after day.

Dry mouth from dehydration (De Conno et al, 1989; Zerwekh, 1983)

Instruct care giver to:

Give patient frequent oral hygiene, removing debris (food, dried sputum) from the mouth and brushing tongue, gums, and teeth with a soft toothbrush, using toothpaste or dipping the brush in diluted mouthwash (avoid the drying effects of lemon and glycerin)

Clean any debris from lips and corners of the mouth, and coat lips with Chapstick, Vaseline, or other protective coating

Offer frequent mouth rinses (with water or mouthwash, diluted to reduce the drying effects of the alcohol)

Offer ice chips, chips of frozen juice, or tonic water

Offer tart hard candies

Increase the air humidity with a humidifier or other moisture-releasing devices

Evaluation   Patient response to nursing treatment may be evidenced in the status of:

Adequacy of self-care in procuring and preparing food or adequacy of assistance in providing nutrients when self-care is no longer possible

Knowledge needed to understand and manage changing body responses to food and eating

Skill in shopping and food preparation

Access to equipment to expedite preparation and storage of food in a usable form

Nutritional goals

Comfort and satisfaction with food-related interactions, including shopping, food preparation and serving, and skill of the person feeding the patient

Quality and adequacy of food and fluids available to or being offered to the patient

Intake of nutrients and fluids commensurate with capacity and goals

Congruence of nutritional goals of patient, health care providers, and care givers

Resolution of control issues over patient eating and fluid intake, including the option for untreated dehydration in the terminal phase

Satisfaction with social aspects of eating and meals

Family response to nursing treatment can be evidenced by status of family member's or care giver's:

Use of feeding as a support to their current denial of the patient's advancing cancer

Knowledge about the patient's changing pathophysiology and its effect on eating, digestion, and food assimilation

Capacity to translate the above knowledge into food preparation, serving, and eating-related interaction with the patient

Skill in shopping, preparing, and serving food and fluids appropriate to the patient's needs and capacities

Equating feeding with love and patient eating with reciprocation of love or appreciation

Responses to patient's eating patterns, such as frustration,
anger, or guilt

Satisfaction with role rewards as food preparer

Resolution of control issues related to patient eating and fluid
intake

Strategies to minimize physical or emotional distancing associated with patient's symptoms or status when meals are
shared

Unresolved interpersonal issues interfering with genuine
companionship in food-related activities

Participation in decisions about management of patient's
terminal dehydration and satisfaction with decisions

Living With Chronic Pain and Suffering

The presence of pain in people experiencing advancing cancer is a common and
feared occurrence; 60% to 90% report pain as a disturbing symptom (Bonica, 1984;
Cleeland, 1985; Foley, 1986). Pain can be a constant experience, an unrelenting
companion in daily living.

Left untreated or undertreated, chronic cancer pain can affect all aspects of daily
living, including sleep, work-related activities, social interactions, mobility, eating, and
sexual activity (Meinhart and McCaffery, 1986). Already facing uncertainty and
disappointment because of the advancing disease, people with unrelieved chronic
cancer pain can experience even greater emotional suffering. This, in turn, can adversely affect the desire and ability to carry out daily living.

Medical Perspective

From the medical perspective, chronic cancer pain is often associated with tumor
progression. It can indicate that the patient's tumor is not responding to treatment or
that earlier treatment is causing iatrogenic pain. The goal of medical treatment in
chronic cancer pain is relief from pain or palliation. Expertise in pharmacologic approaches alone is thought to have the potential to relieve about 70% of cancer pain
(Portenoy, 1988).

Opioid analgesics are the most frequently prescribed because of their recognized
effectiveness (McGivney and Crooks, 1984). Morphine sulfate, the prototype of opioid
analgesics, is prescribed using many routes of administration (Howard-Ruben et al,
1987):

Oral: Elixir, liquid, or tablet form (including sublingual and sustained release tablets) are
available.

Rectal: Morphine suppositories are used when there is nausea and vomiting. No measuring is required, so they may be easier to administer for some care givers.

Intramuscular: This is the least favored route. Patients with advancing disease lose muscle mass and may have hemopoietic factors contraindicating ongoing use of this route.

Intravenous: Intravenous morphine may be given as a bolus by staff or by patient with a patient-controlled analgesia machine, or as a continuous infusion.

Epidural: Epidural morphine may be given as a bolus or as a continuous infusion. Smaller amounts are required by this route. Epidural morphine can give relief for 8 to 24 hours; however, it can result in delayed respiratory depression 12 to 24 hours after injection.

Decisions about the route of delivery depend on several factors: whether the patient is in an institution or in a home setting, the functional capacities of the patient or care giver, and the dosage of morphine sulfate required.

Other pharmacologic interventions include the use of nonsteroidal anti-inflammatory drugs (e.g., aspirin, ibuprofen, indomethacin, or acetaminophen) in conjunction with opioids. This combination results in effective analgesia for many patients, especially those with bone pain (Ferrer-Brechner and Ganz, 1984).

Physicians may also use radiation directed to tumor sites to decrease tumor bulk and relieve pressure, or surgical severing of nerves associated with the pain site. Another technique involves neural blockade with injections of anesthetic or alcohol.

Nursing Perspective

Whereas medicine tends to focus on pain, nursing's focus encompasses the larger problem of pain plus the associated suffering. Suffering is an affective state that includes not only the somatic pain, but also the negative affective perceptions associated with physical disability, isolation, financial concerns, loss of role, and fear of death (Portenoy, 1988).

Nursing is concerned with the effect of daily living on the patient's pain, and the effect of the pain on the patient's and family's daily living. Nursing seeks to prevent or minimize pain and suffering. When total pain control is not possible, nursing diagnosis and treatment concerns management of daily living as effectively as possible in the presence of pain for the patient, family, and personal care givers (Ferrell and Schneider, 1988).

Nature of Chronic Pain and Suffering

Chronic cancer pain may begin gradually, but tends to persist and recur. For most patients the pain is in the moderate to severe range. Its constancy, even when the levels of pain are not severe, tends to make it intolerable after a time. It no longer serves a protective function, but becomes a destructive disease in itself.

When uncontrolled or undercontrolled, this type of pain is unremitting and intractable (Meinhart and McCaffery, 1986). (See Table 6-5 for the nature of tumor-related pain and Table 7-1 for post-treatment pain patterns.)

Patients and family members who closely share the daily living have been found to be competent in describing the patient's pain when they are given credibility, permission, and the instruments to do so (e.g., analogue scales, pain descriptor forms, pain–analgesia logs), (Molbo, 1986; O'Brien and Francis, 1988).

Suffering is a personal experience that occurs as a result of the composite of all noxious stimuli and unpleasant factors in a person's daily living and the meanings assigned to them. It will vary with the individual and will be influenced by religious and cultural beliefs and by past and current experiences. It is shaped not only by somatic problems, but also by the person's interpretation of the meaning and significance of the somatic problems (Benedict, 1989). Suffering is heightened when the person experiences sorrow, dissatisfaction, fear, anxiety, uncertainty, threat, pain, and dependency. Suffering is inescapable in the face of death (Duclow, 1988).

Chronic pain in advancing cancer is a major contributor to suffering, but it is rare that pain is the only source of physical discomfort. The suffering from cancer pain is compounded by other concurrent physical problems, such as nausea, vomiting, diarrhea or constipation, dysuria, sleep disruption, fatigue, and dyspnea. The suffering generated by the totality of physical discomfort may be greater than the sum of the parts. Chronic cancer pain plus the other problems of the advancing disease result in greater, more rapid physical deterioration than that which occurs in people with noncancer chronic pain (Bonica, 1984).

Emotional suffering is another dimension of the patient's experience of advancing cancer. The emotional status of the patient is both a consequence of and a contributor to chronic cancer pain. People with uncontrolled cancer pain tend to respond in ways that could be given psychiatric labels; however, psychiatric diagnoses are not assigned unless the symptoms continue after pain has been adequately controlled (Derogatis et al, 1983; Massie and Holland, 1987).

The Meaning of Chronic Cancer Pain

The meaning of chronic cancer pain is different from that experienced in the acute phase. The patient and family tend to manage even severe pain associated with treatment because of hope for cure and an expectation that there will be an end point to the discomfort (Foley, 1987). The pain associated with advancing cancer conveys quite a different message—a loss of hope. Chronic cancer pain brings regular reminders that cannot be ignored—the cancer is not going away; it is advancing. This in turn can create a dark emotional shadow of sadness, fear, anger, depression, and despair that pervades attitudes toward life and living.

Chronic cancer pain goes beyond physical suffering. Once-pleasurable activities require painful effort to initiate and sustain. Relinquishing those pleasures to avoid aggravating one's pain can represent a significant loss that unleashes the emotions of grief.

Manifestations of Chronic Cancer Pain

The person experiencing chronic cancer pain does not exhibit the physiologic signs common to acute pain. The autonomic nervous system adapts to the chronic pain. The patient's report of pain is the only real measure of its existence (Coyle and Foley, 1985). Other indirect manifestations of chronic cancer pain include depression, fatigue, withdrawal, disinterest, inability to cheer up at the prospect of pleasure, uneasiness, anger, disturbed sleep, loss of appetite, loss of ability to concentrate, shortened attention span, repetitive speech, muscle rigidity, bruxing (grinding one's teeth), restless legs, holding tight to someone or something, decreased social interaction and conversation, emotional lability, and increased sensitivity to noise, censure, or indicators of decreased support from others (Kerr 1987–1988; Massie and Holland, 1987; Molbo, 1986; Noyes and Kathol, 1985). Engaging in pain-controlling behaviors may also be indicative of pain (e.g., taking analgesics; guarding, immobilizing, or repositioning body areas; rubbing or adjusting pressure on painful areas).

Major depressions are a common corollary to chronic cancer pain (Massie and Holland, 1987). While acute pain is accompanied by anxiety, chronic pain is linked to depression (Sternbach, 1974).

Responses to the Experience of Pain and Suffering

People who experience chronic cancer pain and the associated suffering in their lives can ultimately respond in several ways (Copp, 1985). Some become apathetic and allow events to wash over them. Those who take a more active approach can be perceived as responding in two different ways—by *resistance* or by *transformation* (Duclow, 1988).

Resistors continue to struggle against the disease and its manifestations despite the reality that aggressive therapy cannot produce a cure (Duclow, 1988). In their resistance they continue to hope for and seek recovery. Such patients may see adequate analgesia as diminishing or defeating their capacities to resist further encroachment of the cancer.

Those who deal with the chronic pain and suffering of advancing cancer by transformation engage in a different struggle. They strive not against the disease, but with their own attitudes of acceptance of the reality of their situation and for areas for control (Duclow, 1988). Such patients and families may accept analgesia more readily as a means of sustaining quality of life and permitting more effective management of daily living and achievement of life goals when cure is no longer possible.

Underlying Mechanisms

The underlying mechanisms for chronic cancer pain and for the associated suffering and difficulties in managing daily living are multiple. They encompass the pathology, medical patterns of treatment, other discomforts, pain-related physical limitations, losses that are anticipated or occurring, and emotional responses to all of these.

Pathophysiologic and Iatrogenic Factors

Tumor-Related Factors   The incidence and severity of pain varies with the location of the tumor. Tumors involving the pancreas, bone, stomach, and cervix create more pain than do leukemias and cancers of the kidney, colon, or breast (Meinhart and McCaffery, 1986). (For specifics refer to Table 6-5.) Tumors that invade nerve complexes (e.g., the brachial plexus or single nerves) or those in hard enclosed spaces (e.g., bone) cause severe pain.

The rate of tumor growth can also affect pain control. Some tumors, such as Burkitt's lymphoma and other lymphomas, can grow at a phenomenal rate. At the same time, it can take 15 hours to achieve a steady state of 90% serum opioid levels for a designated level of pain control. By the time one level of pain control has been reached, the tumor can have grown so much that higher serum opioid levels are needed. A situation of ineffective "catch up" can result.

Treatment-Related Factors

Medical treatment of chronic pain associated with advancing cancer is directed toward relieving pain, not creating iatrogenic pain, as occurred in the initial treatment phase. However, medical treatment of chronic cancer pain often leaves it uncontrolled or undercontrolled. A variety of factors, singly and in combination, contribute to inadequate medical treatment to obtain pain control. These include:

Failure to recognize the difference between the patient's growing tolerance for analgesics and the quite different problem of psychologic and physiologic addiction to drugs that occurs among people not experiencing chronic cancer pain

Unwillingness to accept the patient's perceptions of pain as the authoritative criteria for the level of pain that is present

Failure to consider the diminished physiologic manifestations of pain associated with the body's having adapted to the ongoing presence of the pain

Inadequate knowledge about equianalgesic dosage, routes of administration, and drug tolerance

Differences in beliefs about the level of pain that is considered acceptable or tolerable on a day-to-day basis for patients (e.g., one resident-level physician indicated that a 5 level of pain on a scale of 10 was "quite acceptable,"* while the nurse caring for the same patient believed that 3 was the acceptable maximum and that lower levels than that were highly desirable, given the highly eroding qualities of persistent, unrelieved pain).

False ideas that the patient who can sleep is not experiencing pain (McCaffery, 1979)

Daily Living Factors

Activities in Daily Living

Activities in daily living can both affect and be affected by chronic cancer pain and suffering. Physical activities and the time of day when they occur can affect the amount of pain experienced and the need for a particular pattern of analgesia

---

*Among 101 patients assigned psychiatric labels in a study looking at the prevalence of psychiatric diagnoses among patients experiencing pain, 39 rated the severity of their pain >50 on a scale of 0 (no pain) to 100 (worst possible pain). Among the 114 who were not given psychiatric labels only 19 rated their pain >50 (Derogatis et al, 1983).

(e.g., preparations for an evening meal, going for an appointment, or work).

The activities of others in the household can also affect the patient's pain experience (e.g., sensory overload from the activities and noise of young children or adolescents; grief over one's husband moving out of the bed and bedroom that the couple have shared for 30 years).

There may be times in the day when relative freedom from pain is particularly important (e.g., when quality time is desired with particular members of the family, such as when the children come home from school or the spouse comes home from work).

The activities in daily living (both care giving and other activities) of the primary care giver or support person can also play a part in determining the comfort of the patient. For example, if the care giver must also work outside the home to provide the family's income, then pain management is left to the patient. The care giver may have little energy left over to support the patient in the pain and suffering being experienced, and may also require adequate sleep to be able to function on the job. Thus the patient may have long, lonely hours with the suffering, both at night and in the daytime.

Events in Daily Living

Events in which the patient wishes to participate may dictate particular temporary needs for comfort and pain control, requiring supplementation of the usual dosage.

Demands in Daily Living

The person who has pain has self-expectations regarding personal behavior in response to the pain experience and also has expectations about how others will respond in their daily living toward the person in pain. In turn, others who share the patient's daily living have expectations about the atttitude and activities of the person in pain and how they should behave and respond to the pain and the person (Franklin, 1988; Levin et al, 1985). The expectations of family members, employers, or coworkers may exceed or underestimate the patient's capacity to function in the presence of pain; they may support or negate the patient's emotional and physical approach to the pain experience. Lack of congruence in expectations and demands between the patient and those who share the daily living can contribute to the patient's suffering.

The demands of the patient and the health care system that care givers and family members manage the analgesic technology and the patient's pain experiences may exceed their cognitive, emotional, and physical capabilities.

The inability to adjust role requirements to accommodate increasing pain and associated functional restrictions is also an area for consideration. (See Chapter 6, section on Role.)

Environment for Daily Living

The physical and sensory aspects of the environment are considered in terms of the barriers to effective management of daily living, given the pain patterns the patient is experiencing. Mobility restrictions suggest consideration of stairs, railings for support, and distances to frequently used facilities. Lighting and potential for controlling noise and odors are other considerations. Opportunities to be with others and to experience diversion and sensory stimulation or to limit participation and sensory input can make a difference in management of daily living with chronic cancer pain.

The nature of the neighborhood and any concerns for personal safety in purchasing, transporting, or storing prescribed narcotics in the home may be an area for investigation in some circumstances.

Changing one's environment, as in moving from one hospital to another or to home or a long-term care facility, may mean changing the technology for adequate pain control. Even changing from one unit to another within a hospital can result in different approaches to the analgesia regimen. For example, on surgical units bolus administration of analgesics is most common, while on oncology units continuous infusions are not uncommon. If a patient moves from the oncology unit and continuous infusions to a surgical unit and the bolus pattern, pain control can be radically changed.

Values and Beliefs

Patient comfort and patterns of use of analgesics will be affected by values and beliefs of the patient, family members, and care givers (personal or professional). Values and beliefs that can be involved include:

The level of pain or comfort believed to be acceptable on an ongoing basis

Belief in the appropriateness of an analgesic protocol that seeks to maintain steady-state serum levels of the drug by administration of the analgesic agent at regular intervals around the clock, rather than giving analgesics only after the patient's pain becomes severe

Belief in the redemptive qualitities of pain

Belief that dosages of analgesics sufficient to control current pain will preclude adequate control of pain as the cancer advances, as opposed to the belief that there should be no upper limit on the amount of analgesics that can be given to achieve ongoing pain control

Belief that drug tolerance and drug addiction are the same and that both are either immoral or criminal

Valuing of courage and stoicism over comfort

Functional Health Status

Strength and Endurance
Chronic cancer pain will affect strength and endurance. Uncontrolled cancer pain is debilitating. It reduces the desire to move, to be active, and to eat. It causes patients to draw into themselves—to withdraw from external events. Pain also contributes to sleep deprivation. Uncontrolled or undercontrolled chronic cancer pain can produce stress sufficient to exhaust the patient's physical and emotional resources for managing the requirements of daily living.

At the same time, weakness and fatigue make enduring chronic cancer pain more difficult.

Analgesics used to control the pain can contribute to losses in physical energy through their sedative effects; however, the comfort derived with pain control can contribute to the maintenance of emotional resources.

Personal care givers can develop deficits in their own strength and endurance as they share the patient's pain experience around the clock, day after day. Sleep deprivation can be a problem for family members or care givers as well as the patient.

Sensory Responses
Chronic cancer pain can cause the individual to become increasingly sensitive to sensory overload and to cues that are perceived as indicative of censure, lack of support, and physical or emotional separation.

Cognition and Communication
Pain is distracting and disorganizing. It interferes with thinking and processing of other stimuli. It causes the person to be less willing to participate.

It has been suggested that, as cancer progresses, the adaptive response makes individuals become more passive and less verbal, to the point where they fail to adequately identify to others the pain they are experiencing (Abrams, 1966).

The capacity to communicate the nature of the pain experience in a credible way may also be limited by not having a common vocabulary with physicians and nurses. If central nervous system tumors or metastases further impair cognition, it can be increasingly difficult to communicate the reality of the pain experience.

Personal care givers may be so desirous of improvement that they seek to deny the patient's pain and its significance. Patients may not wish to hurt or disappoint their health care providers and care givers and may seek to disguise or hide their suffering.

Mood
Depression is a common mood with chronic pain. There is a frightening, negative significance to the pain of advancing cancer—that the disease is not being controlled. This can lead to despair. Passiveness and apathy may occur (Abrams, 1966).

Post-treatment pain may continue despite the reality that the treatment was not effective. The post-treatment pain may have been unanticipated, or may occur long after the treatment was completed. Anger at health care providers may emerge. Easy irritability may occur.

Care givers, both personal and professional, can experience continuing fear, anxiety, frustration, helplessness, anger, and sadness at seeing the patient suffer and at being ineffective in their comfort measures.

Skills   Ongoing control of escalating pain as cancer advances often requires skill and coordination in administration of the analgesics, in use of high technology equipment, and in documentation.

External Resources

Managing daily living with the chronic pain of advancing cancer is highly dependent on external resources. The availability, accessibility, expertise, and skill of physicians and nurses in utilizing the most effective, current knowledge and technology for pain control can be major factors in effective daily living with cancer pain. The availability of technology and equipment in the health care setting (e.g., hospital, nursing home, or home) is also important. Pain control achieved in one setting can be lost when the locale of health care changes. Money for analgesics and transportation to pick up medications and supplies are important external resources. Another important external factor is the availability of home care nurses skilled in addressing the pain control need of the cancer patient and family. Some home health care agencies have especially trained and designated cancer home care nurses.

Nursing Diagnosis and Treatment

Diagnostic Targets   The targets for nursing diagnosis and treatment include the patient, care givers (including nurses and physicians as well as personal care givers), family, and others who may share the patient's suffering).

Risk Factors   Factors that increase the risk of not managing daily living in the face of the pain of advancing cancer include:

Having tumors that cause the greatest pain (e.g., invasion of neural plexes, bony metastases)

Living alone

Lacking consistent, competent care givers

Living in a geographic area that lacks professionals skilled in pharmacologic, surgical, and anesthetic techniques for controlling the pain of advancing cancer

Having care givers (professional or personal) whose knowledge deficits, attitudes, or beliefs interfere with adequate pain control

Having inadequate or impaired capacity to communicate the pain experience (patient, family member, personal care giver)

Being dependent on others to pick up or administer narcotics or other analgesics

Being severely depressed or highly anxious

Experiencing other concurrent manifestations of the advancing cancer or post-treatment discomforts and difficulties

Having had inadequate pain management in the past that generates fears of failure to control present and future pain (Molbo, 1986)

Living in a setting with sensory overload or underload

Having role obligations that cannot be shifted to others

Fearing addiction (McCaffery, 1979)

Diagnostic Areas

PATIENT

Inadequate pain management R/T:

Knowledge deficit about the effect of the drug

Physiologic tolerance for current drug dosage

Inappropriate concern about addiction in end-stage cancer

Failure to accept analgesia now for fear of subsequent loss of pain control

Knowledge deficit regarding need to maintain steady state of serum levels of the analgesic and strategies for doing this

Transition from hospital to nursing home or home setting with less skilled pain managers

Lack of skill in pain assessment and management skills among care providers

Inadequate equipment or skill in using equipment to maintain an optimum regimen

Limited reporting of the level of pain R/T:

Lack of vocabulary or availability of analogue guide

Fear of disappointing the physician or care giver

Need to be stoic

Attribution of redemptive qualities to pain

Impaired mobility, self-care, or care of immediate environment R/T anticipated or unrelieved pain

Difficulties in asking for or accepting assistance R/T unacceptability of being dependent on others

Disrupted social, family, or marital relationships R/T unmanaged pain

Difficulty in carrying out of role responsibilities (specify role—e.g., parent, homemaker, employee) R/T uncontrolled or undercontrolled pain

Unrealistic planning for daily living R/T failure to include pain as a factor

Fear of picking up and transporting narcotics from the pharmacy or of having them in the home R/T the possibility of assault or robbery

CARE GIVERS   Difficulty in helping to manage patient's pain R/T:

High level of anxiety and feelings of helplessness, L/T reluctance to be available to the patient

Knowledge deficit of the need to maintain adequate, steady serum levels of the analgesic agent

Lack of (specified) skills in administering analgesics to the patient

Inability to interpret patient's pain signals

Ineffectiveness in communicating the patient's pain experiences to the physician or nurse

Values and beliefs that preclude adequate pain control

Exhaustion from sleep deprivation and long hours of care without respite

Difficulty in relating to patient in a satisfying way R/T discomfort at being in the presence of the patient's pain

Manifestations   Signs and symptoms that daily living is being disrupted or not effectively managed in the presence of present or threatened pain will focus on the patient, family, and care givers.

PATIENT   Reported:

Fear of anticipated pain

Experiences of unrelieved pain

Increasing pain-related mobility restrictions

Decreased eating related to pain

Sleep loss; long, lonely nights

Inability to think or concentrate

Unusual irritability

Inability to function in usual or desired activities because of pain

Neglect of basic self-care

Difficulties with analgesic-related constipation

Observed:

Becoming more withdrawn and introspective than usual

Deterioration of personal appearance, grooming, and self-care

Reducing eating and drinking in order to minimize trips to the bathroom

Napping in the daytime, but restless at night

Becoming less active

Having difficulty with engaging in usual functions associated with work, home maintenance, parenting, cooking, sexuality, relating to others, and so on

Becoming more easily irritated

Reluctance to participate in family or group gatherings, telephone conversations, or other social activities

Failure to replenish analgesics and other supplies

Refusal of pain medications despite the recognized existence of pain and suffering

FAMILY, CARE GIVERS

Reported:

Feelings of helplessness and frustration at not being able to bring comfort to the patient

Difficulty in being around the patient and witnessing the pain experience

Not knowing how to talk to the patient

Not knowing how to recognize signals of pain

Not knowing how to help the patient to describe the pain experience or how to communicate the patient's pain experience to the doctor or nurse in a useful way

Lacking the skills or desire to administer the prescribed analgesic regimen

Fear of moving the patient or giving personal care R/T reluctance to cause more pain or lack of knowledge and skills on how to carry out tasks with the least amount of patient discomfort

Chronic sleep deprivation related to the patient's discomfort and restlessness at night

Inability to prevent or deal with the patient's increased irritability, depression

Personal depression over the meaning of the patient's pain pattern

Observed:

Avoidance of being with the patient or unusual superficiality in relating to the patient

Lack of skill in administering analgesics, moving the patient, or giving personal care in the least painful way

Failure to follow the analgesic regimen in ways that promote stable serum values

Growing fatigue

Growing sadness or depression

Prognostic Variables

A poor prognosis for managing daily living with the pain of advancing cancer is associated with:

A pain management regimen that is not adequate to afford pain relief as defined by the patient

Tumors that grow so quickly that control is difficult if not impossible

Pain management technology that is difficult or impossible to transfer from one hospital to another or to home or nursing home

Care givers who fail to follow the prescribed pain regimen and do not give as much medication as has been prescribed

Patient or family beliefs that it is not possible to control chronic cancer pain

Complications

Complications associated with ineffectiveness in managing daily living with chronic cancer pain include:

Unnecessary immobilization and restriction of activities

Disruption of relationships with family, close friends, and support persons

Increased suffering and self-absorption

Decreased eating, sleep disturbances, and increased fatigue

Physical, cognitive, and emotional deterioration

Suicide or active euthanasia by a family member who can no longer witness the patient's suffering

Treatment Guidelines

Treatment will be directed toward the patient's internal resources for managing pain, suffering, and the associated daily living activities and relationships. It can also be directed to care givers and family members as they seek to deal with the patient's pain-related difficulties and their own responses.

Lack of knowledge about the effect of drug tolerance on drug dosage requirements

Give information about drug tolerance with confidence and sincerity. These attitudes are as important as the content.

Use confidence-building initial phrases such as "Research has shown..."; "Our experience has shown us that..."; or "There's one thing we know for sure and that is that...."

Provide the information in an easily understood manner (e.g., "The body gets accustomed to the amount of drug it is receiving and then eventually the pain breaks through. This tells us that it is time for more medication. It is not the amount of drug being received that is important, but the body's response to it. We have seen patients receiving 250 mg of morphine each hour who were awake, talking, responding, and doing what they wanted to do" or "Morphine is a good drug when it is properly used to treat certain types of pain, just as aspirin is a good drug for other types of pain").

Use the American Cancer Society pamphlet "Questions and Answers about Pain Control" (1983).

Inappropriate concern about addiction

Provide information that:

Addiction is rarely a problem for patients with cancer pain (if they were not addicts before the cancer)

Patients whose pain has decreased or been managed by other medical treatments have been found not to want any more morphine

At this time, comfort is more important than concern about addiction

Indicate that others may be concerned about the patient's addiction because of their lack of correct information. Help the patient to develop some scripts (e.g., "My nurse (or doctor) tells me that addiction to morphine is a rare problem with their patients who have pain because of their tumors. At this point maintaining comfort and quality of life is the important concern" or "Research has shown that the body does become accustomed to a certain amount of morphine in the body and then the pain can break through. This is a signal to the doctor that the body needs an additional amount of the medication. But this body response is not addiction").

Failure to accept adequate analgesia for fear of inadequate pain control if it is needed more later

Ask if their concern arises because they have known of other patients who had cancer whose pain was not controlled.

Explain that there are now many more options for controlling pain than there were even 5 years ago.

Use such reassuring statements as, "I'm not worried that we will be able to manage your pain."

Failure to take analgesics on a schedule that maintains steady serum levels because of lack of knowledge

Explain that with analgesics taken by mouth it is essential to maintain a round-the-clock routine because it is necessary to maintain a steady level of the medication in the bloodstream—just as one does when one takes penicillin to control an infection.

If the patient is being started on analgesia by infusion, explain that the concentration of the medication in the fluid is much lower than when it is taken by mouth and that it takes about 15 hours to arrive at 90% effectiveness, and that therefore during that initial period, additional amounts will be given to keep the patient comfortable until the blood level has been achieved.

Don't make assumptions about the knowledge level of care givers in other settings. Gather information and then make the plan for pain management so that the patient's comfort is maintained in the transition.

When a patient is being transferred from the hospital to a long-term care facility where the personnel's expertise in cancer pain management is unknown, write a discharge summary to be sent with the patient in which the pain management schedule and its rationale are specifically discussed, and follow up with a phone call to explain the patient's situation and any special problems or techniques that may be helpful in the new care setting.

If a patient is being discharged to home care or to a nursing home where there is some concern about the capacity to manage the pain regimen, several days (more than 48 hours) prior to discharge, work with the physician to change the analgesia regimen to one that is within the capacity of patient or care givers (e.g., sustained-release oral morphine).

If the patient is being discharged to a home setting, work through contingency plans for common problem areas with the patient:

If one day you find that you hurt every time you move, what will you do? (Suggest phoning the doctor.)

What will you do if your care giver has to be away for 8 hours? (This may give data on the patient's willingness to skip doses of analagesia.)

What will you do if your family or friends express concern about addiction? (See scripts offered earlier in the treatment guidelines.)

What will you do if you notice a pattern that you begin to feel pain before the next dose of analgesia is due? (Suggest that if it is 30 minutes or less, to try taking the medication early; if the pain is relieved for only 2½ hours and the patient is on an every 3 hour schedule, suggest phoning the doctor—it may be time to adjust the dosage or the frequency.)

Lack of skill in pain assessment and management by care providers

Use the McGill–Melzack pain questionnaire or other pain description forms to help patient and care givers develop verbal skills for locating, describing, and quantifying pain (Melzack, 1975; Molbo, 1986).

Legitimize use of the patient's words to describe the pain experience and use of the care giver's own words to describe observed patient responses to the pain (Copp, 1985). Demonstrate how to give such descriptions and offer to help them as they begin to do so.

Provide a pain log. Demonstrate how to communicate about the patient's pain pattern from information care givers gather.

Suggest that they need to contact the doctor or nurse if the pain is not controlled or if the patient becomes unable to take anything by mouth and is on an oral analgesic, develops unmanageable constipation, becomes nauseated, or becomes confused.

Inadequate equipment or lack of skill in using the technology to maintain adequate pain control

Arrange for a secure method of financing the use of the equipment and supplies.

Train the patient and care giver in the skills of using the equipment on several occasions before discharge.

Make a home visit to assure that the skills have transferred from the hospital to the home setting.

Offer support via the telephone as needed.

Limited reporting of level of pain and pain patterns

Provide the patient and care giver with logs that include analogue scales, pain descriptors, and places for documentation.

Use pain descriptors in data gathering about the patient's pain. If the patient says, "Yes, that's the pain I have" (e.g., burning pain), follow with questions such as:

Where is it located?

Does it move?

When does it change?

Is it there when you wake up? Does it waken you?

Instruct the patient that using these words and descriptions in telling health care providers about the pain will help them to understand. Offer an example of a clear pain description (e.g., "You have a steady burning pain on the inner aspect of your left arm. It doesn't move and doesn't change. It is there when you wake up, and you notice it when you turn in bed during the night").

Underreporting of the true severity of the pain

If the patient does not tell the doctor about pain that the nurse has observed or denies pain when asked by the doctor, make the following type of comment, "I was surprised you didn't tell the doctor about the pain you have been having." Pause to allow time to offer an explanation should the patient wish to do so. Point out that the doctor needs to know about the pain in order to give proper medical care.

Document the pain patterns the patient has been having and make a follow-up contact with the physician.

Speak to the family separately, asking about the patient's pain and its management:

Do you think the patient is getting adequate relief from the pain medications?

Is the patient accepting all of the pain medications that are offered?

Do you have any idea as to why the patient may not wish to let others know how much pain is actually being experienced (e.g., fear of loss of control)?

When the nature of underreporting has been confirmed, negotiate with the family to speak for them in a family conference with the patient. Go in and see the patient together and tell the patient of the family's concern that he is having discomfort and suffering when it could be managed. Point out that when the patient is suffering those who care about him are also hurting. Negotiate for some mutually acceptable strategies for reporting pain and receiving relief.

Need to be stoic about the pain experience

First attempt to build a trusting relationship with the patient. Determine whether the stoicism is based on a personal preference (e.g., male machismo image), a cultural norm, or other factors.

With male machismo it is often possible to use a teasing approach (e.g., "We really don't need another super tough guy on this unit" or "We'll enjoy your male macho in other respects, but let us at least make you a bit more comfortable").

With culture-based stoicism, acknowledge and respect the cultural values, but offer the option of managing at least a portion of the pain. Give sound reasons for this option (e.g., "If we can keep you more comfortable, you will be able to eat better, enjoy what you want to and relate more comfortably with your family").

Difficulty in asking for or accepting help associated with the pain experience

Gather data on the basis for difficulty in asking for assistance.

Discuss options and strategies that might be more comfortable, such as:

Mutual planning of schedules and of activities in which help is needed with the care giver or family member, followed by carrying out of the activities as planned (eliminating the need to request help) and regular times of evaluating and readjusting the schedules and activities

Setting up of the patient's immediate surroundings so that objects, medications, fluids, phone or signal device, diversions, and so on are comfortably available for daytime and nighttime use

Explore with the patient the possibility of the patient or the nurse talking with others about the difficulties the patient is experiencing in being dependent, with the idea that others could make specific offerings of assistance (e.g., "I would like to come over on Tuesday and help to...," not "If you need anything, just give me a call"). (Wendy Bergren, a cancer patient, identified 20 suggestions for ways to help. They can be obtained by writing to Focus on the Family, Box 500, Arcadia, CA 91006.) Or, negotiate with care givers, family, or friends to tell the patient that they need to know what the patient would find helpful and ask how the patient would feel comfortable in providing this information.

When the patient makes the transition from one care setting to another, provide information about the patient's reluctance to request assistance and indicate strategies that have proven successful. Follow up with a phone call to patient or family when this is possible.

Disrupted social or family relationships R/T pain

Determine the relationships that have been affected and how they have been changed by the presence of pain (e.g., the family member or friend who cannot stand to see someone in pain discontinues face-to-face or even phone contacts). Note particular events or times when the difficulties occur (e.g., at mealtime; when the children come home from school; during infrequent or special visits from friends or relatives who have travelled some distance).

Try to adjust the pain medication regimen to provide comfort at critical times (e.g., modify the dosage, propose a period of rest prior to important activities).

When others' relationships toward the patient become disrupted because they cannot bear to see the patient in pain, ask a health care provider whom the family members would trust, respect, and listen to (e.g., chaplain, physician, head nurse, clinical nurse specialist) to offer guidelines for the family's and friends' behavior based on what the patient needs at this time, followed by expectations for the behavior the patient will exhibit. Follow up to determine how the situation is progressing from the patient's and family's perspective.

Difficulties with role responsibilities because of pain

See Chapter 6, section on Role, under Treatment Guidelines.

Realistic fear of transporting narcotics to the home or having them in the home

Mobilize a service to have the narcotics brought or delivered to the home rather than having the patient or a family member pick them up.

Evaluation

Patient response to nursing interventions can be evaluated in terms of the status of:

Comfort within care settings or in transitions between care settings

Capacity and willingness to accurately and credibly describe the pain experience

Satisfaction with the pain regimen

Capacity to participate in daily living activities and events at a level commensurate with other functional capacities

Management of side-effects of analgesics

Access to analgesics and associated technology

Participation in the prescribed analgesic regimen

Congruence between beliefs and values, pain experienced, and analgesic regimen

Family or care giver response to nursing treatment can be evaluated in terms of the status of:

Comfort with the level of pain control achieved by the current regimen

Skills, willingness, and credibility in describing patient's pain experiences to health care professionals

Congruence between beliefs and values of appropriate levels of pain control and actual or planned analgesic approaches

Competence and comfort with the skills needed to administer the analgesics and associated technology

Alterations in relationships with the patient associated with patient's pain and pain-related behavior

Living With Dyspnea

Dyspnea can be a presenting symptom with some cancers, but it is more common during advanced stages. At this point it is often only one of several concurrent dysfunctions and may be overlooked in terms of its particular impact on daily living.

Medical Perspective

Medicine's perspective is to determine the etiology and pathology of the ventilatory deficit. Medical management tends to be pharmacologic, using expectorants, narcotics, sedatives, steroids, antimuscarinic agents, or oxygen to improve the airway, gaseous exchange, and patient comfort (Billings, 1985).

Nursing Perspective

Nursing diagnoses and treats situations that tend to trigger dyspneic attacks as well as the disruptions, problems, and dysfunctions in managing daily living arising from the associated loss of strength and endurance. The dyspnea-related anxiety of the patient and family members or care givers is also a focus for nursing diagnosis and treatment.

Nature of Dyspnea

Dyspnea is a demand for ventilation that cannot be met by the individual (West, 1985). It is also a subjective sensory experience of difficult, uncomfortable, labored breathing that can only be described and rated by the person experiencing it. The patient's reported experience does not necessarily correlate with measures of pulmonary function or blood gases (Janson-Bjerklie et al, 1986; Zerwekh, 1987).

In advanced cancers dyspneic episodes show a distinctive, consistent pattern of a slow onset, a lengthy plateau, and a gradual decrease (Brown et al, 1986). Problems in daily living increase as the episodes of dyspnea occur more frequently, to the point that there are few or no intervals between them (Brown et al, 1986).

Underlying Mechanisms

Pathophysiologic and Iatrogenic Factors

Ventilatory deficits are created by mechanical, chemical, and emotional factors. Advanced cancers can contribute to all three.

Mechanical Factors

Mechanical impediments to breathing result from tumor involvement of airway receptors located near the carotid arteries. There is associated bronchospasm, obstruction of airflow in and out of the respiratory system, restriction of movement of lung tissue, and weakening of respiratory muscles.

Advancing lung cancers can cause *obstructive dyspnea* when the neoplasms partially or totally obstruct the main bronchi (this is noted most on inspiration), or when large cell tumors create diffuse obstruction of peripheral lung tissue or small bronchi (this is noted most on expiration). Lymphangitic metastases to the mediastinum can cause central obstruction.

Restrictive dyspnea results when tumors reduce the elasticity of lung tissue or pleura and chest wall, or create space-occupying pleural effusion. Pleural effusion usually arises from metastatic pleural involvement, lymphatic involvement, infection, and hypoproteinemia. Earlier treatment of the thoracic area with radiation and chemotherapy can create fibrosis that compounds restrictive breathing problems (Wickham, 1986). Pain also causes restriction in breathing and can be associated with neoplastic-caused inflammation of the pleura, destruction of ribs, or involvement of nerve roots in the chest wall.

Weakness in respiratory muscles has been found to be related to two neoplastic phenomena. Malnutrition, often a concomitant condition to advancing disease, reduces respiratory muscle strength needed for breathing (Openbrier and Covey, 1987). Persistent hypercapnia has been found to decrease the contractility and endurance of the diaphragm (Juan et al, 1984).

Chemical Factors

Dyspnea also results from abnormal blood gases. Shallow, ineffective breathing associated with obstruction, pain, atelectasis, pneumonitis, and pneumonia can result in abnormal blood gases.

Emotional Factors

Air hunger or feelings of suffocation and shortness of breath provoke emotional responses of anxiety and fear. Further, the awareness of dyspnea tends to change the usually unconscious activity of breathing into a conscious one. The individual can become preoccupied with maintaining as high a level of ventilation as possible. Body position, physical activity, and emotional demands (both pleasant and unpleasant), are modified to keep requirements within the available breathing capacity. Increasing the rate and depth of respiration is a frequent response to dyspnea-related anxiety, and this, in turn, can contribute to the ventilatory deficit by increasing the muscular workload (Foote et al, 1986).

The anxiety, fear, and helplessness experienced by those who share the dyspneic attacks and want to help is important. Their anxiety can feed into the patient's tension, creating even more difficulties.

Daily Living Factors

Daily living is closely and pervasively involved with dyspnea. Requirements for physical, mechanical, and emotional activity can exceed the patient's ventilatory capacity. The environment in which daily living takes place affects the air quality available.

The daily living of the patient is not the only area for consideration. Those who closely share the experiences 24 hours each day also experience major changes in their daily living and functioning. If they become less functional or dysfunctional because of anxiety, fatigue, or chronic sleep disruption, their capacity to provide needed support for the patient is reduced.

Activities and Events in Daily Living

The patient's role requirements and schedule in terms of daily activities and events can exceed ventilatory capacity in specific areas and at particular times. Progressively, even the most basic activities and responses can be impaired. The capacity to react to situations with laughter, crying, or anger may be diminished (Brown et al, 1986). Eating, chewing, and swallowing must be synchronized with breathing. Sleep can be disrupted, and position changes limited to those that will accommodate breathing. Even the needed activity of planning in order to economize on expenditure of effort can become impaired (Molbo, 1986). Sudden precipitous attacks of exhaustion can appear with few prodromal indicators; such episodes can make the patient fearful of leaving home (Molbo, 1986).

Emotional responses in daily living can be sufficient to bring on dyspneic episodes (e.g., anxiety about the inability to work or carry out responsibilities, anger or tension in disagreements with others, frustration with one's situation, worry over the trajectory of the disease, and anxieties caused by family members or others) (Brown et al, 1986).

Care givers' or family members' daily living can be disrupted as it becomes increasingly difficult to leave the patient unattended. Sleep disruption and deprivation may become chronic.

Demands in Daily Living

Self-demands tend to involve expectations of the degree to which one will attempt to maintain role obligations in daily living in the face of decreasing ventilatory capacity. There may be a tendency to conceal breathing difficulties and associated loss of capabilities in order not to burden others (Brown et al, 1986). Women may have a more difficult time in shifting responsibilities in daily living to others, both because of their own patterns of expectations and those of others (Green, 1986).

Self-expectations of the patient's *care givers* may exceed their own physical and emotional capacities as they seek to make the patient feel secure and well cared for around the clock.

Demands of others that exceed the patient's resources may reflect the effectiveness of the patient's disguising of symptoms, or may communicate denial and wishful thinking about the patient's condition. Where family and friends are perceptive of patient deficits the expectations may be congruent; however, solicitude may be seen by the patient as being overprotective or the result of pity.

Health care providers may have expectations for the patient coming to the clinic for appointments that exceed patient resources because patients have not shared accurate information about their reduced capacities.

Environment for Daily Living

The environment, particularly as it relates to air quality (e.g., bad weather, high pollen counts, crowded places, or smoke), can throw the compromised person into dyspneic episodes. Distances, stairs, or inclines between the patient's usual resting place and other needed facilities (e.g., bathroom or kitchen) can be factors in managing daily living. The availability of distractors in the environment—view, television with remote control, radio, books, and telephone—can make a difference in passing the time with dyspnea.

Functional Health Status

Areas of functional health status commonly affecting and affected by dyspnea include physical strength and endurance, cognitive capacities, and mood. (See also Chapter 6, sections on Role and Sexuality.) These functional capacities should be considered when assessing, diagnosing, and treating care givers and family members as well as the patient.

Strength and Endurance

Strength and endurance for all forms of physical work are most affected by ventilatory deficits. When there is slow onset, there may be time to initiate activities to relieve the dyspnea, unless the episodes have little interval between them (Brown et al, 1986). Increasing time is needed to recoup enough oxygen and energy to undertake more work as pathology progresses.

Cognition

Loss of ability to concentrate, to plan ahead, and to remember occurs with dyspnea. Eventually, even the planning needed to conserve energy is impaired (Molbo, 1986).

Mood   Patients report that trying to maintain a positive attitude, accepting the situation, and accepting assistance are useful approaches (Brown et al, 1986). Anxiety, fear, and panic can precipitate and heighten dyspnea.

Nursing Diagnosis and Treatment

Diagnostic   Diagnostic targets include the patient, those who either offer
Targets   assistance or set expectations for patient activities and re-sponses, and those whose emotional interactions with the patient can alter the patient's emotional responses.

Risk Factors   Patients who are more likely to have difficulties in managing daily living with ongoing episodes of dyspnea are those who:

Have ongoing responsibilities and deficits in external resources or an unwillingness to accept assistance

Are women, with or without a partner, who have family responsibilities (Green, 1986)

Experience concurrent maturational or situational crises in addition to the cancer (e.g., children acting out, menopause, retirement, divorce, children moving out of the home, death of a relative or close companion)

Lack financial and personal resources to gain assistance with requirements in daily living

Live in areas with poor air quality or high pollen counts, or with persons who smoke

Are unable to take a positive attitude toward their presenting situation

Live alone

Care givers or family members who are likely to have difficulty in managing daily living with the patient's dyspnea are those who:

Are emotionally close to the patient and therefore share the suffering

Feel dependent on the patient for particular services or emotional support

Have little knowledge of and skill in dealing with dyspneic episodes and feel helpless

Are highly anxious or frightened

Are increasingly sleep-deprived and fatigued, physically and emotionally, due to lack of respite care

Have other conflicting role responsibilities

**Diagnostic
Areas**

PATIENT

Dyspnea-related problems in management of activities of daily living R/T:

Difficulty in scheduling tasks and rest periods

Responsibility-laden roles (e.g., single mother, employee, care giver to other or self)

Lack of assistance from personal network

Reluctance to reveal dyspnea or to accept help

Living alone and lacking a competent personal care giver

Emotional strains between patient and *——————
(*children, spouse, personal care giver, physician, nurse—specify)

Air pollution, pollen, smoke

Worry and preoccupation with symptoms and illness

Environmental barriers (specify—e.g., stairs, distances to bathroom, kitchen, laundry, garage, or supermarket)

Contagion of anxiety or panic in personal care givers or those who share daily living

Ineffective management of dyspneic episodes R/T:

Knowledge deficit of preventive strategies

Knowledge deficit of treatment strategies

Persistent sleep disruption R/T dyspnea, L/T long, lonely, anxious nights and increased fatigue

Inadequate nutrition R/T:

Lack of food in the consistency the patient can chew and swallow given the rapid respirations

Lack of strength or endurance for self-feeding

Lack of coordination between breathing and swallowing

Lack of assistance for shopping and food preparation

FAMILY, CARE
GIVERS

Helplessness in dealing with dyspneic episodes R/T lack of knowledge or skill in managing daily living with the patient's dyspnea

Burnout R/T inadequate respite from care giving or the stress of sharing the patient's suffering

Manifestations

PATIENT

Dyspnea is manifested by reported:

Shortness of breath

Difficulty in breathing

Difficulty in "moving the air"

Feeling of suffocation, tightness, filling up, drowning, or smothering

Associated symptoms, including poor concentration, loss of appetite, and loss of memory (Brown et al, 1986)

Dyspnea is manifested by observed:

Increased respiratory rate

Flaring nares, use of accessory muscles

Change in duration of inspiration or expiration

Resting more

Moving more slowly

Eating less

Resting between bites of food

Sweating

Orthopnea

Increased frequency of episodes of dyspnea

Cognitive changes associated with cerebral hypoxia (e.g., disorientation and confusion)

Associated difficulties in management of daily living are manifested by reported:

Being too short of breath to undertake or complete usual or desired tasks, including food preparation, eating, personal hygiene, urinary and bowel elimination, care of bedding, home maintenance, and keeping up on relationships with others

Difficulty in sleeping; long, lonely nights

Eating foods that require less chewing

Eating less at a time, snacking instead of preparing meals

Reducing fluid intake to decrease the number of trips to the bathroom

Fear of being alone, of choking

Reluctance to let family or friends know of the difficulties—to be a burden to them

Wondering how to manage, because the breathing difficulties are getting worse

Associated difficulties in management of daily living are manifested by observed:

Deterioration in personal appearance and upkeep of surroundings

Decreases in the usual tasks undertaken, slowing of pace of work and movement, interrupting of work for rest periods

Loss of affect in response to others (responding requires increased ventilation)

Withdrawal (emotional or physical) from social and family gatherings; less participation in conversations

Denial to others of observed breathing difficulties or need for assistance

Difficulty in coordinating eating with rapid breathing

Reduced fluid intake and more concentrated urine

FAMILY, CARE
GIVERS

Reported:

Fear, anxiety, or helplessness in the presence of the patient's dyspneic patterns

Concern about lack of knowledge and skill in helping to manage the dyspnea and the patient's emotional responses

Sleep deprivation

Fatigue

Observed:

Deterioration in grooming and appearance or in relationship with the patient, care of the patient, or home environment

Constant attendance of the patient with no known periods of respite or opportunities to share their difficulties

**Prognostic
Variables**

Poor prognosis for managing daily living with dyspnea is associated with:

Rapidly increasing dyspnea

Deteriorating cognition

High levels of anxiety

Difficulty in accepting the situation

Lack of a personal network or financial resources for needed services and emotional support

Lack of knowledge about the nature of dyspnea and its management

Environmental barriers to ease of mobility

High levels of stress and discord in daily living

Air quality with pollution levels that are intolerable to the patient

Lack of respite for care givers

Complications

Failure to manage daily living in the presence of dyspnea can result in:

Increased malnutrition

Altered fluid balance

Sleep deprivation

Inordinate fatigue

Fractured ribs with uncontrolled coughing

Increased fatigue or nausea and vomiting associated with coughing

A negative spiral in physical and emotional well-being

Treatment Guidelines

Lack of knowledge regarding precipitating factors for dyspnea

Gather data on patterns of activities, responsibilities, priorities, and factors in home or work environment that increase physical demands, and on any situations creating emotional tension.

Provide information (orally or in writing) about situations that precipitate episodes of dyspnea, including physical activities that exceed compromised ventilatory capacity; laughing or crying; getting angry; air pollution, pollen, and smoke; and emotional stressors (self-generated—e.g., worry about health situation, frustration with behavior of others; or generated by others—e.g., disagreements, failure to take patient's needs into consideration). Tailor teaching to patient's own situation by using the precipitants identified in the data gathering as the examples.

Explore feasible options and strategies for managing the precipitating factors more effectively. Where the patient is a woman, with or without a partner, do not take for granted that physical assistance with home responsibilities will be taken over by others (Green, 1986). Check regularly with the patient and family members. If patient is unable to mobilize support from family or others to keep workloads and emotional stressors within ventilatory capacity, seek permission to make contact with one or more significant persons in the personal network to plan for appropriate assistance in reducing workload and stressors. Where health care providers are part of the problem, negotiate for changes in scheduling, behavior, or attitudes to promote patient sense of support and well-being.

Take extra precautions to protect the patient from interpersonal stressors whenever possible.

Where air quality is a factor, recommend that the patient remain indoors when pollution is high. Make some "No smoking" signs available. Check with physician regarding the possibility of ordering oxygen for days when bad weather or air pollution increases dyspnea. For patients receiving third-party reimbursement provide the following information (required for Medicare reimbursement): medical diagnosis, laboratory values on arterial blood gases or ear and pulse oximetry (to document the hypoxia),* and the medical order, including liter flow per minute, oxygen concentration, estimated number of hours of use per day, and duration of use (a p.r.n. order will not suffice, but an estimate of hours per day will) (US Department of Health and Human Services, 1985).

Lack of knowledge regarding care during episodes of dyspnea and long-term adaptive strategies

During dyspneic episode

Teach the following strategies to the patient to manage dyspneic episodes:

For resting or sleeping, keep upper body elevated, whether in bed or in a recliner.

Try the position of sitting with the thorax inclined forward, the knees apart, and the forearms resting on the thighs, on a pillow on the thighs, or on a table (Foote et al, 1986; White, 1987).

Move more slowly, change position (Brown et al, 1986).

Teach the patient and family members or care givers about coached breathing when the patient becomes anxious during a dyspneic attack and hyperventilates. Instruct the coach to seek to get the anxious patient's attention by commanding in a low, calm voice, "Listen to me. Focus on what I am saying," then at *a rate the patient can actually follow* repeating, "Slow breath in... slow breath out." Teach the patient to breathe in through the nose and to purse the lips when exhaling. In practicing, teach the patient to make a soft whistling sound when exhaling. Exhalation should be about twice as long as inhalation.

Give instructions on the importance of maintaining fluid intake to keep secretions thin. Recommend use of humidifiers for this same reason. Non-narcotic cough syrups (those containing benzonatate or dextromethorphan) can be useful for reducing the cough.

Note that low-flow oxygen may not alter the blood gases, but can have a placebo effect of breaking up the dyspnea–anxiety cycle. Mention that some patients and families use their own funds to pay for standby oxygen when the medical necessity cannot be documented to the satisfaction of third-party payers.

---

*The patient's sensations of inadequate oxygen may not be matched by the blood gas values; that is, the blood gases may not be abnormal enough to seem to warrant use of oxygen, yet the patient may complain of extreme dyspnea and be highly anxious.

Note that the use of prescribed tranquilizers and low doses of narcotics can reduce the respiratory drive and increase comfort without causing respiratory depression (Zerwekh, 1987).

Instruct the patient or care giver to be certain that medications and oxygen are conveniently within reach wherever the patient is resting. Indicate that whenever inhalant oxygen is used, the instructions must be clear and concise, both in their oral and written form.

Instruct the patient and family about when it is important to call for help (e.g., when there have been several severe episodes of dyspnea in a row). Make calling a legitimate behavior (e.g., "Make sure you call (the clinic or 911) if you feel you can't handle what is happening").

Long-term adaptive strategies

Instruct the patient to make the following adjustments to manage ongoing dyspnea:

Seek assistance or transfer activities beyond one's capacity to others.

Eat smaller amounts; eat more frequently; eat foods that are easier to chew.

Wear clothing that is easy to put on (e.g., slip-on shoes) and is nonrestrictive. Wear a short, easy-care hair style.

Plan activities in advance to minimize expenditure of effort. Include planned rest periods, particularly with more demanding activities. Schedule more demanding activities at hours of the day when breathing is the easiest. Set priorities (what is important to the patient, including something really pleasant) and omit low-priority activities.

Avoid situations that the patient finds precipitate dyspnea. (Where these are interpersonal situations, help the patient to develop prepared scripts or behaviors to minimize risks. Offer to role-play the scripts with the patient so he or she gets a feel for it.)

Balance the need to reduce the demands of interacting with groups of people with the need to avoid being alone for long periods of time. (Help others learn how to be with the patient without causing undue fatigue. Start by gathering data on what the patient says is comfortable.)

Seek acceptance of the breathing limitations as reality and focus on strategies for managing life to achieve the best quality possible.

Use breathing techniques (see above) that have been found to be useful.

Difficulties in scheduling tasks and rest periods

Gather data on deterrents (e.g., inability to plan and factors that make scheduling and rest difficult).

Work with patient or care giver to:

Determine real priorities

Determine what can and cannot be changed

Look at acceptable options and strategies for obtaining help through their personal network, resources in the community, or care, respite, and chore services, and seek possible assistance in payment from insurance plans. Help in developing an initial tentative plan. Ask for feedback by phone or in a clinic visit to evaluate its effectiveness. Modify the plan accordingly.

Lack of assistance from personal network†

Gather data on the nature of the personal network, past patterns of assisting one another, the extent to which the patient has revealed or is willing to reveal symptoms and difficulties, and the extent to which the patient or care giver will request or accept help.

Explore the possibility of negotiating agreements for specific assistance with tasks that are becoming difficult or for respite.

Negotiate among care giver, family members, and patient about who is going to worry about what—don't worry about the same things or there will be no one to intervene. For example, the care giver can take responsibility for making sure that we don't run out of medications, inhalers, or oxygen. The patient can take responsibility for knowing how to get help if the care giver is not present.

Explore options for patient (or care giver) to provide positive feedback or other rewards in exchange for the attention and services of others in order to maintain services.

Help patient and care giver to plan strategies, in advance, for dealing with situations where agreements to help are broken. Plan a repertoire of possible responses.

Negotiate with the patient and care giver or family members about the necessity and legitimacy of adequate rest and respite for the care giver. (If the care giver becomes ill, the patient will be even further disadvantaged. Therefore, care givers are serving the patients at the same time that they gain rest and respite for themselves.) Understand that family members may be reluc-

---

† This treatment may be needed for the patient or for the care giver, who may be at risk of burnout.

tant to experience pleasure themselves when the patient continues to suffer, and that the patient may be frightened at having to deal with a less experienced or comfortable care giver for a period of time. Emphasize that it is important to adequately train the surrogate care giver and to help that person to become comfortable with the primary care giver and the patient.

Emotional strains between patient and others

Gather data on high-risk situations or encounters.

Explore options for avoiding the situation or taking action before the strains become full-blown.

Plan a repertoire of responses from which the patient and family members can choose.

Wherever possible, protect the patient from emotional tensions.

Worry and preoccupation with symptoms

Gather data on times and causes of greatest worry, and on feasible factors that would reduce the worry.

Teach the patient about the link between worrying, anxiety, and respiratory difficulties.

Explore what alternatives there might be to the worrying that might produce a more positive outcome (e.g., diversion, looking for some positive experiences that could be created within the limitations of breathing), and discuss ways to make these happen.

Sleep difficulties

Gather data on the kind of chair or bed in which the patient is spending time during the days and nights. Seek ways to make them more comfortable for the relatively upright position the patient must maintain. Note that many patients find that a recliner is most comfortable for both days and nights. It can be made the patient's headquarters, where it is possible to be involved, see what is going on with the family, watch TV, and do diversionary activities. Medications and supplies may also be kept there. With such a situation it may be possible to use the radio or TV as distraction if the patient is wakeful at night.

If the patient spends most of his time in bed, help arrange an effective means of support to keep the upper body in the raised position, with a foot board or box to prevent sliding down.

If the care giver does not sleep in the same room, help arrange an effective call system (e.g., a bell) for peace of mind for both patient and care giver.

If the care giver sleeps in the same bed or the same room, determine how the care giver's sleep and rest are affected by the mechanisms used to keep the patient's upper body elevated, the sounds of the patient's breathing or restlessness, or fear of going to sleep in case the patient stops breathing. Encourage the care giver that getting adequate rest is an important factor in the ongoing capacity to provide care to the patient. Suggest that the inexpensive dual listening and speaker system used by parents to monitor infants can provide peace of mind for both patient and care giver if they sleep in separate rooms. Note that it is important to consider the impact of changing long-established sleeping arrangements of couples (e.g., moving out of the double bed or to a separate bedroom; this can be seen as another loss and cause increased symptoms). (See section on Separation in Chapter 11.)

Environmental barriers

Gather data on the barriers in the home and work setting and the impact they are having on keeping activities within ventilatory capacity.

Explore other options for managing the activities involved.

Evaluation

Patient response to nursing treatment aimed at improving management of daily living in the face of increasing dyspnea can be evaluated in terms of *the patient's:*

Behavior in avoiding situations that make the dyspnea more severe (e.g., emotional tensions, physical activities that exceed ventilatory capacity)

Degree of acceptance of the changed ventilatory capacity and willingness to adjust to changed capabilities

Self-care related to dyspneic status (e.g., effective self-administration of medications or oxygen, mobilization and acceptance of the assistance of others as physical and cognitive capacities to meet daily living requirements diminish)

Organization of requirements in daily living and environment to adjust to dyspneic status

Patient response may also be evaluated in terms of *the care giver and family's:*

Level of acceptance and understanding of the patient's changing ventilatory capacity

Level of knowledge and skill in managing the patient's symptoms and requirements in daily living to maintain the patient's comfort and emotional well-being

Status of organization of the environment to accommodate decreased physical capacities and to promote safety

Understanding of their own needs for regular respite and rest in order to serve the patient's best interests and be able to provide ongoing care over time

Degree of skill in handling stressors and interpersonal tensions in order to minimize their impact on the patient and maintain their own mental health

---

Other Problems

Living With Confusion

While the patient's decreased levels of consciousness place additional burdens on the care giver to take over the most basic of self-care activities, the symptoms of confusion probably cause care givers and family members greater emotional and physical problems in daily living. Patients themselves may or may not be distressed by the symptoms.

Confusion can be caused by many variables present in advanced cancer, including primary or metastatic brain tumors, liver or renal failure, drug side-effects, drug intoxication related to impaired hepatic and renal capacity to excrete drugs normally, pain, sleep deprivation, grief, anxiety, and preexisting conditions (e.g., organic brain syndrome) (Billings, 1985).

Manifestations of Confusion That Create Difficulties in Daily Living

Symptoms that make it increasingly difficult for care givers and family members to manage daily living with the patient and provide care include apathy, emotional lability, lack of inhibition, shallow affect, selective inattention, irritability, forgetfulness, self-neglect, lack of insight, inability to reason, inability to recognize family members or care givers, fear of familiar persons, agitation, restlessness, combativeness, uncooperativeness, and random or bizarre gestures. Symptoms that may add to the distress of the patient include agitation, disorientation, misinterpretation of the environment, suspicion, terror, nightmares, and inability to focus attention (Billings, 1985).

Help for the Patient in Managing Daily Living With Confusion

The following strategies may be useful in helping the patient to manage daily living more effectively or comfortably in the presence of confusion:

Take over the tasks and functions previously carried out by the patient, including basic hygiene and safety measures, as needed.

Provide a safe environment (e.g., padded side rails for the agitated, restless patient, posey belts or other barriers to prevent wandering or injury).

Provide a friendly, well-lit environment using familiar and orienting objects (e.g., clocks, calendars), familiar faces, and consistent care givers.

Minimize distractions and disturbances such as loud noises, unfamiliar sights, sounds, or people, and frightening procedures.

Ask those who enter the room to identify themselves and to describe what they are going to do before and as they are carrying out activities.

Avoid interrupting sleep or sudden intrusions into the patient's space.

Gently correct patient's inaccurate perceptions or misinterpretations. Provide opportunities for patient to touch and examine misperceived objects. Explain that the illness causes the difficulties (e.g., "When a person is sick as you are, sometimes the mind plays tricks on you" or "That tumor is really making things seem peculiar for you today"). If the patient can tolerate it, help to find some humor in the situation, but direct the humor at the tumor or the situation, not at the patient.

Direct the conversation to reminiscences involving pleasant memories of earlier times.

Help for Care Givers and Family Members in Managing Daily Living With Patient Confusion

Help the family members and care givers to:

Realize that some forms of confusion are reversible (e.g., drug toxicities)

Understand that the illness is creating the behavior—it is often not under the control of the patient. (Make an analogy to other symptoms that result from the cancer. Indicate that it is more difficult to accept subtle or serious behavioral changes as being symptoms of the tumor because of a lifetime of expectations regarding responsibility for one's own behavior and role relationships with others. This may require repeated explanations or role modeling, for example, regularly associating the tumor with the behavior. Encourage the family to use humor to refer to or deal with the behavior if it helps the family and does not distress the patient.)

Accept and plan for equipment and strategies for protecting the patient from injury should agitation and restlessness increase the risk of bruising or falling (e.g., padded side rails, posey belt, other restraints)

Plan strategies to protect themselves from injurious patient behavior (e.g., being bitten, struck, or kicked)

Realize that the demands on the physical and emotional stamina of the care givers are greater with the symptoms of confusion than with many other symptoms because of the constant need for surveillance and the lack of expected, needed, or logical feedback from the patient, and that, therefore, regular opportunities for adequate rest or respite are crucial

Realize that most third-party payers do not pay for respite care; however, it is possible that the patient's symptoms can be medically evaluated and that the patient could be admitted for some form of medical care that would also provide the home care givers with the respite they need

Living with Risks of Oncologic Emergencies

Symptoms associated with oncologic emergencies can occur at any time in the cancer experience; however, many tend to occur with metastatic disease and in the more advanced stages of the disease. Treatment of oncologic emergencies is primarily a medical responsibility. However, since most of daily living with advanced cancer occurs in the home rather than in an acute care setting, the patient and care giver need to have some degree of preparedness for the oncologic emergencies that are a high risk in their particular situation. Preparedness involves knowledge of what to expect and what to do, and decision making concerning the level of medical treatment to seek or accept.

Being Prepared with Knowledge

In advanced cancer, the patient is usually experiencing some symptoms on a regular basis. It becomes important, then, for the patient and care giver or family to recognize changes and know which changes or new symptoms should be reported quickly because they represent the onset of an emergency situation. They also need to know to whom the information should be communicated in order to achieve the desired response (e.g., dialing 911, notifying the doctor or home nurse). They also need to know what action to take until professional help arrives on the scene.

While patients or care givers may need this information, being given knowledge about potential problems carries its own risk. The imparting of this information may cause greater anxiety and stress, rather than lead to the security of contingency planning.

Many family members and care givers wonder about the course of events that will lead to the patient's dying. It is possible to provide information keyed to the patient's specific cancer situation that will give them the information they need. The oncologic emergencies, the types of neoplastic conditions in which they are likely to occur, and their symptoms are shown in Table 10-2.

Knowledge about these and other conditions can be shared in ways that tend to seek to minimize their stressfulness. The choice of words will be important, for example:

Medical words	could become	Lay language
Arrhythmia or dysrhythmia		Irregular pulse
Cyanosis		Dusky color
Tachycardia		Increased pulse rate
Cold and clammy		Skin cool and moist
Severe petechiae		Increase in small red spots under the skin
Paraplegia		Weakness in the lower part of the body
Carotid blowout		Heavy bleeding from the tumor area in the neck
Hematemesis		Retching and vomiting of blood
Hemoptysis		Blood flowing from the mouth without retching
Renal shutdown		Decreased or no urine output

Table 10-2. Oncologic Emergencies: Underlying Pathology and Manifestations

Condition	Underlying Pathology	Symptoms
Cardiac tamponade	Pericardial tumor involvement, late effects of mediastinal radiation	Shortness of breath, chest pain, anxiety, restlessness, cough
Disseminated intravascular coagulation	Leukemia, sepsis, hepatic failure, mucin-secreting adenocarcinomas of lung, pancreas, stomach, or prostate	Severe petechiae, gastric bleeding, shortness of breath, pallor, cool and clammy skin
Hemorrhage		
Upper or lower gastrointestinal tract hemorrhage	Uncontrolled tumor growth with erosion of vascular walls	Retching and vomiting of blood; passing of blood rectally
Lung hemorrhage	Uncontrolled tumor growth with erosion of vascular walls	Blood coming from mouth without retching
Carotid blowout	Uncontrolled tumor growth with erosion of vascular walls	Sudden massive flow of blood (spurting or steady flow) from tumor area on neck
Hypercalcemia	Breast or prostate cancer with bony metastasis; lung or renal cancer; multiple myeloma	Increased fatigue, irritability, lethargy, nausea and vomiting, increased urination, thirst, irregular pulse
Septic shock	Leukemia, lymphoma, neutropenia, gram-negative bacterial infection	*Early (warm shock)* Irritability; restlessness; lethargy; disorientation; inappropriate euphoria; temperature subnormal, normal, or elevated; skin warm; rapid, bounding pulse; widening pulse pressure; rapid respirations; normal urine output, but possible glucosuria; normal bowel sounds *Late (cold shock)* Irritability; restlessness; confusion; cold, clammy skin; rapid, shallow breathing; rapid, thready pulse; abdominal pain; decreased urine output

(continued)

Table 10-2.   Oncologic Emergencies: Underlying Pathology and
Manifestations (continued)

Condition	Underlying Pathology	Symptoms
Spinal cord compression (70% thoracic)	Metastatic tumors from breast, lung, prostate, or kidney; lymphoma	Pain localized in back or referred to chest, abdomen, or upper extremities; muscle weakness; paralysis (paraplegia); tingling; loss of bowel and bladder control; decreased temperature and pain in affected areas; sexual dysfunction
Syndrome of inappropriate antidiuretic hormone (SIADH)	Small-cell lung cancer, lymphoma, pancreatic, brain, acute, or chronic leukemias, prostate cancers	Confusion, hostility, headache, disorientation, lethargy, weakness, anorexia, nausea and vomiting, diarrhea, weight gain, increased urine output, muscle cramps
Superior vena cava syndrome (SVCS)	Lung cancer, lymphoma, metastases to mediastinum or thrombus	Face, neck, trunk, and arms swollen on waking; dyspnea; chest pain; hypotension; cyanosis; headache; lethargy
Tumor lysis syndrome (occurs 1 to 5 days after initiation of chemotherapy; patient is usually in the hospital)	Non-Hodgkin's lymphoma, leukemias—especially acute lymphoblastic, chronic leukemias in blast phase	Decreased or no urine output, hematuria, flank pain, irregular pulse, cramps, confusion, tetany

(Barry, 1989; Billings, 1985; Dangel, 1985; Findley, 1987; Poe and Taylor, 1989)

To provide the information needed to make contingency plans with the least amount of distress the nurse might say, "When patients have a breast cancer that has spread to the bone the way Mary's has done, sometimes calcium from the bone builds up in the blood stream. This is a treatable condition, particularly when it is recognized early. It would be wise to get in touch with your nurse or the doctor if you notice that Mary is unusually weak and tired but restless, seems a little out of touch with reality, is putting out more urine both in the daytime and nighttime, is thirstier, doesn't want food, and complains of nausea or a stomachache. This combination of symptoms may indicate that the doctor needs to do a blood test and give Mary a special medication to correct the condition." Or, the nurse might say, "Not often, but once in a while we see patients with a lung tumor where the tumor grows into a blood vessel and causes it to leak blood. If this were to happen to Jim, he would begin to cough up blood. This may be very frightening to him so it would be important for you to act calm, even if you don't feel that way. Quickly place a receptacle or towel up to Jim's mouth to collect the blood. See that he is either sitting up or lying on his side. Depending on the prior agreements you and he have made about how you wish to manage emergencies like this, seek help or let it take its course. You could call 911 for immediate assistance, or call your doctor or your home nursing agency to decide what professional help or support you need and want. We don't think this will happen, but it helps to know what to do, if it should."

The hospital or home care nurse needs to make a judgment based on the way the patient, family members, and care givers have responded in earlier stress situations as to whether they will feel more competent or be immobilized if given information about high-risk oncologic emergencies.

Factors Influencing Decisions About Treatment

Another consideration in dealing with oncologic emergencies when the patient has advanced cancer involves some choices about the level of desired medical treatment (Billings, 1985). Medical treatment usually requires hospitalization for a period of time. Some of the conditions described in Table 10-2 lend themselves to improvement with medical treatment (e.g., hypercalcemia) or surgical treatment (e.g., spinal cord compression). The duration of improvement can vary, since often the basic pathology continues or progresses. Depending on the patient's situation, the benefits from the medical intervention may be seen to be worthwhile. On the other hand, the oncologic emergency may be viewed as an "acceptable terminal event" (e.g., hemorrhage may be seen as one of the less distressing ways for a patient with advanced cancer to die) (Billings, 1985).

There may be a decision not to actively treat the pathology, but there may be a separate decision about hospitalization. An earlier decision may have been for the patient to remain at home in the terminal illness. However, oncologic complications may create a new patient care situation in which it is not possible to maintain the patient's safety or where the burden of care exceeds the care giver's resources. For example, the patient may be confused and restless, not recognize the care giver, or even be frightened of the care giver. It may not be possible for the care giver to sustain this type of care through the remaining days or weeks.

Contingency decision making takes into account the real possibility that the potential oncologic emergencies may never arise. The decisions also should be made with the option that patient and family may wish to alter their original decision at a later time as circumstances change. Nevertheless, such advanced planning allows family members and care givers to feel control over decisions and actions.

Other Strategies for Increasing Security about Oncologic Emergencies

Beyond the contingency decision making there are other plans that can offer care givers and family members security.

The Home Health Care Nurse

Having a concerned, expert home care nurse as a case manager, consultant, liaison with medical care providers, and ongoing source of assistance offers a consistent foundation of support to patient and care givers. Should a sudden, serious emergency arise when the contingency plan is hospitalization, a call to 911 and then to the home care nurse can be the planned action. Or, should the plan be that the patient will remain at home, the first call would go to the nurse.

Having Supplies or Equipment

The care giver or family members may be reluctant to assemble supplies or equipment for emergencies. The nurse may find it helpful to make the analogy to the first aid kit that is present in most homes or the emergency carts that are kept on the units in the hospital. Both are rarely needed, but it is comforting to know that supplies and equipment are available should a need arise. They should be kept close at hand, but out of the patient's sight if possible. The nurse who knows the patient's condition and risks could help the family assemble any supplies that might be needed (e.g., receptacles or towels for hematemesis, hemoptysis, or hemorrhage; padding or pillows for side rails if agitation and restlessness occur; restraints to keep the patient from getting out of bed).

Summary

The nurse needs to take knowledge of the risks of oncologic emergencies and combine it with data on the patient's pathophysiologic status, the patient's and family's current plans and goals, and the patient's and family's crisis management behavior. From this it is possible to make clinical judgments about whether and how to present needed knowledge and how to help both the patient and care givers to do contingency planning that can bring greater peace of mind about managing possible emergencies well.

Bibliography

Asthenia

Billings JA. Outpatient management of advanced cancer. Philadelphia: JB Lippincott, 1985.

Brody EM. Parent care as a normative family stress. Gerontologist 1985;25:19.

Brody EM. Women in the middle. Gerontologist 1981;21:471.

Bruera E, Brenneis C, Michaud M et al. Association between involuntary muscle function and asthenia nutritional status, lean body mass, psychometric assessment and tumor mass in patients with advanced cancer. Proceedings of the American Society of Clinical Oncologists 1987;6:261.

Bruera E, MacDonald RN. Asthenia in patients with advanced cancer. Journal of Pain and Symptom Management 1988;3:9.

Bruera E, MacDonald RN. Nutrition in cancer patients: an update and review of our experience. Journal of Pain and Symptom Management 1988a;3:133.

Bruera E, MacDonald RN. Overwhelming fatigue in advanced cancer. Am J Nurs 1988b;88:99.

Copstead LE, Patterson S. Families of the elderly. In: Carnevali D, Patrick M, eds. Nursing management for the elderly. Philadelphia: JB Lippincott, 1986.

DeWys WD. Pathophysiology of cancer cachexia: Current understanding and areas for future research. Cancer Res 1982;42(suppl):721s.

Heard L. Care of the patient with potential for skin breakdown related to pressure ischemia. In: Reiner A, ed. Manual of patient care standards. Rockville MD: Aspen Publishers, 1988.

Holroyde C, Axelrod R, Skutcher C et al. Lactate metabolism in patients with metastatic colorectal cancer. Cancer Res 1979;39:4900.

Kaempfer SH, Lindsey AM. Energy expenditure in cancer: a review. Cancer Nurs 1986;9:194.

Leahey M, Wright LM. Families and life-threatening illness. Springhouse, PA: Springhouse Corp, 1987.

Lindsey AM. Cancer cachexia: effects of the disease and its treatment. Semin Oncol 1986;2:19.

Molbo D. Cancer. In: Carnevali D, Patrick M, eds. Nursing management for the elderly. Philadelphia: JB Lippincott, 1986.

Morrison SD. Control of food intake in cancer cachexia: a challenge and a tool. Physiological Behavior 1976;17:705.

Nail LM, King KB. Fatigue. Seminars in Oncology Nursing 1987;3:257.

Norton J, Brennan M. In vivo utilization of substrate by sarcoma bearing limbs. Cancer 1980;45:2934.

Noyes R, Kathol RG. Depression and cancer. Psychiatr Dev 1986;2:77.

Pines A, Aronson E, Kafry D. Burnout: from tedium to personal growth. New York: Free Press, 1981.

Ritter M. Ostozyme. International Association of Enterostomal Therapy 1982;9:79.

Slaby AE. Cancer's impact on caregivers. Adv Psychosom Med 1988;18:135.

Stetz KM. The relationship among background characteristics, purpose in life and care giving demands on health of spouse caregivers. Scholarly Inquiry for Nursing Practice: An International Journal 1989;3:133.

Theologides A. Anorexins, asthenins and cachectins in cancer. Am J Med 1986;81:296.

Theologides A. Asthenia in cancer. Am J Med 1982;73:1.

Vess JD, Moreland JR, Schwebel AI, Kraut E. Psychosocial needs of cancer patients: learning from patients and their spouses. Journal of Psychosocial Oncology 1988;6:31.

Warmolts J, Petek K, Lewis R et al. Type II muscle fibre atrophy: an early systemic effect of cancer. Neurology 1975;25:374.

Weisman AO. Understanding the cancer patient: the syndrome of the caregiver's plight. Psychiatry 1981;44:161.

Wesdorp RIC, Krause R, von Myenfeldt MF. Cancer cachexia and its nutritional implications. Br J Surg 1983;70:352.

Eating and Feeding Problems

Baines M. Nausea and vomiting in the patient with advanced cancer. Journal of Pain and Symptom Management 1988;3:81.

Bernstein I. Etiology of anorexia in cancer. Cancer 1986;53:1881.

Beutler B, Cerami A. Cachectin and TNF as two sides of the same biological coin. Nature 1986;320:584.

Billings JA. Outpatient management of advanced cancer. Philadelphia: JB Lippincott, 1985.

Bruera E, Chadwick S, Fox R et al: Chronic nausea and anorexia in patients with advanced cancer: a possible role for autonomic dysfunction. Journal of Pain and Symptom Management 1987;2:19.

Bruera E, Chadwick S, Fox R et al. A study of cardiovascular autonomic insufficiency in advanced cancer patients. Cancer Treat Rep 1986;12:1383.

Bruera E, MacDonald RN. Nutrition in cancer patients: an update and review of our experience. Journal of Pain and Symptom Management 1988;3:133.

Caspar R. Food and water: symbol and reality. Health Progress 1988;69:54.

De Conno F, Ripamonti C, Sbanotto A, Ventafridda V. Oral complications in patients with advanced cancer. Journal of Pain and Symptom Management 1989;4:20.

De Wys WD. Anorexia as a general effect of cancer. Cancer 1979;43:2013.

De Wys WD. Weight loss and nutritional abnormalities in cancer patients: incidence, severity and significance. Clinics in Oncology 1986;5:251.

DeWys WD, Begg C, Lavin PT et al. Prognostic effect of weight loss prior to chemotherapy in cancer patients. Am J Med 1980;69:491.

Dolan MB: Another hospice nurse says. Nursing 1983;83:51.

Evans W, Nixon D, Daly J. A randomized study of standard or augmented oral nutritional support versus ad lib nutrition intake in patients with advanced cancer. Clin Invest Med 1986;9:127.

Gargaro W. Cancer nursing and the law: informed refusal. Cancer Nurs 1980;3:467.

Grosvenor M, Bulcavage L, Chiebowski RT. Symptoms potentially influencing weight loss in a cancer population. Cancer 1989;63:330.

Heber D, Byerly L, Chi J. Pathophysiology of malnutrition in the adult cancer patient. Cancer 1986;53:1867.

Horton C. Care of the cancer patient experiencing nutritional deficits. In: Reiner A, ed. Manual of patient care standards. Rockville, MD: Aspen Publishers, 1988.

Koretz R. Parenteral nutrition: is it oncologically logical? J Clin Oncol 1984;2:534.

Lynn J, Childress JF. Must patients always be given food and water? Hastings Cent Rep 1983;13:17.

Micetich KC, Steinecker PH, Thomasma DC. Are intravenous fluids morally required for a dying patient? Arch Intern Med 1983;143:975.

Molbo D. Cancer. In: Carnevali D, Patrick M, eds. Nursing management for the elderly. Philadelphia: JB Lippincott, 1986.

Moseley JR. Alterations in comfort. Nurs Clin North Am 1985;20:427.
Nixon D. The value of parenteral nutrition support. Cancer 1986;58:1902.
Torosian M, Daly J. Nutritional support in the cancer-bearing host. Cancer 1986;58:1915.
Twycross RG, Lack SA. Alimentary symptoms. In Twycross RG, Lack SA (eds). Therapeutics in terminal cancer, p 36. London: Pitman Publishing Ltd, 1984.
Zerwekh JV. The dehydration question. Nursing 1983;83:47.

Chronic Pain and Suffering

Abrams RD. The patient with cancer: his changing pattern of communication. N Engl J Med 1966;274:317.
American Cancer Society. Questions and answers about pain control. New York: American Cancer Society, 1983.
Benedict S. The suffering associated with lung cancer. Cancer Nurs 1989;12:34.
Bonica J. Management of cancer pain. Recent Results Cancer Res 1984;89:13.
Cleeland C. Measurement and prevalence of pain in cancer. Seminars in Oncology Nursing 1985;1:87.
Copp, LA. Pain coping model and typology. Image 1985;17:69.
Coyle N, Foley K. Pain in patients with cancer: profile of patients and common pain syndromes. Seminar in Oncology Nursing 1985;1:93.
Derogatis LR et al. The prevalence of psychiatric disorders among cancer patients. JAMA 1983;249:751.
Duclow D. Into the whirlwind of suffering: resistance and transformation. Second Opinion 1988;9:10.
Ferrell BR, Schneider C. Experience and management of cancer pain at home. Cancer Nurs 1988;11:84.
Ferrer-Brechner T, Ganz P. Combination therapy with ibuprofen and methadone for chronic cancer pain. Am J Med 1984;77:78.
Foley K. The treatment of pain in the patient with cancer. CA 1986;36:194.
Foley KM. Pain syndromes in patients with cancer. In: Swedolow M, Ventafridda V, eds. Cancer pain. London: Hastings Hilderly, 1987.
Franklin D. Just say yes to narcotics. Hippocrates 1988;2:24.
Howard-Ruben J, Mcguire L, Groenwald SL. Pain. In: Groenwald SL, ed. Cancer nursing: principles and practice. Monterey, CA: Jones & Bartlett, 1987.
Kerr N. Signs and symptoms of depression and principles of nursing intervention. Perspect Psychiatr Care 1987-1988;24:48.
Levin DN, Cleeland CS, Dar R. Public attitudes toward cancer pain. Cancer 1985;56:2337.
Massie MJ, Holland J. The cancer patient with pain: psychiatric complications and their management. Med Clin North Am 1987;71:243.
McCaffery M. Nursing management of the patient with pain. 2nd ed. Philadelphia: JB Lippincott, 1979.
McGivney W, Crooks G. The care of patients with severe chronic pain in terminal illness. JAMA 1984;251:1182.
Meinhart N, McCaffery M. Pain: a nursing approach to assessment and analysis. Norwalk, CT: Appleton-Century-Crofts, 1986.
Melzack R. The McGill–Melzack pain questionnaire: major properties and scoring methods. Pain 1975;1:277.
Molbo D. Cancer. In: Carnevali D, Patrick M, eds. Nursing management for the elderly. 2nd ed. Philadelphia: JB Lippincott, 1986.
Noyes R, Kathol R. Depression and cancer. Psychiatr Dev 1986;2:77.
O'Brien J, Francis A. The use of next-of-kin to estimate pain in cancer patients. Pain 1988;35:171.
Portenoy R. Practical aspects of pain control in the patient with cancer. CA 1988;36:327.
Sternbach RA. Pain patients: traits and treatment. New York: Academic Press, 1974.

Dyspnea

Billings JA. Outpatient management of advanced cancer. Philadelphia: JB Lippincott, 1985.
Brown ML, Carrieri V, Janson-Bjerklie S, Dodd M. Lung cancer and dyspnea: the patient's perspective. Oncology Nursing Forum 1986;13:19.
Foote M, Sexton DL, Pawlik L. Dyspnea: a distressing sensation in lung cancer. Oncology Nursing Forum 1986;13:25.
Green CP. Changes in responsibility in women's families after the diagnosis of cancer. Health Care for Women International 1986;7:221.

Janson-Bjerklie S, Carrieri VK, Hudes M. The sensations of pulmonary dyspnea. Nurs Res 1986;35:154.

Juan G, Calverly P, Talamo C et al. Effect of carbon dioxide on diaphragmatic function in human beings. N Engl J Med 1984;310:874.

Molbo DM. Cancer. In: Carnevali D, Patrick M, eds. Nursing management for the elderly. 2nd ed. Philadelphia: JB Lippincott, 1986.

Openbrier DR, Covey M. Ineffective breathing pattern related to malnutrition. Nurs Clin North Amd 1987;11:225.

US Department of Health and Human Services, Health Care Financing Administration, Medicare Program. Coverage of oxygen for use in a patient's home. Federal Register 1985;50:13742.

West JB. Respiratory physiology: the essentials. 3rd ed. Baltimore: Williams & Wilkins, 1985.

White E. Home care of the patient with advanced lung cancer. Seminars in Oncology Nursing 1987;3:236.

Wickham R. Pulmonary toxicity secondary to cancer treatment. Oncology Nursing Forum 1986;13:69.

Zerwekh JV. Comforting the dying dyspneic patient. Nursing 1987;87:66.

Other Problems

Barry SA. Septic shock: special needs of patients with cancer. Oncol Nurs Forum 1989;16:31.

Billings JA. Outpatient management of advanced cancer: symptom control, support, and hospice-in-the-home. Philadelphia: JB Lippincott, 1985.

Dangel RB. Injury, potential for, related to disseminated intravascular coagulopathy. In: McNally JC, Stair JC, Somerville ET. Guidelines for cancer nursing practice. Orlando: Grune & Stratton, 1985.

Findley J. Nursing management of common oncologic emergencies. In: Ziegfeld C. Core curriculum for oncology nursing. Philadelphia: WB Saunders, 1987.

Poe CM, Taylor LM. Syndrome of inappropriate antidiuretic hormone: assessment and nursing implications. Oncol Nurs Forum 1989;16:373.

11

Daily Living With Terminal Illness and Dying

Those who have managed daily living through the diagnostic, treatment, post-treatment, survival, and recurrence phases of the cancer experience have experienced multiple losses and feelings of separation. With the movement to the terminal phase, the patient and family face the ultimate loss and separation, loss of life for the patient and loss of a loved one for the family.

There may be some variation in interpretation of when the terminal phase of the cancer experience begins. For medicine it begins when treatment shifts from curative to palliative. For patients, families, and nurses the beginning is less definitely marked. Unlike the diagnostic or treatment phase, often no major event signals the movement into the terminal phase. It is heralded by a change in patient status. Both the patient and the family become aware of it at some intuitive level (Seravalli, 1988). Physical symptoms become exacerbated. There is greater restlessness, less verbal communication, and more nonverbal communication—the knitted brow, sighs, wet eyes, smiles, hand gestures, perhaps an empty or astonished look (Kubler-Ross, 1969). One nurse who observed the transition to the terminal stage many times said the patients have a "pre-peaceful look."

Communication between the patient and family may become more difficult for a time. The awareness of the transition and its significance has come, but the words for dealing with the change have not. There may be ambivalence in wanting release from suffering for all of the participants, yet each may desire not to let go, given the irreversible nature of this separation.

The terminal phase varies in duration. It may be quite short, lasting only days, or it may last for weeks, seeming interminable. Whether long or short, the terminal stage intensely affects the daily living of all participants. As in the other phases, some patients and families manage terminal illness, dying, and death with remarkable effectiveness. They grow in the midst of the stresses and crises. Other patients and families are ill-prepared to handle the extreme and often prolonged stresses of terminal illness and its demands.

Medical Perspective

Although some oncologists will continue to attempt to control neoplastic processes with all the technology available for as long as possible, for most the medical perspective in diagnosis and treatment in the terminal phase focuses on palliation. Contacts with the patient become more attenuated as the patient is less able to travel to the doctor's office. Once the patient is unable to go to the office, except for periods of hospitalization patient contact tends to occur by telephone, and eventually the contact is with care givers rather than the patient. Data come from the observations and descriptions of others (e.g., home care nurses, care givers, family members) rather than from direct observation, which dominated in earlier phases.

Medical judgments concern differential diagnosis of symptoms as a basis for treatment (e.g., Is the situation an oncologic emergency requiring immediate medical treatment? Is the nausea and vomiting from a treatable electrolyte imbalance, an obstruction in the gastrointestinal tract, or remote tumor effects?). Some complications of advancing cancer lend themselves to treatment; others do not. The goal is to manage symptoms effectively in order to help the patient move through the final stages of the disease as comfortably as possible (Wanzer et al, 1984).

It has been suggested that physician education and conditioning may cause physicians to be most effective and comfortable when they can be actively involved in treating the neoplasm or managing the symptoms (Wanzer et al, 1984). Many are less prepared for situations when all that can medically be done has been done and their role is that of being relatively "helpless bystanders," unable to further forestall the patient's dying (Seravalli, 1988).

Nursing Perspective

Daily living and its requirements continue for both patient and family members while life ebbs and dysfunctions mount. Nursing responsibilities grow in complexity and intensity as the patient and family face crises in which they have little experience and expertise and as they move into the uncharted aspects of daily living with dying.

One nursing goal is to help the patients and families retain decision-making capacity and control as long as possible and to help them achieve the goals and tasks that are important to them at this point in their lives (Lewis, 1982). A second is to help them to move through the dying process in a manner they see as suitable (Benoliel, 1985).

Nature of Terminal Illness and Underlying Mechanisms

The Dying Role

Just as society has developed behavioral expectations for the person in the sick role, it has expectations for the person who is dying. They are not the same. Patients in the dying role are expected to (Noyes and Clancy, 1977):

Want to live

Arrange for orderly transfer of property and responsibilities

Use available support persons and services but decrease dependence on physicians

Accept decreased freedom and privileges

Adapt to rules and routines of care givers

Be as independent as functional status permits

Dying patient's rights include (Noyes and Clancy, 1977):

Disengagement from the world

Exemption from social responsibilities

Continuing care and support from family and health professionals

Maintenance of status despite declining functioning

Patients may cling to the sick role instead of making the transition to the dying role and may be supported in this by the behavior of family members and the continued active treatment orientation of health care professionals. They may also be hampered in managing the role of the dying person through lack of role knowledge and skills (Williams, 1982).

Symptom Progression

The terminal phase of cancer is marked by the progression of existing symptoms and dysfunctions as well as the appearance of new ones. Management of them becomes more difficult and less effective. New evidences of the tumor may appear in the form of visible lesions, fistulas, pressures on organs, obstructions, and neurologic deficits. The cancer and its manifestations become a focal point in daily living.

The patient's symptoms cannot be adequately managed unless the treatment takes into account the tenor of the patient's days—the requirements, self-expectations and goals, unfinished business, needs of others that have an impact on the patient's waning resources, environment, and status of the patient's external resources. This is true whether the patient is in the hospital, in a nursing home, or at home. External resources also will affect patterns of symptom management. Some treatment options may be possible in certain treatment centers where staff are highly trained and experienced with the technology, but not in others.

Symptom progression and the associated suffering affects not only the patient, but also those who share daily living. Their suffering and their feelings of anger and helplessness at being unable to protect the patient from the final ravages of the cancer can affect the care they are able to provide to the patient. Some not only cannot help the patient, but find it difficult to remain in the immediate environment. Family members and care givers vary in their desire and capacities to participate in the complex and demanding requirements of day-to-day living with a terminally ill patient, whether the patient is in the home or in the hospital. Many patients fear abandonment and are particularly sensitive to any cues that might indicate emotional or physical withdrawal of those upon whom they depend for love or care. Symptom management plans need to take these factors into account.

Monotony and Boredom

Being sick with cancer is monotonous and boring (Billings, 1985). Days and nights can be very long for patients when they are so dysfunctional that they are confined to limited spaces and when their bodies bombard them with symptoms. The increasing symptoms and dysfunctions reduce the capacity to participate in activities. They also sap the capacity to initiate desired and feasible activities and even the motivation to be involved with those that are made available. The world shrinks and becomes more egocentric as the patient limits contacts with others. The suffering can become the focus of attention; time passes slowly. Still, the minutes and hours of the day remain to be managed in ways that either bring comfort and meaningful involvement or monotony.

Where the patient becomes more lethargic and moves toward lower levels of consciousness there is a tendency among others to further limit sensory stimulation. Often there is evidence that seemingly out-of-touch patients are still able to hear and respond to auditory stimuli and touch. It becomes important to maintain an appropriate level of stimulation for the patient by avoiding an environment that is barren of auditory and tactile stimuli, continuing to communicate normally with the patient, providing auditory stimuli that the patient previously enjoyed, and using touch and presence as a means of communicating comfort and caring.

Separations

Some forms of separation have occurred earlier in the cancer experience (e.g, the feeling of separation of the person with cancer from those who don't have it, physical separations associated with treatment or the location of treatment, separations associated with disfigurement or dysfunction, sexual separations, divergence in goals and priorities). However, with the realization that death is near, the specter of final separation looms large.

Many terminally ill persons experience an almost overwhelming need for contact with others (Seravalli, 1988). There is often less desire for sexual intimacy but more for nongenital contacts and emotional intimacy (Billings, 1985).

The patient's affectional needs may be complicated by others' emotional responses to the patient's terminal status (e.g., anger, anxiety, fear, resentment, guilt, exhaustion, and revulsion, as well as love, affection, and the desire to help) (Billings, 1985). Terminally ill cancer patients may be unusually sensitive to cues that they correctly or incorrectly interpret as withdrawal. This can create additional burdens for family members and care givers who have difficulty being in contact with the patient's suffering or who have other responsibilities that keep them from attending totally to patient needs. There are some exceptions, however. Nurses do report having cared for the occasional patient who seems to have accomplished tasks of separation earlier and who chooses to face dying alone. Partners, care givers, and family members of terminally ill persons have their needs for attention and affection too. Purposefully providing for affectional needs of care givers and grieving family members as a part of daily living is an important element in the terminal phase of the cancer experience.

Lack of readiness to separate from particular *roles* seems to be a factor affecting the trajectory of dying. Patients hang on because they feel that role obligations have not been completed. For example, a mother hasn't completed preparation of the children for roles they will need to assume on her death. An adult child has not completed arrangements for the care of dependent parents. The single parent with distant relatives hasn't found a satisfactory arrangement for long-term care of the children. A wife's prolonged denial of the husband's impending death has prevented him from preparing her to assume responsibility for some important duties related to their business and family finances.

Spouses, partners, or other family members too may be unready to separate from the patient. They may beg the patient not to leave them yet. One nurse illustrated this difficulty in separation in a situation where the husband was begging his wife not to die yet, "Mary, please don't leave me; you've got to try to stay." The wife's response was, "I'm so tired, Floyd, I don't know if I can stay." After a time the husband seemed ready to release his wife, "It's OK, Mary. I know how tired you are, you can quit trying to stay for my sake. I love you and I'll miss you, but I'll be all right." At this point the wife became fearful and the nurse turned her attention to helping the wife let go. "Mary, you've done all the things you needed to do and done them well. You're tired now. It's time to rest. Floyd will be OK. Floyd and I are here with you. It's all right to let go."

Unfinished Business

Some patients and families come to the final stage of the cancer experience with increasing tensions associated with unfinished business. Sometimes this involves wanting to tell another person about feelings that haven't been shared earlier (e.g., "I always wanted to tell you about how I felt when... but I didn't know how"). Another common situation is the desire for reconciliation and forgiveness for wrongs that were committed or perceived at earlier times.

The health care provider often senses the tension arising as opportunities for dealing with unfinished business become more limited. Therapy may involve helping the patient or other person to talk about their concerns. It can also involve arranging for desired encounters by making the patient as comfortable and functional as possible and providing privacy for the encounters. Therapy may also involve legitimizing the concerns being described and helping the patient or other person to think through strategies for approaching the subject. For example, a patient was moving into a comatose state and her husband was distressed that he had not been able to adequately tell his wife about some of his feelings and how important she had been to him through all the years. The nurse indicated that she could arrange for them to be undisturbed and that he might want to go in and talk to his wife as if she were fully conscious: "Even though she isn't speaking much now, we really think that she can hear and understand. She's told me about all the good years you've had together. It could make her more at peace and satisfied if she were to hear you say these things."

Taking steps to achieve reconciliation is not always easy. It may require motivation, courage, and skill in larger measures than would seem to be available. Individuals may need help in identifying small, safe steps to initiate the process. They also can be helped by acknowledgement of actions they do take (e.g., "You did a nice job of bringing up Jim's problems and making it easy for him to speak his mind. I'm sure that helped him")

Lack of Knowledge About Dying

Uncertainty about the experiences leading up to death can produce fear and anxiety. Some patients have a need to talk about the feelings they are experiencing. Others genuinely want knowledge about what symptoms and experiences will occur as a prelude to death. Appropriate treatment is contingent on making an accurate differential diagnosis between the need to ventilate feelings and the desire for knowledge.

It is a nursing goal to support the participants through the experiences associated with terminal illness and dying with as much comfort and control as possible. This means providing information when it is genuinely wanted in ways that convey the information but do not increase the discomfort. Since it is difficult to predict what will actually occur, absolutes are avoided. Expertise and experience enable the nurse to know the common complications that are associated with dying, given the patient's type of cancer and metastatic configuration (e.g., infections, hemorrhage, abnormal electrolytes, renal failure, liver failure). By developing scripts for each of these that focus on symptoms with which the patient is already familiar and using the patient's own language it is possible to describe potential scenarios that give the patient or family information they are seeking without creating panic.

Sometimes patients or families are faced with having to decide whether to further treat some complication or to face dying without treatment. They may then want to have some idea about the course of events that may occur with treatment and without. For example, when uremia occurs, dialysis is an option for prolonging life for a time. The question then arises as to what it is like to die from the uremia (e.g., growing lethargy progressing to coma, with the heart stopping as a result of accumulation of potassium in the body) and what is involved for patient and family if the patient is placed on dialysis (Hoffart, 1986).

Another area of uncertainty that emerges relates not to the dying process, but to death itself and the hereafter. Given the various belief systems and religious backgrounds, it is wise to encourage patients to talk about what they believe, have heard, or think the death experience is like in order to utilize words and ideas that are familiar and not frightening. Discussions in this area may lead to a direct or disguised request to have contact with a minister in the faith of their choosing.

Sometimes existential questions arise. For those whose background has not included development of a strong belief system associated with life after death, thoughts now move beyond the dying and death experience: "Is there a heaven? Do you think I will go there?" This reflects another uncertainty, the need to know where they are going.

Powerlessness

Many aspects of terminal cancer contribute to the patient's feelings of powerlessness and helplessness. These include the inexorable progression of the cancer and its effects, pain that at times can be managed but not controlled, the often total dependence upon the good will and expertise of others, and the awareness that death is inexorably approaching. Family members and care givers too feel helpless, immobilized, and angry as they watch the patient suffering and losing ground yet feel they have little expertise to intervene.

Where patients and families are immobilized and overwhelmed, therapy involves helping them find specific strategies that make parts of the situation more manageable. Areas for management are focused. Goals are concrete and limited. A nursing goal is to find areas in which both the patient and the family experience success in achieving control (Lewis, 1982).

Nursing Diagnosis and Treatment

Diagnostic Targets   In addition to the patient, the care givers and close family members are an important focus for nursing diagnosis and treatment. This is particularly true when the terminally ill or dying patient is cared for in the home.

Risk Factors   Patients who may experience difficulty in managing daily living during the terminal phase of the cancer experience are those who:

Have had difficulty in adapting to previous stress situations

Have unmanaged or poorly managed symptoms

Experience a prolonged terminal illness and dying

Are agitated and anxious about unfinished business

Have difficulty in articulating their goals

Are illiterate or have language barriers

Have professional and personal care givers who do not accommodate the patient's wishes and goals related to daily living in the terminal and dying phases of the illness

Distrust care givers

Are forced by severity of symptoms or lack of care givers to go to undesired care settings

Have limited financial resources

Fear abandonment or experience some degree of abandonment by significant others

Have a highly distressed and anxious family

Are cared for in an understaffed environment or one that lacks capable personal care givers

Are cared for by personal or professional care givers who do not espouse a hospice philosophy and lack the hospice knowledge and skills, or who have a distaste for caring for patients who are dying

Fear death

Family members who are likely to experience difficulties in managing daily living with the patient's terminal illness and dying are those who:

Have unfinished business with the patient

Have been emotionally, physically, or sexually abused by the patient

Are the primary care givers and lack the physical strength and stamina, desire, or expertise to manage the requirements of the role

Have health problems of their own

Are alone or feel alone in the care giving role

Are illiterate or have language barriers

Have not managed previous crises effectively

Have alcohol or drug abuse problems

Are still seeking to support their denial of the patient's terminal status

Are highly anxious and fearful

Are immobilized or repulsed by the patient's symptoms

Have conflicting role obligations that interfere with being with the patient (e.g., need to work to maintain health insurance, child care, care of other dependent family members)

Feel guilty because they are geographically distant and can maintain contact only by telephone or letter

Fear death

Diagnostic Areas

PATIENT

Suffering R/T:

Inadequate symptom management or fear of inadequate symptom management

Fear of abandonment by personal or professional care givers

Physical or emotional neglect

Lack of skilled, hospice-oriented care

Loss of control over body

Loss of control over decisions

Dissatisfaction with quality of life R/T:

Difficulty in communicating goals

Lack of ability or capacity to negotiate for goals

An unpleasant environment

Uncaring or ineffective care givers

Anxiety R/T:

Inability to maintain personal contact with the physician

Lack of reconciliation; need to forgive or seek forgiveness from family members or friends

Desire to share some previously uncommunicated thoughts or feelings

Incomplete arrangements for care of children, dependent relatives, business, personal assets, or objects of personal significance

Uncertainty about the events, experiences, and feelings that will accompany dying

Uncertainty about the death experience

Uncertainty about the hereafter

Ambivalence R/T conflict between fear of loss of control and desire for pain control

Sensory deprivation or monotony R/T:

Restricted, barren environment

Impaired ability to initiate desired activities

Impaired capacities to participate in activities

Failure of others to talk to or touch the patient appropriately because of patient's lowered level of consciousness

FAMILY, CARE
GIVERS

Impaired ability to manage patient's symptoms R/T:

Being immobilized by the nature of the patient's symptoms and suffering

Knowledge deficit of the basis for the patient's symptoms and strategies of management

Illiteracy or language barriers

Deficit in technical skills

Inadequate strength and endurance for the physical or emotional requirements of the care giving (e.g., having own health problems)

Lack of supportive equipment and supplies

Lack of adequate, predictable professional support

Burnout

Missed opportunities for interaction R/T:

Failure to attend to patient cues

Misinterpretation of nonverbal communication

Anxiety R/T concern over not having the opportunity to resolve or reconcile interpersonal problems

Discomfort with patient R/T:

Difficulty in talking to or touching a terminally ill or dying person

Uncertainty about how to respond when the patient unpredictably shifts from acknowledging terminal status to seeming not to recognize it (Billings, 1985)

Difficulty in talking to a comatose person

Anxiety or resentment R/T:

Uncertainty about the trajectory of the patient's terminal illness and dying

Patient's inability to fulfill care givers' or family members' expectations or goals for the dying experience

Prolonged dying phase and the impaired capacity to fulfill other critical role obligations

Helplessness at being unable to relieve the patient's prolonged suffering

Frustration R/T environmental constraints on grieving according to their customs, traditions, and preferences

See also Chapter 10, section on Asthenia, under Diagnostic Areas for Family, information on burnout.

Manifestations

Indications that the patient or family are not meeting challenges of daily living effectively can be observed in a variety of ways.

PATIENT

Reported:

Inadequate relief from pain, nausea, vomiting, diarrhea, constipation, itching, dry mouth, weakness, shortness of breath, lack of air, noxious odors, pressure, immobility, incontinence, insomnia (Billings, 1985)

Inadequate or ineffective care; inability to get professional support needed

Worrying about how the spouse or children will manage, who will care for children or dependent parents, how the business will be managed, how to dispose of assets or personal treasures

Wanting to remain at home, but fearing that care givers will not be able to manage the symptoms, the burden of care will be too much, or professional support will not be available

Worrying that there won't be enough time to teach other family members what they need to know to manage specific roles and tasks in daily living

Feeling uneasy that there has been no reconciliation with particular family members over past differences or that particular messages or feelings have not been adequately shared with another person

Fear that goals for living with terminal illness and the approach to dying will not be respected by health care providers or family members

Feeling torn between wanting relief from pain and yet wanting to be in control of daily living

Finding the days and nights too long; having too much time to think and focus on the discomforts

Wondering what is to come

Feeling that others are withdrawing; feeling very alone

Being angry at life, fate, events, or people

Being frustrated with the care received

Feeling misunderstood

Having no one to "really talk to" or lacking energy to talk

Observed:

Pain-related behavior, vomiting, constipation or diarrhea, hiccups, ascites or lymphedema, skin breakdown or contractures, inability to change position, incontinence of urine or feces, presence of debris of sputum or food in the mouth, cracked lips, dried secretions on the eyes, noxious odors from fetid breath or infected wounds, drainage from wounds or fistulae, scratch marks, breathing in a labored manner, rales or rhonchi, confusion, lowered level of consciousness

Being unkempt (unshaven, hair not recently shampooed or combed, soiled clothing or linen)

Having an environment that does not place needed objects in convenient places, is untidy or unclean, lacks options for sensory stimulation, has barriers to ease of care, lacks options for privacy or, conversely, limits contacts with others, or lacks equipment to communicate with others

Having unpredictable, unskilled, or highly anxious personal care givers

Lack of contacts with family or friends

Being withdrawn and apathetic, not engaging in any activity

Refusing narcotic analgesia

Avoiding talking about any remaining goals in life or about impending death; refusal to participate in any planning

Being angry at family, care givers, or health care providers (Kloer and Stricklin, 1981)

Seeming tense and worried

Attempting to control all elements in daily living

FAMILY, CARE
GIVERS

Reported:

Difficulty in being with the patient and seeing the suffering

Not knowing what is going on, why the patient is having the symptoms, what can be done

Feeling helpless

Not knowing how to talk to the patient

Wishing it were over

Being angry at the patient

Being physically and emotionally exhausted

Being sleep-deprived

Wondering what will happen, how death will come, how long the patient will live

Being afraid that they won't recognize symptoms or emergencies until it is too late

Being afraid that they won't be able to abide by patient's wishes for no resuscitation but may call 911 for help

Wanting to bring up unfinished business or unexpressed feelings, but not knowing when or how to do it

Observed:

Being immobilized by the situation and unable to identify problems, set goals, or take action

Lacking the physical strength, endurance, dexterity, or knowledge to provide effective care

Physically distancing themselves from the patient or engaging in superficial conversation; not touching the patient

Not talking to but talking about the patient as if he or she were no longer able to hear or understand

Making the patient the totality of their daily living and neglecting self in the process

Exhaustion

Criticizing other family members who are not as directly involved in patient care

Having no respite plan or resources

Refusing offers of help or assistance

Venting anger and frustration on each other or the care system

Prognostic
Variables

Effective management of daily living with terminal illness and dying is more likely when:

The patient's symptoms can be and are well managed in the context of the patient's daily living

Care is skilled and congruent with patient goals

The patient and family have met crises effectively in the past or have assistance in crisis management in the present situation

Unfinished business is resolved for significant participants

The patient has been able to tell his story and review his life

Patient, family, and care givers are able to articulate their goals and help each other achieve them

Expressions of the range of emotions associated with terminal illness and dying are accepted

The important people in the patient's life continue to maintain an effective relationship

The patient and family are able to learn about what to expect in dying and death to the extent that they wish to know and at a pace and in ways that are comfortable

The patient and family maintain a sense of some control over their daily living and choices

The environment offers the patient sensory stimulation and diversion in quality and quantity appropriate to wishes and capacities

Care givers have adequate respite and support

The patient and family feel cared about as well as cared for

Patient, care givers, and family receive appropriate professional support and access to equipment and resources

Treatment Guidelines

PATIENT   *Fear of inadequate symptom management*

See index for specific symptoms and nursing management.

Provide information about the options for management of symptoms the patient has or fears. For patients and families who are literate, supplement oral instructions with clear, written, specific instructions whenever possible (e.g., "Take methadone hydrochloride every 8 hours around the clock. If you have pain between the regular methadone doses, place 1 tablet SL morphine under the tongue every hour. If the morphine does not adequately take the pain away, call the home care nurse or the physician").

Suggest keeping a log of symptoms, medications used, and activities engaged in as a basis for providing health care providers with specific data on the symptoms and the relative effectiveness of current treatment. Provide a form or give suggestions for columns and headings in making their own form.

Provide physician with data on patient symptoms, effectiveness of current regimen, patient goals, and requirements in current daily living, and negotiate for a medical regimen that takes both symptoms and daily living into account.

Arrange for scheduled feedback on the effect of any changes in the medication or treatment regimen.

Offer options for activities the patient can engage in to contribute to control of symptoms (see index for treatment of specific symptoms).

Indicate to patient how you will work with personal or professional care givers to achieve skill and consistency in symptom management behavior.

Fear of abandonment

Gather data on the basis for the patient's concerns from the patient and those who are involved.

Discuss the hospice option as a support system for the patient, care givers, and other family members, in the home, inpatient, or hospice setting.

Alert care givers and family members to the patient's concerns and discuss ways of reducing that fear (e.g., scheduling care, visits, and phone calls; always fulfilling the scheduled encounters; conveying warmth and caring verbally and through touch in patient contacts). Alert physician and the person who takes physician's phone calls to the patient's fears so that they can respond in ways to build confidence and trust in their availability.

If need be, confront the spouse or family member about their leaving (Forsyth, 1982); for example, "How soon will you be coming back? Your wife will be asking" or "We think you'd better stay—your father really wants you with him".

Provide resource phone numbers (e.g., for physician or home nursing agency) and assure them that someone is available on call 24 hours each day.

Neglect

Determine the areas of neglect and the causes.

If neglect is due to the care giver's lack of knowledge, skill, or confidence in symptom management or basic hygiene, arrange for appropriate knowledge and skill teaching with supervised practice or (if financially feasible) arrange for assistance in the form of home nursing and chore services.

If neglect is due to the care giver's inattention to or inability to accurately interpret the patient's nonverbal cues, help the person to build skill in observing and interpreting patient cues.

If neglect is due to lack of a personal care giver, arrange with physician or social worker for home care or placement that is compatible with patient's financial resources and wishes.

If neglect is related to the care giver's burnout, determine options for respite and professional support (see Chapter 10, section on Asthenia, treatment guidelines for burnout).

Vacillation between acknowledging and "not knowing" of impending death

Recommend encountering the patient without assuming what the current state of mind is about impending death, and accepting the patient's current thinking, even though it represents a change from the last contact.

When there are issues in which failure to make decisions can result in prolonged harm (e.g., failure to make arrangements for minor children, resulting in foster home placement), confront the patient with the need for decisions. Explore patient wishes and follow up on the discussion with those who are involved.

Ineffective goal achievement

In the first encounter with the patient who is in the terminal stage of illness, gather data on patient goals (e.g., "It would help me to know what is important to you"; "Is there something you really want to accomplish?"; "What do you truly want?"; or "How would you like to spend your time?"). If the patient hasn't thought this way, suggest that he or she write down a list of wishes and goals so that they can be discussed in the home nurse's next visit or with the hospital nurse the next day (McCorkle, 1984).

Where goals are unrealistic, try to shift to more immediate goals—for the day or for this week, where the patient (or care giver or family) has better knowledge of the capacities and opportunities. Model the use of smaller, achievable goals.

Encourage the patient and those who share the patient's daily living to think and talk about their goals and to look toward ways of achieving them.

As needed, help the patient (or others) to think of options and strategies for achieving wishes and goals.

If appropriate, suggest that the patient keep a running list of achieved goals. Give warm acknowledgment when goals, strategies, and options are identified or goals achieved.

Point out the importance of experiencing a sense of satisfaction and achieving an area of control by acknowledging goals and seeking to achieve them.

Unfinished business

Attend to cues (e.g., tension, increased worry, disguised messages) or direct expressions about family disagreements, misunderstandings, or the need for forgiveness.

Legitimize the concerns by indicating that realization of the need to deal with unfinished business occurs with many families and friends at this point in an illness. Indicate that it is a problem that lends itself to solution, and that reconciliation, forgiveness, and the conveying of long-overdue messages are important to gaining peace of mind.

If the patient or a family member desires it, talk through strategies for approaching the situation and dealing with it (e.g., using picture albums or reminiscences of events surrounding the misunderstanding or missed opportunity to express feelings). Offer some scripts (e.g., "Do you remember when we...? I was so upset that I said some things I was sorry for afterwards. It has bothered me ever since. I'd like to ask your forgiveness"; "Do you remember when...? I don't know if you knew it, but I was really hurt when you..."; "I've wanted to tell you for a long time..."; or "I never told you how proud I was of you when you...").

Suggest that reconciliations can be taken in small steps.

Arrange for a desired meeting by assuring that the patient is as symptom-free and rested as possible. Arrange for privacy and freedom from interruption.

Ask the patient if there is anyone else they wish to talk with.

Acknowledge the person's achievement when steps are taken to deal with unfinished business.

If the patient wants to plan for giving away special objects and is physically capable, suggest labeling each object with the name of the person for whom it is intended. If strength is limited, suggest that a friend or neutral volunteer be asked to come in, make a list of the patient's wishes, and then label the objects with the names of the persons for whom they are intended. Add a codicil to the will indicating that this action has been taken.

If the patient is able and wishes to, suggest writing letters or making an audio or video tape for children or grandchildren who are too young to talk or remember.

Loss of control over decisions

Inform the patient and family of their rights to choose among the medical options or to refuse treatment. Identify the choices they can make. Serve as an advocate with the physician if patient choices are likely to create interpersonal difficulties.

Provide information about living wills or physician directives (see sample physician directive and chart label in Figure 11-1) as well as about power of attorney for health care (see sample power of attorney for health care in Figure 11-2).

Determine areas in daily living in which the patient can make choices. Incorporate these into the nursing orders. Arrange with care givers to check with the patient in advance about preferences and goals.

PATIENT'S INSTRUCTIONS IN THE EVENT OF INCURABLE INJURY, DISEASE OR ILLNESS

Directive made this_____ Day of_____
(Month, Year)

I, (Print) _____ , being of sound mind, wilfully, and voluntarily make known my desire that my life shall not be artificially prolonged under the circumstances set forth below, and do hereby declare that:

(A) If at any time I should have an incurable injury, disease, or illness certified to be a terminal condition by two physicians, and where the application of life-sustaining procedures would serve only to artificially prolong the moment of my death and where my physician determines that my death is imminent whether or not life-sustaining procedures are utilized, I direct that such procedure be withheld or withdrawn, and that I be permitted to die naturally.

(B) In the absence of my ability to give directions regarding the use of such life-sustaining procedures, it is my intention that this directive shall be honored by my family and physician(s) as the final expression of my legal right to refuse medical or surgical treatment and I accept the consequences from such refusal.

(C) If I have been diagnosed as pregnant and that diagnosis is known to my physician, this directive shall have no force or effect during the course of my pregnancy.

(D) I understand the full import of this directive and I am emotionally and mentally competent to make this directive.

Signed _____

VMMC Number: _____

Address: _____
(Street)

_____
(City)   (County)   (State)

Witnesses: This directive must be signed by two witnesses. The following persons _may not_ serve as witnesses: A) Anyone related to the declarer by blood or marriage; B) Anyone entitled to a part of the declarer's estate, by will or otherwise; C) Anyone with a claim against the declarer's estate; and D) The employees of a health facility (hospital or nursing home) in which the declarer is a patient.

The Declarer has been personally known to me and I believe him or her to be of sound mind.

_____   _____
Witness   Witness

_____   _____
Address   Address

FM - 18   **This directive complies with the Natural Death Act, Chapter 112, Washington Laws of 1979 However, additional specific directions may be included by the declarer.**

A

B

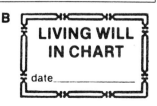

Figure 11-1. (A) *Example of physician directive ("Living Will") communicating incurable illness.* (B) *"Living Will" identification sticker for patient's chart.* (Courtesy of Virginia Mason Medical Center, Seattle, Washington)

POWER OF ATTORNEY FOR HEALTH CARE

I appoint _____, whose address is _____, and whose telephone number is _____, as my attorney-in-fact for health care decisions. I appoint _____, whose address is _____, and whose telephone number is _____, as my alternative attorney-in-fact for health care decisions. I authorize my attorney-in-fact appointed by this document to make health care decisions for me when I am incapable of making my own health care decisions. I have read the warning below and understand the consequences of appointing a power of attorney for health care.

I direct that my attorney-in-fact comply with the following instructions or limitations: _____

In addition, I direct that my attorney-in-fact have authority to make decisions regarding the following:

Withholding or withdrawal of life-sustaining procedures with the understanding that death may result.

Withholding or withdrawal of artificially administered hydration or nutrition or both with the understanding that dehydration, malnutrition and death may result.

_____
(Signature of person making appointment/Date)

DECLARATION OF WITNESSES

We declare that the principal is personally known to us, that the principal signed or acknowledged the principal's signature on this power of attorney for health care in our presence, that the principal appears to be of sound mind and not under duress, fraud or undue influence, that neither of us is the person appointed as attorney-in-fact by this document or the principal's attending physician. Witnessed by:

_____   _____
Signature of Witness/Date   Printed Name of Witness

_____   _____
Signature of Witness/Date   Printed Name of Witness

ACCEPTANCE OF APPOINTMENT OF POWER OF ATTORNEY

I accept this appointment and agree to serve as attorney-in-fact for health care decisions. I understand I have a duty to act consistently with the desires of the principal as expressed in this appointment. I understand that this document gives me authority over health care decisions for the principal only if the principal becomes incapable. I understand that I must act in good faith in

---

Figure 11-2.   *Sample power of attorney for health care.*

Suggest that the patient think about specific goals for the day, the week, and so on and share those goals with care givers so that schedules and medications can be implemented in ways that enhance goal achievement. Help the patient to formulate goals if this is a new behavior and to plan scripts for sharing the goals if this may prove difficult.

xercising my authority under this power of attorney. I understand that the principal may revoke ιis power of attorney at any time in any manner, and that I have a duty to inform the principal's ttending physician promptly upon any revocation.

_____
Signature of Attorney-in-fact/Date

_____
Printed Name

_____
Signature of Alternate Attorney-in-fact/Date

_____
Printed Name

WARNING TO PERSON APPOINTING A POWER OF ATTORNEY FOR HEALTH CARE

'his is an important legal document. It creates a power of attorney for health care. Before signing ιis document, you should know these important facts:

'his document gives the person you designate as your attorney-in-fact the power to make health are decisions for you, subject to any limitations, specifications or statement of your desires that ɔu include in this document.

ɔr this document to be effective, your attorney-in-fact must accept the appointment in writing. 'he person you designate in this document has a duty to act consistently with your desires as stated ι this document or otherwise made known or, if your desires are unknown, to act in a manner ɔnsistent with what the person in good faith believes to be in your best interest. The person you esignate in this document does, however, have the right to withdraw from this duty at any time.

'his power will continue in effect for a period of seven years unless you become unable to articipate in health care decisions for yourself during that period. If this occurs, the power will ɔntinue in effect until you are able to participate in those decisions again.

ɔu have the right to revoke the appointment of the person designated at any time by notifying ιat person or your health care provider of the revocation orally or in writing.

)espite this document, you have the right to make medical and other health care decisions for ɔurself as long as you are able to participate knowledgeably in those decisions.

 there is anything in this document that you do not understand, you should ask a lawyer to κplain it to you. This power of attorney will not be valid for making health care decisions unless it signed by two qualified witnesses who are personally known to you and who are present when you gn or acknowledge your signature.

Identify any incongruences between patient and care givers' goals. Help them to find "win—win" resolutions (Forsyth, 1982).

Monotony or deficits in external stimuli

Determine the sensory experiences the patient is having and those that would be seen as pleasant and helpful.

Observe the patient's environment and suggest options for changes (e.g., moving the chair or bed to a different position so that the view is better, putting pictures and snapshots on the wall, putting "treasures" within view or reach, making room for the family pet, plants, fresh flowers from the garden, or a small aquarium).

Recommend creating a patient "center" with objects and options for sensory stimulation within reach (e.g., radio, tape recorder and favorite tapes, remote control for TV, books [with big print if needed and a book holder], books on tape that can be checked out from the public library, crafts if the patient has the energy and interest).

Determine what will help the patient to pass the long hours of the night if sleep is a problem (e.g., night talk shows on the radio, old movies on TV, video tapes of movies or family gatherings, a volunteer [other than the usual care giver] to sit with the patient or read to the patient for part of the night).

Plan for visits from people the patient wants to see, or for a talk on the telephone. Prepare visitors to sit quietly and hold the patient's hand or just "be there," if this is as much as the patient can tolerate. Suggest to a friend or family member mobilizing friends and relatives to send cards and letters. Arrange for a dog or cat to visit if the patient has no pets and enjoys animals.

Uncertainty about the future

When the patient wonders aloud or asks what is likely to happen, determine whether the patient really wants to talk about feelings and fears or genuinely wants to know (e.g., "You seem upset these days. Is there something in your situation that is bothering you?"). If the patient indicates that there is no specific concern, indicate that you are available if there is anything that you can do to help. If the patient asks directly about what it will be like to die, validate the request (e.g., "What would you really like to know?").

If it is determined that the patient wants to know the condition or symptoms that are likely to precede death, provide the information in neutral, nontechnical language, using familiar words and, if it is realistic, symptoms the patient has already experienced. Avoid absolutes, since the exact cause of death may be hard to predict, but link the possible antecedent to death to the high-risk complications associated with the particular cancer this patient has. (For example, John has lymphoma. The nurse might say, "We have found that lung infections are a fairly common complication that lead to death among our patients who have your type of cancer. If you were to get such an infection you would feel more short of breath and feel a need for more oxygen. You'd feel restless and it might be hard to get comfortable. You'd likely have a fever and sweating. You might become confused. You would sleep more and gradually become less and less conscious of what is going on around you. Eventually you would stop breathing, then your heart would stop." Some of these symptoms have already been experienced by the patient, so they feel familiar rather than new and frightening.)

If the patient is asking about what death itself is like, try to learn what they have heard or imagined and what they believe. Then use their words and ideas. If it seems appropriate, consider drawing on the reports of people who have had near-death experiences. Common descriptions include moving toward a warm light at the end of a tunnel or road, being free of pain and any other symptoms, and being welcomed by people the patient knows who have already died. People who have had these experiences reportedly have no fear of death afterward, but instead see it as a positive experience.

If the patient is concerned about life after death, seek to learn about their belief system and background. Support the patient's beliefs. Ask if it would make them more comfortable to speak with a minister or person representing their own or a particular faith.

FAMILY, CARE GIVERS

Ineffective management of patient symptoms

Determine the deterrents to effective management of patient symptoms (e.g., ineffective communication with the doctor about the patient's situation; being overwhelmed and immobilized by the patient's symptoms; knowledge deficit of the basis for the symptoms, what symptoms to expect, and strategies for dealing with them; lack of equipment or technical skills; care giver exhaustion or dysfunctions; lack of desire to care for the patient; poor communication between care giver and patient; denial of the patient's symptoms).

If the care giver does not have the skills to report to the doctor, provide language (e.g., a written list of variables and descriptive words) and suggest keeping a log of patient symptoms and medications or treatments given and patient response. Create or provide a form if necessary.

Provide information about the patient's situation in neutral, nonthreatening language. Indicate the meaning of the symptoms and how to be prepared to deal with them. For example, if the patient has episodes of vomiting, instruct having available a big enough receptacle, a cloth to cover it, a damp washcloth to wipe the patient's face, some dilute mouthwash to rinse the patient's mouth, and a hard mint to suck on (Moseley, 1985). If the problem is odor from a draining and infected wound, demonstrate how to cleanse the wound and suggest cleaning it and putting on fresh dressings if needed several times per day. Note that spraying wounds or draining areas every 2 hours with safe, nontoxic, hypoallergenic Ostozyme is an excellent way to control odors (Moseley, 1985). Provide written instructions.

Where the care giver does not know how to go about obtaining needed equipment or supplies, make contact with the appropriate agency or provide a contact point for the care giver.

For exhaustion and burnout, see Chapter 10, section on Asthenia, treatment guidelines for care giver burnout.

Frustration with the trajectory of the patient's terminal illness and dying

Determine the difficulties being experienced by the person because of the pattern of the patient's illness and dying.

If the difficulty is that the care giver has taken a leave from work and the time is almost up, explore the possibility of another person assuming the responsibilities of care, freeing the first care giver to return to work.

If the conflict is that the care giver has to work to maintain the family's health insurance or finances and is exhausted from trying to be with the patient and carry out other responsiblities, help the person to recruit other friends or family members (acceptable to the patient) to be with the patient more of the time so that there is some respite. Suggest development of a planned schedule for family members or friends, rather than relying on people to "drop by."

If the difficulty is emotional upset with watching the patient's suffering for those keeping vigil with the patient, regularly affirm the importance of their presence. Indicate how they contribute to the patient's well-being and peace of mind.

If the problem is feeling helplessness to prevent the patient's death, engage in values clarification (e.g., "Why do you think that you need to change things for Sally?" or "What is it that so distresses you about Fred's dying?").

Frustration with constraints on preferred pattern of grieving

Determine the customs of grieving, any deterrents to following these patterns in the present situation, any possible disturbance to others, and the possible need for a private room or other arrangements.

Arrange for a consistent care team that can be committed to accept the activities and family responses.

Arrange for protected time for mourners to undertake their activities.

Evaluation   To the extent that nursing had the opportunity to be involved in the patient's care during terminal illness at home, in the hospital, or in the nursing home, effectiveness of nursing therapy in assisting the patient to manage daily living through the terminal phase of cancer and dying can be evaluated by gathering data on the status of:

Symptom management as it permits and promotes comfort, effectiveness in participation in daily living, and maintenance of control over decisions and daily living for as long as possible or desired, and as it prevents complications that could be avoided by expert nursing care

Congruence of options for control in treatment decisions and in daily living with the desire and capacity for control

Consistency of care giving

Knowledge and expertise of care givers

Congruence of sensory and interpersonal environment with patient desires, capacities, and well-being

Patient satisfaction in encounters with care givers, family members, and significant others

Capacity and resources to manage unfinished business and reconciliations

Dying in a way that the patient deemed suitable

The response of care givers, family members, and significant others to nursing intervention can be evaluated in terms of the status of:

Appropriate knowledge about the patient's pathophysiology, symptoms, and treatment

Capacity to deliver safe, skilled care

Confidence in their care giving capacities

Knowledge of what to do should an oncologic emergency arise

Capacity to report credibly and accurately to health care providers on patient status

Feelings of being supported, offered opportunities, and given additional expertise in trying to address unfinished business with the patient

Feeling supported in meeting patient needs and their own when the terminal illness phase and dying is prolonged

Their own physical well-being

Preparation for the impending death

Participation in the dying process

Satisfaction with their care of or relationship with the patient in the final stages of the illness

Bibliography

Benoliel JQ. Loss and terminal illness. Nurs Clin North Am 1985;20:439.

Billings JA. Outpatient management of advanced cancer symptom control, support, and hospice-in-the-home. Philadelphia: JB Lippincott, 1985.

Forsyth DM. The hardest job of all. Nursing 1982;82:86.

Hoffart N. Chronic renal failure. In: Carnevali D, Patrick M, eds. Nursing management for the elderly. Philadelphia: JB Lippincott, 1986.

Kloer P, Stricklin W. A good death and the lives it affected: a story, in words and photos, of family, faith and hospice. Florida Times Union, March 30–April 2, 1981.

Kubler-Ross E. On death and dying. New York: Macmillan, 1969.

Lewis FM. Experienced personal control and quality of life in late-stage cancer patients. Nurs Res 1982;31:113.

McCorkle R. Diagnostic reasoning in nursing care of advanced cancer patients in the home. In: Carnevali D, Mitchell P, Tanner C, Woods N. Diagnostic reasoning in nursing. Philadelphia: JB Lippincott, 1984.

Moseley JR. Alterations in comfort. Nurs Clin North Am 1985;20:427.

Noyes R, Clancy J. The dying role: its relevance to improved patient care. Psychiatry 1977;40:41.

Seravalli EP. The dying patient, the physician, and fear of death. N Engl J Med 1988;319:1728.

Wanzer SH, Adelstein SJ, Cranford RE et al. The physician's responsibility toward hopelessly ill patients. N Engl J Med 1984;310:955.

Williams CA. Role considerations in care of the dying patient. Image 1982;14:8.

Index

A _t_ following a page number indicates tabular material and an _f_ following a page number indicates an illustration. Drugs are listed under their generic names. When a drug trade name is listed, the reader is referred to the generic name.